Parkinson's Disease For Dummies®

Cheat Sheet

Managing Your Medication Routine

- Carry a complete list of current prescription (Rx) and over-the-counter (OTC) medications. Give a copy to your care partner as well.
- Tell all doctors of allergies or other problems.
- Ask the doctor:
  - Name of medicine
  - Purpose
  - Dosing schedule (how much, how often)
  - How to take and how long to take
  - Side effects
- Ask the pharmacist to:
  - Check new Rx with your current Rx and OTC meds for possible interaction
  - Print label in large print
  - Provide easy-to-open cap
  - Explain how to take med
- At home:
  - Add new med to list of meds you carry with you
  - Read and file information print-out
  - Take med exactly as prescribed

Words and Acronyms to Know

- akinesia: Inability to move spontaneously
- ataxia: Impaired balance and coordination
- bradykinesia: Slowed movement
- carbidopa/levodopa: Medication to relieve PD symptoms
- dopamine: Acts as one of the brain's messengers to signal movement and maintain balance and coordination
- dyskinesia: Abnormal involuntary movements
- PD: Parkinson's disease
- PWP: Person (or people) with Parkinson's disease
- T.R.A.P.: Acronym for 4 primary PD symptoms:
  - Tremor: Shaking of limb (usually hand) while at rest
  - Rigidity: Muscle stiffness and resistance to movement
  - Akinesia/bradykinesia: See above
  - Postural instability: See *ataxia* above

Bookmark These Web Sites

- American Parkinson Disease Association, Inc.: www.apdaparkinson.org
- The Michael J. Fox Foundation: www.michaeljfox.org
- National Parkinson Foundation: www.parkinson.org
- Parkinson Action Network: www.parkinsonsaction.org
- Parkinson's Disease Foundation: www.pdf.org
- National Institute of Neurological Disorders and Stroke: www.ninds.nih.gov

Red-Flag Medications

The following classes of medications may be incompatible with routine PD meds. Provide the following list to all medical professionals before they prescribe any new medicine (Rx or OTC), and review any new medications with your neurologist before you begin taking them:

- Antinausea dopamine agonists
- Gastrointestinal anticholinergics
- Antipsychotics
- Postoperative pain-management drugs (Demerol in particular)

Contact the National Parkinson Foundation (www.parkinson.org or 800-327-4545) for a wallet-sized card that lists drugs that may be contraindicated.

For Dummies: Bestselling Book Series for Beginners

Parkinson's Disease For Dummies®

Your Daily CHECK-IN

Here's a quick and easy way to remind yourself that living *well* with PD is possible. Read this list once a day – twice if it's a rough day.

- ✔ **C**hallenge — acknowledge and face the facts
- ✔ **H**umor — find and revel in the absurd
- ✔ **E**mpowerment — refuse to surrender your life and relationships to PD
- ✔ **C**ollaboration — team with your family, friends, and healthcare providers
- ✔ **K**nowledge — know the difference between myth and fact and keep up with the latest developments
- ✔ **I**ntegration — treat the body, mind, and spirit
- ✔ **N**ever — give up!

When You Go to the Hospital or ER

- ✔ Have copies of the following information ready; give them to the Admissions office, the doctors, and ER or floor staff:
  - • Your neurologist's contact information – phone, pager, e-mail, and fax info
  - • Your doctor's written instructions for stopping and starting your PD meds during ER or hospital treatment
  - • A list of all Rx and OTC medications you currently take
  - • A list of the red-flag medications (see previous page)
- ✔ Examine meds you are given in the hospital. If you don't recognize a med, ask what it is, who prescribed it, and why you're taking it.
- ✔ Make sure your care partner has copies of all personal info (as noted in Chapter 9) including insurance info and copies of your advance directive and living will.
- ✔ Have your care partner monitor all ER- or hospital-administered meds.
- ✔ Before leaving the hospital, get a list of medications you're now taking.
- ✔ After you're home, contact your neurologist to review the list of new meds.

Emergency Contacts

Fill in these blanks to keep important phone numbers close at hand:

Primary care partner: _____

(h)_____ (w)_____ (cell)_____

Secondary care partner: _____

(h)_____ (w)_____ (cell)_____

Neighbor: _____

(h)_____ (w)_____ (cell)_____

Support group member/leader _____

(h)_____ (w)_____ (cell)_____

Primary doctor: _____

(h)_____ (w)_____ (cell)_____

Neurologist: _____

(h)_____ (w)_____ (cell)_____

Pharmacist: _____

(w)_____

For Dummies: Bestselling Book Series for Beginners

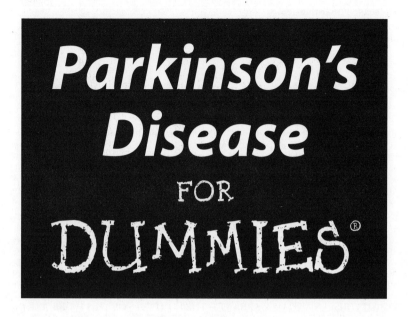

Parkinson's Disease FOR DUMMIES®

by Michele Tagliati, MD; Gary N. Guten, MD, MA; and Jo Horne, MA

Foreword by Deborah W. Brooks
President and CEO of The Michael J. Fox Foundation for Parkinson's Research

BICENTENNIAL
1807
WILEY
2007
BICENTENNIAL

Wiley Publishing, Inc.

Parkinson's Disease For Dummies®

Published by
Wiley Publishing, Inc.
111 River St.
Hoboken, NJ 07030-5774
www.wiley.com

Copyright © 2007 by Wiley Publishing, Inc., Indianapolis, Indiana

Published by Wiley Publishing, Inc., Indianapolis, Indiana
Published simultaneously in Canada

For general information on our other products and services, please contact our Customer Care Department within the U.S. at 800-762-2974, outside the U.S. at 317-572-3993, or fax 317-572-4002.

For technical support, please visit www.wiley.com/techsupport.

Wiley also publishes its books in a variety of electronic formats. Some content that appears in print may not be available in electronic books.

Library of Congress Control Number: 2006939494

ISBN: 978-0-470-07395-7

Manufactured in the United States of America

10 9 8 7 6 5 4 3 2 1

1O/QZ/QR/QX/IN

WILEY

About the Authors

Michele Tagliati, MD, is a movement disorders specialist with extensive experience in the diagnosis and treatment of Parkinson's disease. As Director of the Parkinson's Disease Center at Mount Sinai Medical Center in New York, he follows hundreds of patients at several stages of disease progression. He dedicates his professional life to caring for PD patients and developing research protocols that will ultimately improve their condition. In particular, Dr. Tagliati is a leader in the field of deep brain stimulation for PD and dystonia. He currently serves as teaching faculty at the annual courses given on DBS programming at the American Academy of Neurology and the International Movement Disorders Society. He has published over 40 peer-reviewed articles and 20 book chapters. A medical graduate and neurologist specialist from the University of Rome in Italy, he moved to New York in 1991 with a PD research scholarship. After completing a second neurology residency at Mount Sinai Medical Center, Dr. Tagliati served as a faculty member at Albert Einstein College of Medicine and then moved back to Mount Sinai to become Division Chief of Movement Disorders. He is currently Associate Professor of Neurology at Mount Sinai School of Medicine and a diplomate of the American Board of Psychiatry and Neurology.

Gary N. Guten, MD, MA, is qualified to contribute to this book for three reasons: He's a sports medicine orthopedic surgeon, author, and Parkinson's patient. As an orthopedic surgeon, he specializes in sports medicine, exercise, and nutrition. He was the founder of Sports Medicine and Orthopedic Center in Milwaukee, Wisconsin. The center now has eight doctors. As an author, he has published six books on sports medicine and 27 medical journal publications — 14 are on the Web site of the National Library of Medicine accessible at www.pubmed.com. As a Parkinson's patient, his insight and understanding of Parkinson's disease comes from the fact that he developed PD in 1995. He had to stop doing surgery — but continues to actively do office practice and consultations. Gary received his medical degree from the University of Wisconsin, and as a lifelong learner received a Master of Arts degree in 2005 in Bioethics from the Medical College of Wisconsin. His master's thesis subject was *Placebo Surgery* with a critical analysis of stem cell surgery for PD.

Jo Horne, MA. Many factors came together to lead Jo to this project. After receiving her master's degree in communications from the University of Cincinnati, she spent the early years of her career as a college lecturer. Later as she began an eight-year journey as the long-distance caregiver for her parents, she became aware of the need for a comprehensive guide for caregivers. Over the next several years she wrote three such guides, all published by AARP. At the same time, she left teaching to work with her husband as he and others pioneered the concept of adult day care in the state of Wisconsin. She was also a fellow of the Midwest Geriatric Education Center's initial class and was tapped to deliver the keynote address at the national meeting of the Association of University Professionals in Health Administration for her work in developing curriculum on professional/patient interactions in long-term care. Her work as a communications manager in the dual corporate worlds of long-term care insurance and later the pharmaceutical industry further prepared her to research and write on the effects of Parkinson's on patients and their care partners. Finally when her sister was diagnosed with PD, Jo found herself up close and personal with the impact PD can have. Her unique combination of personal and professional experience has made her a popular speaker and workshop leader as well as a guest expert for national television and radio talk shows.

Dedication

Michele Tagliati, MD — In memory of my father, Silvano Tagliati, who suffered with great dignity from Parkinson's disease, and my beloved wife, Tracy, who greatly inspired my life as a man and a doctor.

Gary N. Guten, MD, MA — This book is dedicated to the lasting memory of my neurologist, Dr. Steven Park, who died in 2006 from a tragic accident. Not only was he a Parkinson's disease maven, but he was my medical mentor, respected colleague, and golfing buddy.

Jo Horne, MA — Every book is for Larry, whose belief in me has never wavered. This one is also especially for Patsy Horne DeBord — my sister and friend — whose fight with PD brought our family closer in spite of the years and miles separating us. It is also for my siblings, Betsy and Earle, and in-laws, Tom and Carole, who took on the demanding role of care partner for Patsy without hesitation and — learning on the job — performed it with love.

Authors' Acknowledgments

Michele Tagliati, MD — I would like to thank Jo, whose enlightened spirit envisioned and inspired this book, and all my patients, who teach me a great deal about their disease every day. In addition, I would like to thank the Department of Neurology at Mount Sinai Medical Center and the Bachmann-Strauss Dystonia & Parkinson Foundation for their continuous support.

Gary N. Guten, MD, MA — One person stands out as being responsible for my insight, knowledge, and fight against Parkinson's disease. That person is my piano teacher — Rita Shur. She has taught me to play the piano (or write) — not with my fingers — but with my heart and my head.

Jo Horne, MA — Without the unique expertise and indefatigable dedication of Michele and Gary, this project would still be on the drawing board. I am indebted to both of them for their insights and humor as we made this journey. I am also deeply indebted to my agent Natasha Kern and everyone on the project team at Wiley Publishing. But as Willie Loman said in the Arthur Miller play *Death of a Salesman,* "Attention must (also) be paid" to the dozens of PWP, their care partners, and healthcare professionals who contributed to the work just by showing me what it means to live with PD. Finally I am profoundly indebted to those fearless and tireless warriors at the foundations and organizations who daily wage the battle to find a cure. My deepest wish is that they make this book obsolete in a very short time.

Publisher's Acknowledgments

We're proud of this book; please send us your comments through our Dummies online registration form located at www.dummies.com/register/.

Some of the people who helped bring this book to market include the following:

Acquisitions, Editorial, and Media Development

Senior Project Editor: Alissa Schwipps

Acquisitions Editor: Michael Lewis

Copy Editor: Pam Ruble

Technical Editor: Ramón Luis Rodríguez, MD

Senior Editorial Manager: Jennifer Ehrlich

Editorial Assistants: Erin Calligan, Joe Niesen, David Lutton

Cover Photo: © Stockbyte

Cartoons: Rich Tennant (www.the5thwave.com)

Composition Services

Project Coordinator: Jennifer Theriot

Layout and Graphics: Lavonne Cook, Denny Hager, Stephanie D. Jumper, Barry Offringa, Alicia B. South, Erin Zeltner

Special Art: Kathryn Born, Medical Illustrator

Anniversary Logo Design: Richard Pacifico

Proofreaders: Jessica Kramer, Techbooks

Indexer: Techbooks

Publishing and Editorial for Consumer Dummies

Diane Graves Steele, Vice President and Publisher, Consumer Dummies

Joyce Pepple, Acquisitions Director, Consumer Dummies

Kristin A. Cocks, Product Development Director, Consumer Dummies

Michael Spring, Vice President and Publisher, Travel

Kelly Regan, Editorial Director, Travel

Publishing for Technology Dummies

Andy Cummings, Vice President and Publisher, Dummies Technology/General User

Composition Services

Gerry Fahey, Vice President of Production Services

Debbie Stailey, Director of Composition Services

Contents at a Glance

Table of Contents

Foreword

A diagnosis of Parkinson's disease is a life-altering event. There is no one way to deal with it. Everyone has a unique set of circumstances, and every patient experiences Parkinson's differently. That's why one book on PD can never be all things to all people. Whether you are living with the disease or are a caregiver or friend to someone who is, you will come to rely on a wide variety of high-quality books, manuals, Web sites, resources and tools. You may be surprised by the voracity of your appetite for newer, better, and just plain more information about PD. And since Parkinson's is — for now, at least — a disease that stays with you for life, your information needs may evolve and change over time.

This book represents something incredibly important: a place to start. We commend its emphasis on tenets that we at The Michael J. Fox Foundation strive to incorporate into our work: an action orientation, a problem-solving mentality, and the distillation of a great deal of complicated information into clear, logical next steps.

Most importantly, the Foundation shares with the authors of this book a commitment to keep patients front and center in every decision we make. As the largest funder of Parkinson's research outside the federal government, we actively partner with scientists to innovate new funding mechanisms that can maximize the quality, quantity and pace of PD research. With a comprehensive view of the field and proactive management of the grants in our portfolio, we are ideally positioned to bridge the gap between basic research and the clinic. For years scientists have asserted that with sufficient research funding, a cure for Parkinson's is within reach. We are working urgently to prove them right.

I am continually inspired by the patients I meet who are endeavoring to live their lives beyond the potentially limiting effects of this disease, defining themselves by their achievements, not their struggle with PD. But no one who knows Parkinson's would suggest that a positive outlook is achievable all the time. Do everything you can to put the odds on your side: Find doctors you trust and can build relationships with; eat well and exercise as much as possible; appreciate and invest in your family and friendships; investigate ways to reduce stress and practice what works for you.

And know that work is continuing aggressively to make this disease, finally, a thing of the past.

Debi Brooks
President and CEO, The Michael J. Fox Foundation for Parkinson's Research

Introduction

*I*f the very idea of a Parkinson's disease diagnosis scares the bejeebers out of you, take a deep breath and pay attention. Although Parkinson's is a chronic and progressive condition with no cure (yet), the strides made in just the last decade to control and manage symptoms are impressive and hopeful. Also the number of national organizations (not to mention big-name celebrities) that are placing the spotlight squarely on the need for a cure is unparalleled.

And we're here to help: An experienced neurologist and lecturer on the treatment of Parkinson's disease (PD); another physician — not a neurologist but rather one who has been living with his own PD (and finding new and innovative ways to maintain control over his life) for over a decade; and a writer of books on aging and giving care whose oldest sister has PD. Together we give you the facts you need, resources you can rely on, and tips on how best to structure your life so that — to paraphrase the popular slogan — you have PD, but it doesn't have you.

This book is your guide to understanding and living with PD. While you — the person with Parkinson's (PWP) are the primary audience — feel free to share *Parkinson's Disease For Dummies* with family, friends, and especially that person who will most likely make this journey with you — your care partner.

We — the doctor-athlete who's fought PD for over ten years, the writer who's seen dozens of people triumph over their PD, and the neurologist who's not in the business of giving up — wish you the strength to persevere, the will to keep fighting for a cure, and the physical and emotional stamina for a long, productive life.

About This Book

At first glance the idea of a *For Dummies* guide to Parkinson's disease may seem ludicrous or even downright insulting. But those of you who have used these guides understand that the dummies reference indicates a guide that presents its topic in simple, straightforward terms. Although PD doesn't have a cure, it can be well managed for years before a person faces its more challenging aspects. And that's what this guide is about — practical ways you can control and manage the symptoms of your Parkinson's so you can get on with your life!

Now, this is not some sugar-coated Pollyanna guide to living with PD. It's a realistic look at what you're facing. It provides solid information and resources to help you and your family come to terms with PD as a factor in all your lives. It offers proven techniques and tips to help you prepare for the future without projecting the worst. And most of all, it reminds you that living a full and satisfying life — in spite of PD — is definitely possible, even probable.

We designed each chapter of *Parkinson's Disease For Dummies* to be self-contained so that you don't have to read the book sequentially or read the first parts to understand any later chapters. You can dip in and out wherever you please and concentrate only on what you need. The table of contents and the index can help guide your search.

Conventions Used in This Book

The following conventions are used throughout the text to make the info consistent and easy to understand:

- All Web addresses appear in `mono font`.

- New terms appear in *italic* and are closely followed by an easy-to-understand definition. We also clearly define the terms in the handy glossary at the back of the book.

- **Bold** is used to highlight the action parts of numbered steps.

- This book has several sidebars (shaded in gray). These aren't essential to your understanding of PD or your use of this guide, but we hope you'll find them interesting and, in some cases, even inspiring.

This guide has a few special conventions that are widely accepted by Parkinson's researchers and advocates as well as by people with PD and their families:

- Parkinson's disease is often abbreviated *PD*.

- A person diagnosed and living with PD is often referred to as *PWP*, or person (or persons) with Parkinson's.

- Because PWP are fully capable of making decisions and planning their care for many years following diagnosis, we refer to their primary caregivers as *care partners*. There may come a day when you need more hands-on care and assistance. Should that day come, that's when your *care partner* takes on the additional role of *caregiver*.

✔ Although we hope your family and close friends will read many portions of this guide, some sections are do-not-miss for these folks. Several chapters have a section titled "A Word for the PD Care Partner" at the end. Be sure to share these sections with the person (or persons) most likely to be your support and eventual caregiver.

Foolish Assumptions

In putting together this guide to living with PD, the three of us have assumed the following about you:

✔ That you have (or suspect you have) PD yourself or are close to someone who does.

✔ That you want reliable information about PD, and you're looking for proven ways (techniques and resources) to treat and manage its symptoms.

✔ That you intend to take a proactive role in facing this challenge and not simply (blindly!) do everything the first healthcare provider you see tells you to do.

✔ That you're open to lifestyle adjustments and complementary or alternative techniques that are proven to manage symptoms and prolong functions.

✔ That you realize PD is not just a physical condition that affects only you; it has elements that impact you — and everyone who cares about you — physically, mentally, and emotionally. You all need to be proactive in preparing for and meeting those challenges head-on.

How This Book Is Organized

All *For Dummies* books are divided into parts and chapters. The goal is for you to easily move from one part or chapter to another without having to read a gazillion pages of information that aren't essential at the moment. Clever, right? The following sections describe each part.

Part 1: Understanding PD

The chapters in this part explain what PD is and isn't. Chapter 1 gives an overview: statistics and background information plus the differences between primary PD and other conditions that can look like it. Chapter 2 gets into the potential causes — genetic and environmental — that researchers study to find new treatments and even a cure. You also find out who's at risk for getting PD. In Chapter 3 we take a closer look at the four major symptoms and signs that distinguish Parkinson's from related conditions. The chapter concludes with the stages of the disease and why these stages have no clear markers.

Part 11: Making PD Part — But Not All — of Your Life

These chapters walk you through those initial steps following your suspicions of PD. We begin with guidance on getting an accurate diagnosis, finding a specialist, and understanding the tests and techniques that confirm your diagnosis. We explain how to connect with other health experts — therapists, counselors, and such — who will play a vital role in managing your PD. In addition, you need to focus on sharing the news with people around you. Chapter 7 gives you tips on how, when, and who to tell. The final chapter in this part addresses the special needs of people with young onset PD (before age 50).

Part 111: Crafting a Treatment Plan Just for You

This is your guide to the current options for treating PD and managing symptoms over the long term. We look at prescription medicines, the possibility of surgery, and proven complementary or alternative therapies that are viable assets. The largest chapter is on diet and exercise, and that's intentional. We include a program of exercises specifically designed to enhance flexibility and build muscle strength. We also insist that you show this program to your physician and physical therapist before trying it on your own! Because PD is a neurological condition (affecting the brain), we include a separate chapter on depression and anxiety, which can be treatable symptoms of the condition itself. Wrapping up this part is a chapter on clinical trials. We discuss how to find such trials as well as the pros and cons of being a participant.

Part IV: Living Well with PD

Because living with PD for many years — even decades — is not only possible but also likely, this part discusses special areas of your life (people, work, and independence) that may need fine-tuning. We explain how people often react differently to a person who now has a chronic and progressive condition and how it's up to you to maintain normalcy with your family, friends, and co-workers. We also address PD and the workplace: the issues you face when you can work as well as the options you have when you can't work. Finally we cover ways to maintain independence and control over your life despite changes in your mobility and mental prowess.

Part V: Coping with Advanced PD

As with any progressive condition, you'll eventually delegate responsibilities and rely on other people to keep you mobile, mentally alert, and emotionally upbeat. This part of the book is as important for your primary care partner as it is for you, so both of you need to read it. We cover important decisions and planning processes that you should address early on, and we discuss the onset of later-stage symptoms that can be incapacitating. We also address the gradual shift of your partner's role from care partner to caregiver, based on ground rules the two of you make. Early discussions on housing, finances, and legal issues are also covered in this part.

Part VI: The Part of Tens

Every *For Dummies* book includes a section of lists, that is, key information that readers can use right away. In *Parkinson's Disease For Dummies,* those lists include ten ways to manage difficult feelings (anger, guilt, sadness, and such), ten ways you (the PWP) can care for your care partner, and — possibly the most important list — ten ways you and your care partner can become active in the fight for a cure.

Part VII: Appendixes

Appendix A contains a glossary of Parkinson's-related terms to use as reference. Appendix B summarizes the many PD resources we mention throughout this guide: organizations, care partner resources, support groups, and assistive devices for making life with PD easier.

Icons Used in This Book

To make this book easier to read and simpler to use, we include icons that help you find (and fathom) key information. Here's what they look like and highlight:

This icon flags essential information that cautions and protects you against potential pitfalls and problems. Do *not* skip over these paragraphs.

This icon signals essential information that's important enough to bear repeating. It's information you should keep in mind.

This icon identifies information that may save you time, offer a resource, or show you an easier way of doing some task or activity.

Where to Go from Here

Where you open this book — Chapter 1, Chapter 18, or somewhere in between — depends on where you are in your journey through Parkinson's. If you suspect PD is the cause behind some troubling symptoms, you may want to start with Chapter 4 for tips on the best way to get an accurate diagnosis. If you've already been diagnosed, then Part III, where we discuss treatment options, may be your first stop.

The point is that this is a *guide,* a roadmap to help you on the path to living with PD. We offer information and resources that you can trust — tools that help you adapt to life with PD without making it your whole life. In the long run, however, it's your resolve to face each day with renewed strength and energy that will see you through. And it's your example that will set the stage for those people who intend to partner with you in the fight.

Part I

Understanding PD

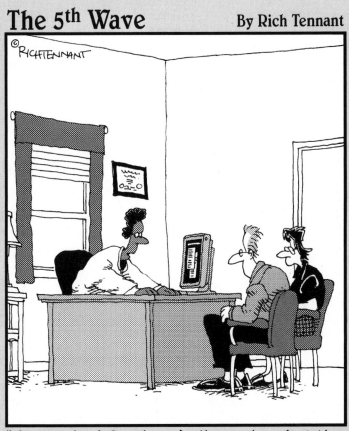

The 5th Wave   By Rich Tennant

"As explained, Parkinson's disease is a depletion of dopamine in the brain. But before you fill up that space with a lot of negative thoughts, let's discuss your treatment options."

In this part . . .

You discover what Parkinson's disease is and how it differs from related forms of parkinsonism. We identify the current theories on causes for the onset of Parkinson's and the risk factors that may play a part for some people. Finally you get a good idea of what symptoms to watch for and what signs doctors look for to diagnose and stage this condition.

Chapter 1

Parkinson's Disease: The Big Picture

*T*he National Center for Health Statistics (a division of the Centers for Disease Control) reports that approximately 1 percent of all Americans over the age of 65 receive a diagnosis of Parkinson's disease (PD). Sixty thousand new cases are diagnosed every year. But you didn't pick up this book because you're interested in mass numbers. You opened it because you're only interested in one number — yours or someone you love. You opened it because you've noticed some symptoms that made you think *Parkinson's,* or you just got a confirmed diagnosis and you're wondering what's next.

What's next is for you to go into action mode — understand the facts (rather than listen to the myths) about PD — what causes it, how it's treated, and, of huge importance to anyone diagnosed with PD, how to live with it. (Notice we said *live,* not just *exist.*) In this chapter, you find the big picture of the rest of the book and (more to the point) where to find the information that you need right now.

Defining Parkinson's — A Movement Disorder

Parkinson's disease is a disease in a group of conditions called *movement disorders* — disorders that result from a loss of the brain's control on voluntary movements. Dopamine (a neurotransmitter in the brain) relays signals from the substantia nigra to those brain regions (putamen, caudate, and globus pallidus — collectively named the *basal ganglia* — in the *striatum*) that control movement, balance, and coordination (see Figure 1-1). In the brain of people with Parkinson's (PWP), cells that produce this essential substance die earlier than normal.

Although a whole group of conditions are known as *parkinsonism,* the one that most people know is called *idiopathic PD*, a Greek word that means *arising spontaneously from an unknown cause*. As the term suggests, the jury is still out as to the underlying cause (though theories do exist).

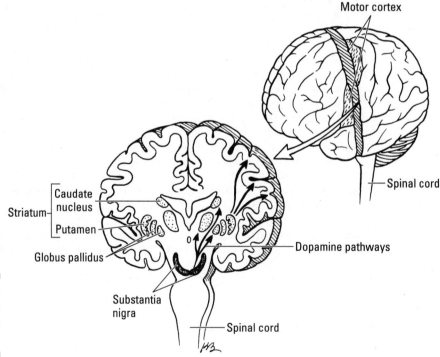

Motor cortex

Spinal cord

Striatum — Caudate nucleus

Putamen

Dopamine pathways

Globus pallidus

Substantia nigra

Spinal cord

Figure 1-1:
The dopamine pathway.

Go into a room filled with 50 people with Parkinson's (PWP) and ask how they first suspected they had PD. You're likely to hear 50 different stories. Take ten of those people who were diagnosed at approximately the same time and you're likely to see varying signs of PD progression — from almost no progression to more rapid onset of symptoms. Similarly, you're likely to experience a variety of attitudes and outlooks from the individuals dealing with their PD.

When you're diagnosed with PD, you set out on a unique journey — one where your outlook, lifestyle changes, and medical treatment can be key directional maneuvers along the way. In truth, this disease is one that you can live with, surrender to, or fight with everything you've got. The road veers and curves differently for each person. Some people may choose one path for managing symptoms, and some people choose another. Sometimes the disease itself sets the course. The bottom line? No clear roadmaps are available. But one fact is certain: Understanding the chronic and progressive nature of PD can take you a long way toward effectively managing your symptoms and living a full life.

Accepting the chronic progressive factors

Chronic and *progressive* can be scary words when you're talking about your health. But keep the words in perspective. Any number of chronic conditions occur with age — arthritis, high blood pressure, and cholesterol management to name three. So, take a realistic look at the terms, accept them for what they are (and aren't), and move on.

Chronic — it's part of you now

In medical terms, illnesses are either *acute* (develop quickly and usually go away with treatment or time) or *chronic* (develop over time, may be managed with treatment, but have no cure at this time). In short, a chronic illness like PD (or arthritis or high blood pressure) is now part of you — a fact that can help or hinder you in the fight.

If you refuse to accept that PD is a fact of life for you, then you're wasting precious time and energy in denial. But, if you accept that most people get challenges in life and PD is yours, then you're ahead of the game. Facing PD is no different than facing any situation that changed the way you thought your life would be.

Progressive — it will get more challenging

Progressive, advancing, worsening — more scary stuff. Here's some good news: For millions of PWP, the progression takes years, even decades. Many PWP live relatively normal life spans following their diagnosis. However, two factors are essential for successfully containing PD's progressive effects: your attitude and your willingness to attend to lifestyle and medical therapy.

Throughout this book we address both factors in multiple ways, but for now, remember:

- ✔ **Your attitude** — refusing to allow this diagnosis to color every part of your routine and life — is a huge factor in coping with the management of new symptoms through the years.

- ✔ **Your willingness to take lifestyle changes seriously** and get involved in the fight to find a cure can make all the difference between you managing the disease or the disease managing you.

To figure out how you're going to live with PD — if you have it — you first need to understand the basics: what it is (and is not), how you get it, what to look for, and how it progresses.

Distinguishing between Parkinson's disease and related conditions

Several neurological conditions may appear to be *idiopathic* (without known cause) PD at first, but they eventually trace back to known causes, progress differently, and respond differently to therapy. (Chapter 3 has more on this.) These other conditions include the following:

- ✔ **Essential tremor** (ET) is perhaps the most common type of tremor, affecting as many as five million Americans. ET differs from the tremor in idiopathic PD in several ways: ET occurs when the hand is active (as in eating, grasping, writing, and such). It may also occur in the face, voice, and arms. The renowned actress, Katherine Hepburn, had ET, not PD. Differentiating ET from PD is very important because each condition responds to completely different sets of medications.

- ✔ **Parkinson-plus syndromes** may initially have the same symptoms as PD. But these syndromes also cause early and severe problems with balance, blood pressure, vision, and cognition and usually have a much faster progression compared to PD.

- ✔ **Secondary parkinsonism** can result from head trauma or from damage to the brain due to multiple small strokes (*atherosclerotic* or *vascular parkinsonism*). Both forms can be ruled out through scans (CTs or MRIs) that produce images of the brain (see Chapter 4).

- **Pseudoparkinsonism** can appear to be PD when in fact the person has another condition (such as depression) that can mimic the inexpressive face of PWP.

- **Drug- or toxin-induced parkinsonism** can occur from taking antipsychotic medications (drug-induced) or from exposure to toxins such as carbon monoxide and manganese dust (toxin-induced). Drug-induced symptoms are usually (but not always) reversible; toxin-induced symptoms usually aren't.

The subtleties of diagnosing idiopathic PD may lead your family doctor to send you to a *neurologist,* a specialist in the treatment of neurological conditions. If that happens, don't panic. Getting the correct diagnosis, discussed in Chapter 4, is the first step toward figuring out what comes next for you.

Debunking some commonly held myths about PD

It's to your advantage to get a grasp on some of the more commonly held myths about PD — what it is and what it isn't.

- PD is not:

    - Contagious

    - Curable (at this writing, but research is hopefully getting closer!)

    - Normal for older people — or impossible for younger people

    - A reason to make immediate life-changing decisions (like assuming you won't be able to work or that you need to move)

    - Bound to get you if you live long enough

- PD is:

    - Chronic (when you have it, you have it — like arthritis or diabetes)

    - Slowly progressive (over time — often years) even with treatment

    - Manageable (often for years) with proper treatment and key lifestyle changes

    - Life-changing for you, your family, and friends (Whether that's good or bad is up to you and how you decide to face it.)

In many ways these debunkers are the key messages we want you to take away from this book. If you have PD, you have an enormous challenge before you, but tens of thousands of people successfully face it every day. You can get through this — and we're here to show you how.

Recognizing symptoms that raise questions

First things first: Do you have PD? Although researchers may not yet have a clear idea of the cause(s) for PD (see Chapter 3), they have established that idiopathic PD starts on only one side of the body and includes one or more of these four key symptoms:

- ✔ Tremor at rest (trembling in the hands, arms, feet, legs, or face when that body part isn't engaged in activity)
- ✔ Rigidity (stiffness in the limbs and trunk)
- ✔ *Akinesia* or *bradykinesia* (lack of movement or slowness of movement)
- ✔ Postural instability (impaired balance or coordination of movement)

Notice how the first letters of the symptoms spell out the handy acronym *TRAP* to help you remember (like you need to be reminded!). You'll have times when the symptoms of PD make you feel trapped inside your body. In this book, we work hard to show you a number of ways to fight back and maintain control of your life in spite of the *TRAP*.

Chapter 3 discusses symptoms (what you report to the doctor) and signs (what the doctor observes) in more detail.

Seeking the Care You Need

Perhaps more than any other chronic condition, managing PD is a team effort. You're going to be working with an entire front line of healthcare professionals (doctors, therapists, and the like) as well as non-professionals like your family and friends and other PWP that you'll meet along the way.

From medical professionals

At least two doctors are likely to be intricately involved: your primary care physician and a neurologist. In addition, you'll possibly connect with several other healthcare professionals along the way: your pharmacist; physical, occupational, and speech therapists; counselors and advisors to help manage any depression, anxiety, diet changes, and exercise regimens; advisors to help manage financial, legal, housing, and other major decisions that'll affect you and your family over the long term. Chapter 6 offers more information about this group.

From loved ones

You'll also have a personal care team: your spouse or significant other; your children (and possibly grandchildren); your close friends and (if you're diagnosed with young onset Parkinson's — YOPD) your parents and siblings. Benchwarmers who may surprise you with their willingness to help out include neighbors, co-workers, members of groups you belong to, and others. In Chapters 7 and 16 we talk more about how to break the news and get these folks involved. Chapter 8 covers questions and situations specific to YOPD.

As your PD progresses

One of the toughest truths you'll face as your PD progresses is that you have to rely on other people's help to some degree. Years may pass before this becomes a factor, but you and your loved ones need to plan for it. In Chapter 18 we discuss the symptoms that can crop up as your PD progresses. Every case of PD is different though; symptoms that occur in another person may never be a problem for you. Knowledge is good, but assuming that you'll have to endure every symptom in this book is just wrong on so many levels.

The more positive approach is to *prepare* without *projecting*. For example, will you have swallowing difficulties? Maybe, but you can have a speech therapist as a part your care team, as we talk about in Chapter 6. She's there on the bench, ready to get in the game if you need help. Will your spouse or significant other have to dress you, feed you, bathe you? Chances are good that he'll need to assist you in these basic daily activities in the advanced stages of your PD. We cover that step in Chapter 19.

Reaching decisions about advanced PD questions before they occur (such as identifying a caregiver and having a family meeting to plan an extended network of support) is just smart planning. (That's in Chapter 19 too).

Treating Parkinson's — Previewing Your Options

After you've educated yourself with facts (not myths or hearsay) and drafted your care team(s), it's time to get down to the serious business of treating your PD and managing symptoms as they appear. In this book we cover the options — in fact, a growing number of options — for treating and managing your PD symptoms. In addition to medications (Chapter 9) and — in some advanced cases — surgery (Chapter 10), you can find relief in complementary treatments (such as physical and occupation therapies) and alternative treatments (such as yoga or acupuncture). See Chapter 11 for more about all of these.

In the beginning your doctor may want you to postpone a prescription-medication regimen in favor of trying some lifestyle changes — for example, diet and exercise (see Chapter 12) and counseling for your PD-related anxiety and depression (Chapter 13). With today's bright spotlight on research for a cure, you may even want to participate in one of the many clinical trials for new treatments (Chapter 14).

As new symptoms appear (usually years after your initial diagnosis), you'll want to check out Chapter 18 to understand the difference between symptoms that can be PD-related and symptoms that can be related to the aging process or another condition entirely(such as high blood pressure).

Starting the Course, Staying the Course

Not surprisingly, for many people and their families, the diagnosis of PD comes as a shock. *Progressive* and *incurable* are likely to be the words that register in these early hours. But as the news begins to sink in, you have choices to make. The following sections provide advice.

Dealing with the here and now

As Debi Brooks, President and CEO of the Michael J. Fox Foundation, notes in the foreword to this book, if you're going to truly have a life with PD, you need to do three things: develop an attitude of action, form a problem-solving mentality, and possess the ability to take a great deal of information coming at you from all directions and distill it into clear, logical next steps.

Here are some tips to get you on the road:

 ✔ Stay in the here and now — not the distant future. PD is a condition you can successfully manage, perhaps for many years, before you must rely on other people.

 ✔ Work with your healthcare team to focus on *your* PD and how you can most effectively manage those symptoms.

✔ Do *not* compare your situation, symptoms, or ability to manage to other PWP. This is not a contest and you are not those persons.

✔ Get organized. What are your questions? Write them down. Who are the best medical professionals to treat your PD? If finding that doctor means traveling to another community, at least consider it. This is your life, after all.

✔ Maintain some sense of control over your destiny by educating yourself. Use only reputable sources such as those we list throughout this guide and in Appendix B.

✔ Use the lingo. Everyone else will — your doctors, the people in your support group, the authors of the articles you read. We define terms as we go, but Appendix A is a glossary for your convenience.

✔ Be a team player by:

- Taking the time to prepare for doctor appointments with questions and information about your current symptoms.

- Taking charge of your own health by making changes to your diet and exercise routine as needed — and sticking with it.

- Understanding that, although you have every right to maintain independence and autonomy over your decisions, you also have a responsibility to care for the people who will care for and eventually speak for you.

- Encouraging innovation in your health team, your family and friends, and yourself. (For example, if you used to love playing jazz saxophone but your tremor makes that impossible, does that mean you have to give up loving jazz?)

- Celebrating even the smallest victory and allowing yourself a decent interval to mourn the greater losses.

- Remembering that your PD is not all about you. Other people are affected, some of them in major, life-changing ways.

- Advocating for new and more effective treatments and a cure. (You can't be more effective than when you're speaking out for those 60,000 PWP who are being diagnosed each year.)

✔ Learn as much as you can, lean on the support of other PWP who have been there (done that), laugh with other people and at yourself, love in return those people who offer love in their support and care, and LIVE with the single determination that you won't be reduced to a PD-only identification ("That's Jack Wilson — he's really an amazing person!").

Working, playing, and having a life

Okay, the medical experts are in place, you're on a regimen customized to manage your symptoms. What's next? How about getting a life — at least getting back to some semblance of the one you had before the diagnosis?

Part IV of this guide is all about living with PD: keeping up with the relationships that are so vital to you as an individual (Chapter 15), maintaining a job (even continuing to build a career if that's important for you; see Chapter 16), and getting out and about — you know, living (Chapter 17).

Making plans for your future

Any diagnosis of a chronic and progressive condition — no matter how slowly it progresses — is a wake-up call for attending to those financial and legal matters everyone needs to address. For you, that time is now. You and your family need to get together with an experienced team of financial and legal consultants and take steps to protect you and your loved ones in the event that you become incapacitated.

If at some point you can no longer speak for yourself or make the complex decisions in managing finances, your care partner must know your choices and have the power to act on your behalf. This advice is just common sense whether a person has PD or not. Chapter 20 offers guidelines and tips that can save you and your family a lot of stress and worry in the future on these matters.

If your current housing become an issue later on (for example bedrooms and the only bath are on the second floor), Chapter 21 takes a look at the growing range of options, including adapting your current residence so you can stay there.

In the course of our individual careers and our collaboration on this book, the three of us have seen case after case of people living full and satisfying lives in spite of PD. We understand that it isn't always easy, but we have seen the incredible results when PWP succeed in living beyond their disease.

Although no single resource can provide all the answers, we believe that in these pages you can find the information you need to make the best decisions for living your life with PD.

Chapter 2

Considering Possible Causes and Risk Factors

Although James Parkinson described the disease nearly two centuries ago and research has been ongoing ever since, the underlying cause — the factor that sets Parkinson's disease (PD) in motion — is still unknown. A number of theories are under discussion and research, any one of which may lead to the breakthrough in managing symptoms or even curing the disease. The medical community has also made progress in assessing risk factors — some more common than others. In this chapter we cover these potential causes and risk factors so you can better understand them as the hunt for a cure continues.

Considering Theories on Causes

The underlying event behind the onset of PD is a loss of neurons (nerve cells) in the *substantia nigra* region of the brain. These neurons normally produce *dopamine,* a neurotransmitter that helps the brain communicate with other parts of the body, telling them to perform common movements (such as walking, handling objects, and maintaining balance) almost automatically.

PD is a little like diabetes because in both diseases

✔ You lose a vital chemical (insulin in diabetes; dopamine in PD).

✔ The chemicals are essential to the body's ability to function properly.

✔ The chemicals can be replaced.

Of course, the diseases are more complex than that, but you get the idea. As we age, all of us lose dopamine-producing neurons, which results in the slower, more measured movements. But the decline of dopamine in people with Parkinson's (PWP) is not normal.

Why PD targets the substantia nigra at the stem of the brain remains a mystery. But the damage results in abnormal protein deposits that can disrupt the normal function of the cells in that area. These protein clumps are called *Lewy bodies,* named for Freiderich H. Lewy, the German physician who discovered and documented them in 1908. The presence of Lewy bodies within the substantia nigra is associated with a depletion of the brain's normal supply of dopamine. For this reason, their presence is one of the pathological hallmarks of PD (although Lewy bodies are present in other disorders).

In reality, Lewy bodies have been found in other parts of the brain affected by PD, which suggests that the problem may be more widespread. This more extensive pathology may explain the occurrence of non-motor and levodopa-unresponsive symptoms (see Chapter 9). Nevertheless, researchers still don't know whether Lewy bodies cause the damage to the nerve cells or are a by-product of damage caused by another factor.

Theories on causes abound — family history, environment, occupation, and so on. Today's researchers generally agree, however, that the onset of PD is a *multi-factorial* process; that is, several conditions are at play in the onset of PD rather than one specific and single cause. But the true causes behind the onset of PD in one person and not another — in one family member and not another — are unknown.

Much of the research today focuses on environmental and genetic factors that may contribute to the onset of PD. This section takes a look at those environmental conditions and then considers genetic issues and other factors that scientists have identified as potential causes.

Taking a close look at environmental factors

According to the National Institute of Environmental Health Sciences, PD is the second most prevalent neurodegenerative disorder behind Alzheimer's disease. Of the three primary risk factors for PD (age, genetics, and environmental exposures), a line of research that began in the 1980s shows an increasing association between environmental factors and PD. The following sections explore the variety of environmental exposures that may play a role in triggering PD.

Free radicals — the internal battle

Free radicals are unstable molecules that lack one electron. In their quest to replace that missing link, they rub against other molecules, seeking a connection that will stabilize them.

Even when the free radical doesn't make a connection, it keeps digging, damaging other molecules in the cell in a process known as *oxidation* or *oxidative stress*. Normally your body has enough antioxidants to stabilize the free radical and repair the damage, but if it doesn't, then those damaged cells die.

Key players in controlling oxidative stress are the *mitochondria* (the part of the cell outside the nucleus that converts nutrients into energy) because they're a potential source of free radicals. In addition, several of the toxins associated with PD seem to damage specifically the mitochondria. Researchers believe a connection may exist between oxidative stress and the death of cells in the substantia nigra, which causes PD symptoms. This theory is one of the main reasons that some doctors recommend a diet rich in antioxidants. (See Chapter 12 for more on diets for PWP.)

Location, location, location

For the overwhelming number of PD patients who get Parkinson's, certain environmental factors seem to put the person at higher risk for getting the disease. Consider that family members share not only a genetic history but also an environmental history — at least for a portion of their lives. They live in the same house, drink the same water, eat the same food from the same sources, have exposure to the same chemical compounds, and so on. Therefore, researchers are studying geographic environmental factors as a possible link to the onset of PD. These factors include living in a rural area and using well water for drinking, cooking, and such.

Exposure to toxins

Toxins that people inhale or ingest can damage the body in many ways, including cell function interference. Research shows that excessive exposure to specific environmental or industrial toxic chemicals such as pesticides and herbicides can increase the risk of developing PD. For example, the damage by the pesticide *rotenone* is directed at the *mitochondria* (the power plant of our brain cells) and can critically reduce the energy produced by the cell until the cell dies. (See the "Free radicals — the internal battle" sidebar for more on this topic.)

In some cases environmental toxicity and genetic factors may operate in tandem. Scientists have discovered that the gene CYP2D6, when functioning normally, produces an enzyme that breaks down the toxicity of pesticides.

But in some people the gene is less effective, leaving those people more sensitive to the toxicity of pesticides. More studies are needed to verify whether there may be a correlation between genetic predisposition to pesticide toxicity and PD.

Links to viral problems

Although PD is not contagious, a viral factor may be associated with its cause. This hypothesis is mainly based on the occurrence of *post-encephalitic parkinsonism* after the influenza pandemic of 1918. More Americans died from this flu in a single year than from the all the wars from World War I through the Vietnam War.

To complicate matters, many patients developed the so-called *sleeping sickness (encephalitis lethargica),* characterized by the progression from severe headache to drowsiness to possible coma and death. Patients who survived the encephalitis (brain infection) often developed symptoms of parkinsonism, including bradykinesia, rigidity, hypomimia, postural instability, and eye movement abnormalities (*oculogyric crises*). The memoir *Awakenings* by Oliver Sacks (Vintage) and the 1990 movie by the same title starring Robin Williams and Robert de Niro provide an insightful and accurate representation of this disease.

In reality, the relationship of a virus (such as influenza) and the brain degenerative lesions causing parkinsonism has not been proven. Furthermore, the pathology described in the brain of patients with post-encephalitic parkinsonism is very different from PD and actually bears more of a resemblance to Alzheimer's disease. So the possible viral link with parkinsonism remains elusive.

Although these environmental factors and cellular interactions appear to significantly contribute to the onset of PD, the Parkinson's Disease Foundation notes "no conclusive evidence that any single environmental factor, alone, can be considered a cause of the disease." (Go to the foundation's Web site at www.pdf.org/aboutPD/ and click on *Causes* for more information on this topic.)

Looking at possible genetic factors

Every human being plays host to a gazillion genes in their DNA molecules. Genes determine everything from the color of your eyes to the possibility of developing a certain disease or condition. Note the use of the word *possibility.* Because you carry genes in double copies, if one of your genes has the propensity for a condition, the other copy may offset that vulnerability.

According to the National Human Genome Research Institute, evidence now shows a genetic factor in the development of PD. People with a close relative (parent or sibling) who has PD are slightly more likely to contract Parkinson's than someone who has no family history of the disease. But, according to the Mayo Clinic, the link is a small one — less than 5 percent — and more common when the onset occurs before age 30, which is also very rare. (For more information on early onset PD, check out Chapter 8.)

So why waste time and money studying genes? Oddly enough, the very fact that PD is one of the most typical nongenetic diseases makes the genetic study of PD patients interesting. In other words, if PD is typically *not* inherited, then what else is going on?

In the last decade, scientists have identified multiple genes with definite links to the onset of PD in families where PD is present in multiple generations. An abnormality in one such gene, *Parkin*, may be a predictor of the onset of Parkinson's at a young age (before age 50). Because Parkinson's is present and progressing for several years before any symptoms become obvious, a gene predictor can mean earlier diagnosis and earlier intervention.

Another recent discovery shows that a *mutation* (change) in the protein-producing gene *alpha-synuclein* may change the gene's amino acid composition and thereby contribute to the development of *clumps* (separate cells bonding together) in dopamine neurons, eventually damaging or destroying the dopamine-producing neuron. Interestingly, alpha-synuclein is part of the Lewy bodies, the hallmark protein deposit in dopamine cells affected by Parkinson's disease. If researchers can find a way to break up those clumps and get rid of the excess proteins, then they may have found a way to slow or even stop the progression of PD. (See the section "Occupational causes" later in this chapter for more about clumping.)

Keep in mind that less than 5 percent of PWP appear to have inherited it; at this writing, any genetic factor seems limited to a relatively small number of families. However, the study of genes enhances the ability to understand which molecules a scientist may target for treatment. If you have a family history of PD or are interested in more information on genetic research, visit www.ninds.nih.gov/disorders/parkinsons_disease.

Checking out other possible causes

If it's not family history and it's not the environment, what caused your PD? Unfortunately, that's a difficult question to answer at this stage. And any time a chronic illness has no definitive cause, theories will fly. At the moment, PD has its fair share of such theories. The following sections describe instances where the jury is still out regarding a link with the onset of PD.

Latent effects of war

Links between PD and Agent Orange (an herbicide used during the Vietnam War) and chemical weapons during the Gulf War continue to be relevant questions for PD researchers. For example, in 2003 the Salk Institute identified a gene (called neuropathy target estrase or NTE). In studies with mice, scientists found that when NTE genes are exposed to organophosphate chemicals (such as those used in the Gulf War), the gene's normal activity was inhibited and even changed. While this discovery has certainly opened new doors (not to mention raised new questions), the evidence is far from conclusive. Remember that age is a consideration in the onset of PD and Vietnam vets are reaching the age that onset of PD is more common simply because of their generation. Whether exposure to Agent Orange may also be a contributing factor is still not clear. The good news is that the Veterans Administration (VA) is conducting ongoing research. If you're a veteran of either war, you can find out more information by contacting the U.S. Department of Veterans Affairs online at www.va.gov.

Overmedication and drug use

Certain drugs taken to excess or over a long period of time may produce the symptoms of PD. Some of the conditions and their drugs include

- Schizophrenia, major depression, or agitation in older people: haloperidol (Haldol) and chlorpromazine (Thorazine)
- Control of nausea: metoclopramide (Reglan) and prochlorperazine (Compazine)

Side effects of such medicines usually subside after the medicine is out of the body's system. *Note:* Symptoms brought on by drug use commonly occur on both sides of your body at the same time, unlike primary PD. The question remains whether a drug reaction of this nature is a predictor for PD.

Illicit drug use may also be a factor. In one case, a group of young people brewed up what they thought was a hallucinogenic drug called *meperidine* and mistakenly produced a heroin-like drug. When injected, this drug, which contained the toxin 1-methyl-4-phenyl-1,2,3,6-tetrahydropyridine (MPTP), headed straight for the substantia nigra, destroying dopamine cells in its path and leaving the youngsters with signs of advanced PD. The tragedy has led to more research on the possibility of a connection between illicit drug use and the onset of PD.

Occupational causes

Many people have theorized that Muhammad Ali's PD was brought on by his years in the boxing ring. "Too many times getting hit in the head," they assert. Indeed some studies suggest an association between head trauma and the development of PD. Possibly Ali's years in the ring brought the underlying presence of his PD to light.

Another class of work associated with onset of PD is the welding profession. At this writing, an absolute connection doesn't exist between prolonged exposure to metallic fumes or dust and the onset of PD-like symptoms. Nevertheless, researchers continue to explore the possibility of a link because studies show that exposure to heavy metals and pesticides — each already linked to a possible cause for onset of PD — can accelerate the clumping of certain protein cells called *alpha-synuclein*. (See the earlier section "Looking at possible genetic factors" for more on this gene.)

Sounds like sci-fi, but a word about neuroprotectors

The brain has two types of cells: *neurons* (nerve cells) and *glia* (cells that respond to injury and regulate the chemical composition surrounding them, among other tasks). Although glia cells are far more prevalent, the neuron cells do the heavy lifting when it comes to brain work. According to the National Institute of Neurological Disorders and Stroke, the three classes of neurons are:

✔ Sensory neurons to carry information from the senses (eyes, ears, and such) to the brain

✔ Motor neurons to carry messages from the central nervous system (comprised of the brain, spinal cord, and network of nerves running through the body) to the body's muscles and glands

✔ Interneurons that communicate only within their immediate location

Within each category, hundreds of neuron types operate with the very specific messaging abilities that make each person unique. But the neurons affected by PD control the body's ability to move. When those neurons die in large enough numbers, the brain's ability to signal the body to move is compromised.

Researchers are working hard to understand the death of these neurons and to develop treatments and therapies that can protect them. One potential value of stem cell research is that neural stem cells may reproduce the variety of neurons in the brain. Scientists could then figure out how to maneuver these new neurons to become

✔ A protector of healthy neurons (preventing or at least slowing further damage or loss)

✔ A replacement for damaged or dead neurons

In addition, ongoing research considers whether certain therapies — such as certain drugs, vitamin supplements, and rigorous exercise therapy — may act as a protector and slow the loss of these vital neurons. For more information on the role of neuroprotection in the battle against PD, check out Chapters 11 and 12.

Oddly enough, in more than one occupational study, teachers and healthcare workers showed a higher incidence of PD — as much as two to three times higher than other professions. Researchers are puzzled because the commonality in the two professions seems to be exposure to infection, even though PD is clearly not a contagious disease.

Weighing Your Risk Factors

Your suspicion that you have PD (or an actual diagnosis from your doctor) can raise all sorts of questions starting with, "How did this happen to me?" It's perfectly normal to look back and consider the risk factors that were present (although unknown at the time) as you also look forward to protecting your children and others around you from those same risks.

Start with what is known for sure:

- ✔ PD is not contagious — you can't get it from or give it to another person.
- ✔ Most cases (at least three-fourths) show up after age 60, and incidence increases every decade after that.
- ✔ Head trauma (a serious fall or accident involving injury to the head) can be a risk factor for PD.
- ✔ Men are more likely to get PD than women.

Your particular risk factors (or family members' risks if you suspect you have PD) are the life and lifestyle details that can increase the chances of developing PD. They may be *multi-factorial.* (You may be at risk from more than one source or situation).

Considering your age and gender

The one concrete risk factor for developing PD is age. Most people develop symptoms in middle age, but the risk for developing PD increases simply because dopamine production declines with age. The average age for onset is 60, and risk increases until around age 75. Some research has shown a significant decrease in the number of people who develop PD after age 75.

At least three studies have confirmed that men are more likely to develop PD than women — in some studies twice as likely. One theory suggests that the production of estrogen may protect women. At the 2006 meeting of the American Academy of Neurology, a research team from the Mayo Clinic presented evidence that points to a possible link between risk for contracting PD and three genes that control the production of estrogen. Simply put, if the presence of estrogen reduces the risk, a decrease in estrogen increases a woman's risk factor for getting PD. However, more studies are needed to confirm a protective role for estrogen in PD.

Taking a look at ethnicity

Studies have shown that non-white populations, such as African Americans and Asian Americans, have a lower risk of developing primary Parkinson's disease but may be more vulnerable to other forms of parkinsonism such as essential tremor and multiple system atrophy (see Chapter 1). However, whether this difference is tied to an economic and class-based imbalance in the delivery of medical care — especially specialized medical care, like seeing a neurologist —has not been fully considered.

Regarding other risk possibilities

Although they aren't definitive causes, some factors we discuss in this chapter may contribute to your risk for developing PD. In a world where pesticides and herbicides have so many uses, it's hard to avoid exposure to chemicals that put you at risk for all sorts of health problems including PD. Similarly, in an eat-on-the-run fast-food society, people may be denying their body's needs for key vitamins and nutrients. And what about the dangers of such evils as smoking and caffeine? Can these all be factors that put people at greater risk for getting PD?

Overexposure to herbicides and pesticides

Your everyday exposure to chemical toxins can range from the chemicals to control weeds on your lawn to the unseen sprays that coat and polish fresh produce from overseas. Because prolonged or consistent exposure to such toxins is a possible cause of PD (check out "Taking a close look at environmental factors" early in this chapter for more on toxins), take the following precautions:

- ✔ Wash all fresh produce thoroughly — even those items like melons or citrus where you normally discard the skin.
- ✔ Limit your exposure to the use of toxins such as pesticides and insecticides.
- ✔ Use all chemical materials in open areas and wear a protective mask.

If your job requires you to work with chemical compounds such as those in industrial pesticides and herbicides, talk to your employer about precautions to protect you and other employees from exposure and contamination.

Factoring in your weight

Face it: Being overweight sets you up for all kinds of health risks. A 2002 study showed that carrying excess weight during your middle and later years can put you at greater risk for PD. A report in the May, 2003 issue of *Psychology Today* magazine shows an increased rate of PD linked to dietary fat and sugar intake. Although the association between weight gain and PD hasn't been proven, the benefits of a diet rich in antioxidants and a regular program of exercise can't hurt. (In some cases, these benefits have prolonged the time before PD symptoms needed to be treated with medication (see Chapter 12).

Reduced levels of B6, B12, and folate

B6, B12, and folate are essential nutrients for maintaining many of the body's functions. Researchers are beginning to explore whether reduced levels of these nutrients may be a factor in PD. Although studies are in preliminary stages to verify any role the nutrients may play in the management of PD, consider asking your doctor about increasing or supplementing your intake of nutrients.

Regardless of the research and the nutrients' potential for managing your PD, people over age 50 are at increased risk for deficiencies of these three essential nutrients. A diet rich in these nutrients and a supplement (if your doctor advises) may be helpful. However, these need to be carefully monitored by your doctor. Too much B6, for example, can cause additional neuropathic problems such as a profound inability to feel your legs.

Check with your doctor before taking any vitamin or herbal supplement. Claims for these products often lack solid research. The overuse of such products may do more harm than good.

Smoking and caffeine

Get this: As many as 50 published studies over two decades have shown that smoking cigarettes reduces the risk of Parkinson's in people who have smoked steadily most of their adult lives. Caffeine also appears to offer some protection.

But these factors are not a guarantee (as Michael J. Fox noted in an NBC *Dateline* interview in 2006). And the negative effects of these factors (such as lung cancer from smoking) that can greatly shorten your stay on this planet are way too grim to think a two-pack-a-day habit may be worth the risk.

Changing Don't Know to Know

The more researchers tackle the problems of PD, the more complex the challenges become. This section takes a quick look at the unknowns of PD and offers ways that PWP and the general public can help PD research move forward.

The need-to-know info

Questions for PD researchers abound, but one of the greatest challenges is simply getting a good handle on the accurate numbers and extent of PD. For example

- ✔ Scientists really don't know how common Parkinson's is.
- ✔ They don't know whether the numbers are changing over time or simply reflecting longevity and an aging population.
- ✔ They don't know whether geographic cluster patterns exist (places in the United States where PD is unusually prevalent or absent).

The Muhammad Ali Foundation has established a voluntary registry where patients may record their PD diagnosis and information. (Register at www. alicenter.org.) However, because this information is random and voluntary, it has limited practicality.

At this writing, PD has no national registry where doctors can report the diagnosis of PD in the United States. (California is the only state where doctors must report cases of Parkinson's.) A mandatory national registry for the diagnosis of PD would be an enormous step forward (a global registry would be even better!) and one of the best ways to help researchers gather the knowledge and data they need. This registry may seem an invasion of your privacy, but information that allows researchers to track patterns is the best way to gain vital knowledge that leads to new treatments and a cure.

The attitude that busts research barriers

At the 2006 World Parkinson's Congress in Washington, D.C., Joan Samuelson (founder of the Parkinson's Action Network) said that when first diagnosed, she believed her job was to be a *patient patient*. That attitude quickly changed as Joan understood more about the known and unknowns of PD. Today her motto is that patients need to be *in the room* — the PD patient community needs to take a vocal and proactive role in helping research move forward.

You may not be ready to take on this larger fight, but keep it in the back of your mind as you use this book. ***Note:*** In many ways you've taken a key first step — you're educating yourself about Parkinson's and what a diagnosis may mean for you and your loved ones. But getting involved with the greater Parkinson's community at a local, state, and national level is one of the most empowering steps you can take to live a full and productive life in spite of PD. (And when you are ready to get more involved, see Chapter 14 for more information on clinical trials and Chapter 24 for ideas on advocacy roles.)

Chapter 3

Sizing Up Symptoms, Signs, and Stages

....

....

*W*henever you have a concern about your health, you've usually taken note of certain troubling (and unexplained) symptoms. Perhaps you seem more clumsy than usual or your joints seem unusually stiff and rigid. If these symptoms are troubling enough, you're likely to make an appointment with your primary care physician (PCP) to have them checked out. After you describe your symptoms, your doctor conducts a clinical exam looking for signs that may explain your symptoms.

In this chapter, we describe the *symptoms* that can signal Parkinson's disease (PD) as well as the *signs* your doctor looks or to reach a diagnosis. Although many chronic, progressive conditions move through defined stages, this chapter stresses how progression in PD is unique for each patient.

Familiarizing Yourself with the Lingo

In the medical world, a *symptom* is

▶ What you feel or perceive before you see the doctor.

▶ The reason you ultimately decide to make an appointment.

▶ The details (vague or specific) you give when the doctor or nurse asks why you've come in.

For example, you may say that you're more tired than usual or moving more slowly because you lack energy. Or perhaps you're depressed or experiencing dizziness or shaking.

In contrast, medical *signs* are what your doctor observes during the examination. The best doctors use their senses in addition to the data from the usual medical imaging techniques and screening tools (see Chapter 4 for more about these instruments). For example, a doctor's touch may sense tightened muscles, or his eyes may observe a fine tremor when your hand's at rest, or he may note a compromised balance or slight shuffle when you walk. His ears may detect softer speech, a searching for words, or unusual sounds in your lungs or intestines.

Simply put, symptoms make up your subjective report of your experiences, and signs contribute to your doctor's objective basis for a diagnosis.

Disease *staging* divides a chronic and progressive illness into levels that usually correspond to the advancement of symptoms and disease. Generally, stages have the following labels:

- *Early stage*: The disease is manageable with little outside assistance.

- *Moderate stage*: The patient needs more assistance and lifestyle changes.

- *Advanced stage*: The disease has advanced to the point that can be difficult to manage; the patient may face the end of life.

The following sections take a closer look at symptoms (what you tell your doctor), signs (what your doctor observes and discovers via tests and examination), and staging (where you are in the progression if you do have PD).

Symptoms — What You Look for

Let's cut to the chase. You suspect that you or someone you love may have PD or you wouldn't be flipping through this book and you definitely wouldn't have turned to this chapter. Ask yourself what's behind those suspicions.

- **A slight shakiness in the hands?** Does it occur in only one hand? If the shaking occurs while the hand is at rest, does it stop when that hand picks up a cup of coffee, a pen, or a tennis racket? If the shakiness is in both hands and doesn't stop when the person grasps something, then PD probably isn't the cause (but get it checked out anyway).

- **A general slowing down of movement?** Does it take longer to walk from one place to another or to get in and out of the car? Has there been an increase in stumbling, clumsiness, or loss of balance? Do you (or does the person) feel tired, stiff, or just *not yourself?*

✔ **A significant change in energy level or outlook?** Everyone experiences days when they're tired or weaker than usual. And everyone has the blues from time to time. But if you've been feeling unusually weak, fatigued, depressed, or anxious for longer than two weeks, those symptoms need attention — even when you have a plausible cause (such as an unusually busy week at work or the death of a loved one).

✔ **Gastrointestinal problems (like constipation) or psychological problems (like increased nervousness or anxiety)?** In some cases, patients show none of the usual symptoms, so don't stop with the more traditional PD symptoms.

These are the symptoms — the feelings, aches, and pains that have made you think something's not right. It may be PD or it may not. Either way, you owe it to yourself to get your doctor's assessment.

Signs — What Your Doctor Looks for

When you see your doctor, she'll listen as you describe your symptoms and then conduct an examination to determine what those symptoms indicate. As you talk about your symptoms, your doctor begins a *differential diagnosis* if your symptoms indicate several possibilities. For example, if your symptoms are in keeping with PD, your doctor also looks for signs that indicate PD. But any doctor worth her salt doesn't offer a firm diagnosis before she's seen the results of several tests and a specialist has confirmed her suspicions.

In addition to four primary signs of PD (which may or may not be evident when you first go to the doctor), your doctor considers several secondary signs and symptoms. And because PD is a neurological condition, it doesn't just affect your physical movement; it can also trigger non-motor or cognitive signs and symptoms. We discuss all of these signs and symptoms in the following sections.

Four primary signs

Although the actual causes and risk factors for getting PD are still mysterious (see Chapter 2 for more on these factors), the primary signs that signal the presence of PD are very clear. You may have noticed one or more of these signs but then dismissed it as something slight, easily explained, or due to an entirely different condition.

Several resources use the acronym *TRAP* to illustrate the four primary signs of PD. And, because PD seems to trap your body with your brain's compromised ability to communicate, the acronym makes the top four symptoms easy to remember.

T = Tremor at rest (uncontrolled shaking)

PD was originally called *shaking palsy* because the *resting tremor* (it goes away as soon as the hand is engaged) rarely occurs in other illnesses. Characteristically, the resting tremor begins in one hand and moves to the other hand years later in the disease. The tremor may extend to the leg or foot on the same side and sometimes to the lips and jaw — or you may have no tremor at all. Tremor in the head and neck, however, is less common in primary Parkinson's disease.

Variations of the resting tremor include:

- Postural tremor (obvious when arms are extended to hold a position or posture)
- Action tremor (present when certain tasks, such as holding, are performed)
- Internal tremor (the patient feels the tremor but can't show it, almost as if it's coming from inside)

While tremor is the most obvious symptom of PD, it doesn't have to be present for diagnosis.

R = Rigidity (stiff muscles)

Rigidity is probably the most ignored and easy-to-explain-as-something-else sign. In plain English, *rigidity* means *stiffness*. (Who doesn't experience stiffness in joints and limbs that makes movement more difficult as they age?) If your doctor observes rigidity (without other signs of PD), he may first suspect arthritis and prescribe an anti-inflammatory medication. But, if medicine doesn't relieve the stiffness, you need to let your doctor know.

A = Akinesia (absence or slowness of movement)

Especially early on, people with PD (PWP) may experience slight *bradykinesia* (unusually slow movement). Much later in the progression, that slowed movement may become *akinesia* (no movement).

Get to know these terms because, if indeed you or a loved one has PD, you'll hear these words again and again. *Kinesia* means *movement* in the sense of knowing what you want your body to do. So *akinesia* and *bradykinesia* indicate problems initiating or continuing an action. For example, to walk across the room, you stand up and your brain tells your foot to step out — but with bradykinesia, your body doesn't move right away.

The problem can extend well beyond simply walking from here to there. Bradykinesia can also affect

- ✔ Facial expression because it slows blinking eye movement and the ability to smile. Read more about this *facial mask* in the next section, "Secondary signs and symptoms."

- ✔ Fine motor movements, such as the ability to manage buttons or cut food because the fingers lack the necessary speed and coordination to perform these detailed actions. In addition, fingers may curl or stiffen because of rigidity.

- ✔ The ability to easily turn over in bed because of lack of coordination between the various parts of the body that need to move in sequence; again muscle stiffness and rigidity may further complicate this normally routine task. (See discussion of secondary signs and symptoms later in this chapter.)

P = Postural instability (impaired balance)

In a healthy person, the natural movement is to alternately swing the arms and step forward with assurance. For PWP, however, the swing slowly decreases; in time the person moves with small, uncertain, shuffling steps. (PWP may adapt by propelling themselves forward with several quick, short steps.) Other PWP experience episodes of *freezing* (their feet feel glued to the floor).

Problems with balance (resulting in falls that can cause major injuries, hospitalization, and escalation of symptoms) are usually not a factor until later stages in PD. In time, PWP may lose the ability to gauge the necessary action to regain balance and prevent a fall. They may grasp at doorways or other stationary objects in an effort to prevent the loss of balance. Unfortunately, these maneuvers can make PWP appear to be under the influence of alcohol or other substances.

Secondary signs and symptoms

Many of the following indicators — although not essential to a PD diagnosis — are observable early on and can contribute to the diagnosis of PD. During your appointment, tell your physician anything that is troublesome regarding these secondary symptoms. They're part of your symptomatic history that helps your doctors see the total picture of your condition.

Facial mask

The mask (lack of facial expression) is a common sign of PD, and it can lead people to assume that you're not listening or not understanding the conversation. The difference may simply be a change in your facial expression due to decreased animation or emotion. Maybe someone has said, "You don't smile as often," and you're thinking, "I'm smiling just as often as before!" Likewise, people may accuse you of staring, but the real problem is that the number of eye-blinks has decreased.

Slowed or slurred speech

You (or other folks) may notice that your voice is softer or fades away after a strong start. Your doctor may further note that your voice lacks normal variations of tone and emotion or that you sound hoarse but report nothing to explain that hoarseness. In some cases you may have trouble saying a word clearly; you slur it instead of enunciating.

As PD advances, other speech issues (such as stuttering or speaking very rapidly) can appear; swallowing difficulties may develop later in the disease. (See Chapter 18 for more info about advanced symptoms of PD.)

Small, cramped handwriting

Handwriting that once was free-flowing and smooth may appear increasingly cramped and jerky. This *micrographia* typically appears as letters that become progressively smaller (for example: Parkinson) and closer together.

Constipation and urinary incontinence

Most people (even some doctors) associate constipation with aging. But PD can also slow the bowels (as it does the rest of the body), so mention any unusual changes in bowel habits or routine to your doctor.

By the same token, *urinary frequency* (having to urinate often) and *urinary urgency* (NOW!) are common sideshows in the aging process. Although these problems may be signs of a totally unrelated condition, they are not uncommon in PD. Definitely bring these symptoms to your doctor's attention.

Increased sweating or oily skin

A sensitivity to heat and cold and excessively oily (or dry) skin are other signs that may indicate PD.

Non-motor signs and symptoms

Although the *TRAP* signs (check out the earlier section, "Four primary signs") are often enough evidence to raise the possibility of PD, non-motor factors may be present before those primary signs appear. Your doctor may ask questions to discover underlying symptoms that you've been ignoring or simply discounting.

It is vital that you keep an open mind and answer your doctor's questions as honestly and fully as possible. Any one of the following symptoms or a combination of them may indicate a condition other than PD. Don't jump to conclusions or try to self-diagnose. Trust your doctor on this!

Anxiety or depression

Anxiety and depression are such an integral part of PD that they get their own chapter (Chapter 13) in this book. For now, remember that these feelings may be some of the earliest symptoms of PD. Anxiety episodes can range from a mild, underlying feeling of uneasiness to a full-blown panic attack. Depression may disguise itself as a general lack of interest in normal activities, or it may be severe enough for you or your family to consider counseling or medication.

Executive dysfunction and cognitive abnormalities

Do you have trouble balancing your checkbook, following directions, or making decisions? In medical terms, these symptoms are examples of *executive dysfunction*. Another term, *cue-dependent function,* is also part of the non-motor symptom package, and it means you need a reminder of some sort. For example, you may need an alarm that tells you to take your medicine or attend a meeting. Or you have labels on cabinets and drawers to remind you of their contents. Of course, many people use these reminders, especially when their lives are jammed with multiple responsibilities and a calendar brimming with appointments and commitments. But if you notice an escalation in the need for such reminders, mention it to your doctor.

In addition as many as half of all PWP experience problems with memory, thought processing, and word finding. These symptoms are usually more pronounced in later stages (see Chapter 18).

Dizziness or lightheadedness

In some cases dizziness or lightheadedness is due to a drop in blood pressure when you stand up, especially in warm weather or over-heated rooms. Although dizziness can be a factor in a number of conditions, don't ignore mentioning it to your doctor if it's one of your symptoms.

Sleep disturbances

PWP usually have no trouble getting to sleep. The more common problems are staying asleep, napping throughout the day, and moving restlessly when asleep. In some cases, the PWP has intense dreams that add to the restlessness and disturbance of normal sleep.

Sexual dysfunction

As with many medical conditions, PD can adversely affect sexual desire and performance. The underlying causes may or may not be related to PD; however, if the problem is part of your PD, it may be relieved with proper medication and treatment.

Visual hallucinations

Visual hallucinations (seeing people or objects that really aren't present) can be a side effect of many medications. In the case of antiparkinsonian meds, hallucinations are usually benign. *Note:* If a patient reports hallucinations before the PD diagnosis and before she begins taking PD meds, the doctor will look for other medications or causes that may be at the root of the problem.

Stages — Understanding the Unique Path PD Can Take

The key to living with any chronic, progressive illness is taking responsibility to maintain your life beyond that condition. We discuss this in much greater depth throughout the book. For now, the significant question is: If this is PD and it does progress, then how fast and to what extent?

Some *chronic* (long-lasting) and *progressive* (advancing or worsening) diseases have clear-cut divisions between *stages* (obvious and even predictable changes in the patient's condition). However, PD isn't one of those — it affects each patient differently. In rare cases, PD can progress rapidly; the person quickly becomes dependent on others for assistance with basic daily activities. However, for most PWP the progression takes years. With proper treatment and management of new symptoms, PWP can live independently for quite some time before they need close care.

Don't let yourself or others try to project the future. *Prepare* — plan for what may happen — yes. *Project* — assume it will happen on a certain timetable — no. Projecting only adds to your anxiety and may actually prevent you from taking some measures that prolong the time between stages.

In spite of PD's lack of clearly defined and timed steps, your doctor may describe your condition in terms of stages. This breakdown is common practice in the medical profession because it permits doctors to use a common and accepted language when making notes about your condition. If you need to change doctors midstream, the new physician's ability to understand the previous doctor's notes can save you valuable time and enhance the new doctor's ability to address your needs.

Although your PD takes a path unique to you and in response to your lifestyle and medical choices, the disease does have some broad outlines of progression. For a fuller discussion of PD rating scales that determine its various stages, turn to Chapter 4.

Early stage PD: When life can be fairly normal

You may have experienced (and ignored) certain warning signals from PD for several years before you went to your doctor. Maybe you were constantly tired or had a vague, don't-feel-good sensation. As your general movement slowed, maybe you dismissed it as *getting older* or *lack of energy today*.

Then you began to notice some troubling (not to mention, annoying!) symptoms: stiffness that was different from the not-as-young-as-I-used-to-be version, shakiness, dizziness, or mood changes. You know the list.

If you have tremor, you may have barely noticed it at first, or maybe you dismissed it as a spasm. It may have appeared in one finger, so you noticed it only when you were performing a certain task, like tying your shoe or buttoning a jacket.

In *early* stage PD, the following conditions may occur:

- ✔ Symptoms are mild and often easily explained.
- ✔ Symptoms are annoying when they occur, but they don't significantly interfere with normal activity.
- ✔ Symptoms occur on only one side of the body.
- ✔ Tremor is present in one limb — usually the hand — and is most noticeable when the hand is at rest.
- ✔ Other people may comment on changes related to appearance, posture, energy, and facial expression.

In the early stages of PD, you can manage for some time with no pharmacological intervention. In other words, you don't need pills to control the symptoms.

Moderate stage PD: When you need to accept help

The defining signal of progression in PD is symptoms on both sides of the body. However, even at this stage, the diagnosis of PD has been missed in some cases simply because the symptoms (rigidity, gait change, tremor) were taken as normal signs of aging.

Other factors that may signal the *moderate* stage include the following:

✔ Your posture becomes stooped; your head is more often bent forward with your chin toward the chest.

✔ Movement of all body parts is significantly slower. When you walk, you often experience *freezing* (your feet feel glued to the floor); your hand tremor may now affect your entire arm, making activities such as shaving or brushing your teeth more difficult.

✔ Cognitive and executive function (see "Non-motor signs and symptoms" earlier in this chapter) is more impaired. Short-term memory, putting thoughts into words, balancing a checkbook, and making decisions are all more challenging.

✔ *Late-moderate* denotes increasing need for anti-dopaminergic medications. Problems with balance and risks of falls (which may result in injuries that require hospitalization) can actually speed the onset of late stage PD. (See Chapter 17.)

✔ PWP must rely on medicines as well as assistance from other people to pursue many of the activities they took for granted before PD. Examples of these activities are driving, getting in and out of a chair or bed, and going to the bathroom.

As symptoms progress, the challenging task for you and your doctors will be to manage your symptoms (see Chapter 9).

After you begin taking them, antiparkinsonian medicines can be amazingly effective. But they also have some serious and unsettling side effects. (For more about PD meds and their side effects, check out the discussion in Chapter 9.) Balancing the dosages and timing is a constant challenge that becomes more difficult as you move from the moderate to the late stage. The good news is that new medicines become available every year, medicines that — ideally — can be more effective without the frustrating side effects.

Late stage PD: When planning keeps you in control

When a PWP reaches the point of serious disability (that is, unable to lead a normal, independent life without major assistance), the medical community describes the stage as *late* or *advanced*. At this stage even the medications that were working so well in the earlier stages start creating problems and complications, and unless the PWP is a candidate for deep brain stimulation surgery (see Chapter 10), he may face unprecedented challenges. This is the stage (for most patients, it's years after the initial diagnosis) when all your planning and preparing (that we preach about throughout this book) pays off for you and your family. In spite of advancing frailty, you are still in control. You have made the decisions necessary to see you through this time, and your family understands and accepts your wishes. You can probably guess the signs:

- ✔ Walking is possible only with a walker and for short distances, if at all.

- ✔ The entire body is stiff and rigid; balance is significantly compromised.

- ✔ The PWP can no longer manage without considerable assistance.

- ✔ Cognitive impairments worsen; physical limitations increase.

- ✔ The benefits of medication wear off earlier between each dose.

- ✔ The PWP is usually confined to bed and requires round-the-clock care (most advanced stage).

The length of each stage is unique to each PWP. With lifestyle and medical therapies and even with certain interventions along the way, PWP can maintain the early-stage status quo for several years.

A Few Words for You and Your Care Partner

If you're living with someone that you suspect has PD, encourage that person to seek a definitive diagnosis. The symptoms may or may not be PD. Many symptoms associated with PD are also factors in illnesses and conditions that are treatable and curable. Neither you nor the other person should jump to conclusions, but you shouldn't ignore the warning signs either.

If the diagnosis is PD, then your first job is to understand that this person you love can continue to live an independent and self-reliant life for some time, even many years.

If you're the person's care partner:

- ✔ Don't assume you need to be Super-Caregiver. Resist the urge to go into full-on nurturing mode; encourage independence and self-reliance.

- ✔ Understand that adding PD to your already busy life can lead to problems if you aren't proactive and don't take the necessary steps to integrate your new role into the rest of your life.

- ✔ Be aware that a decline in the PWP's self-reliance and confidence may be a sign of depression — a common symptom of PD.

If you're the PWP:

- ✔ Maintain your independence and refuse to permit PD to rob you of the normal roles you've always played in all your relationships.

- ✔ Understand that depression is perfectly normal when you first hear that you have PD; however it is not normal for such depression to be prolonged to the point that it actually escalates the progression of your PD and your need for hands-on care.

For each of you, the second task is to realize (and accept) that all the medicines and physician advice in the world can't be effective unless the PWP follows treatment recommendations, including changes in lifestyle. Self-management (the ability to take responsibility through changes in attitude and behavior) is the key to living with chronic illness of any type — and vital for living with PD. If you're the partner, consider what changes you can make in your own routines and habits that support and encourage the PWP to fight this disease.

The following tips may help both of you cope in these early stages:

- ✔ Find out everything you can — from reliable and respected sources — about PD. (See Appendix B for many of the best resources.)

- ✔ Ask questions. Chapters 4 and 5 deal specifically with the diagnosis and the steps immediately following it.

- ✔ Take an active role in partnering with the PWP and medical professionals to consider treatment options and manage symptoms (See Chapter 6 for teaming up with the pros and Chapters 9, 10, and 11 for more about treatment options.)

- ✔ Maintain emotional balance as you each cope with your fears and anxieties about the meaning of this diagnosis for you and other people close to the PWP. (Chapter 7 offers ideas on dealing with other people. Chapters 15 and 19 address relationship questions you may be asking.)

- ✔ Remind each other of times when the PWP faced a difficult situation and didn't just cope, but triumphed in handling it.

- ✔ Whether you're the PWP or the care partner, don't wait to get help for obvious anxiety and depression. (Chapter 13 covers this piece of PD in more detail.)

If the diagnosis is PD, don't panic. You and the PWP are now members of a unique, extraordinarily proactive, well-organized community. If you open yourself to that community, you'll be richer for the friends you make, the information you exchange, and the comfort you share.

Part II
Making PD Part — But Not All — of Your Life

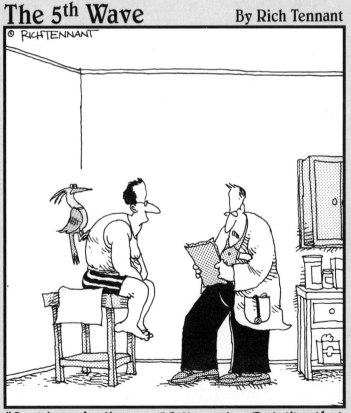

© RICHTENNANT

"Parkinson's disease? Well, maybe. But, like that pain in your shoulder, it could be a lot of things."

In this part . . .

We explore the intricacies of making an accurate diagnosis and why you should see a specialist — a neurologist — to develop a plan for treating your PD and managing your symptoms. You get the basics on how to assemble the healthcare support team you're going to need and the best way (and time) to let other people know of your diagnosis. This part includes a special chapter filled with information for people under age 50 who have young onset Parkinson's disease (YOPD).

Chapter 4

Getting an Accurate Diagnosis

· ·

In This Chapter

▶ Prepping for your primary care doctor

▶ Partnering with a neurologist

▶ Understanding the diagnosis process

▶ Looking for a second opinion

· ·

*O*kay, perhaps you've checked out Chapters 2 and 3 to see the causes and risk factors of Parkinson's disease (PD) as well as its signs and symptoms. And maybe the more you read, the more you worried that you (or someone you care for) may actually have it. Before you freak out, get to a doctor and find out for sure. Your imagination about PD and its consequences is far worse than living with it. In reality, many people with PD live relatively normal and fully active lives for many years after diagnosis. It's your call, but you can set this book aside right now and go bury your head in the sand, or you can take a measured, proactive approach to checking out those symptoms.

Ah, you're still here — great! (Okay, so the book's a little sandy. No problem.) The first step is to get an accurate diagnosis of your symptoms, starting with an accurate list of your current symptoms and medical history. Follow that with a visit to your primary care physician (PCP), who may recommend that you see a specialist. No doubt, you'll be prodded and tested, but you'll finally have a diagnosis. Last step? You want to get that diagnosis confirmed. Ready? Here we go.

Bringing Up the Subject with Your Doctor

This isn't going to be the usual appointment with your doctor. You're not going for an annual check-up or some routine test. You're making this appointment because you have symptoms that you can't explain and that don't seem to be going away. And you're making this appointment because you're concerned something is seriously wrong. An appointment for these reasons needs careful planning all along the way, from scheduling the appointment to gathering information to preparing questions you want to ask. All of this needs to happen *before* the appointment.

Scheduling an appointment

When you call your doctor's office to schedule the appointment, ask to speak to the doctor's nurse or assistant. Tell that person why you're scheduling the appointment. (Yes, go ahead and say it, "I'm concerned that I may have Parkinson's disease.") Then add that you want an appointment when the doctor will have more time — especially if your suspicions are correct. Also ask the nurse what information you should bring with you. When you do make the appointment (usually through the office manager or receptionist), only you can weigh the possible wait (perhaps several weeks until the doctor has this extra time) against the earliest available appointment. *Note:* If you choose the latter, consider booking that later appointment as well in case you want to follow up in more detail with the doctor. In either case, ask to be on the call list. In the event of a cancellation, you can then get to see the doctor sooner.

Preparing for your initial exam

Before seeing your PCP, plan to take the following steps to make that first meeting as productive as possible.

Gathering your medical records

First, be sure that your PCP has copies of all medical records. For example, if you've been seeing a cardiologist, your PCP needs copies of any lab work or stress test results as well as that doctor's notes on observations and treatment.

As soon as you schedule the appointment with your PCP, ask the office staff of any specialist you're seeing to fax copies of recent lab results to your PCP's office. Preparing and transferring such information can take time. So, if time is short, call the clinic where the tests were done or the doctor who ordered the tests and ask for a copy of the results. Then you can pick up these reports and take them with you to your appointment.

Prioritizing your symptoms

Next, make a list of your symptoms and prioritize them. For example, maybe the following is your list of symptoms:

✔ Anxious and not my usual upbeat self

✔ Shaky — especially in my right hand

✔ Unusually fatigued — no get-up-and-go

✔ Not sleeping well

If you suspect PD because you've noticed a slight tremor, you may want to move the second bullet (shaky) to the top of your list.

Keep in mind that the doctor's staff may interview you first. When the nurse asks you why you came in, the first words out of your mouth get her attention. So, if you say, "I haven't been sleeping that well," rather than "Over the last few weeks I've noticed a slight shakiness in my right hand," the nurse writes that your primary issue is *sleep disturbance*. And that statement can take matters in a whole different direction, wasting precious time.

Your doctor refers to the first symptom as your *chief complaint*. When she follows up on your answer with some form of "What makes you suspect Parkinson's?" then you can offer the rest of the symptoms on your list.

For heaven's sake, if you suspect PD, don't be afraid to introduce it into the conversation right away. Life — and doctor's appointments — are too short to beat around the bush!

Compiling your medical history

Writing down your personal medical history helps you prepare for the many questions along the way to your diagnosis. Preparing your history in advance also gives you time to think carefully about the specifics instead of trying to remember details on the spot.

If you've seen a doctor recently, you know that the questions are usually the same — no matter how many times you give the information. First, one or two members of the staff gather your information, and then the nurse or physician assistant (PA) may ask the same questions. But, with a trusty print-out of your history, you can provide a clean copy for their file and still have a copy in-hand (you made two copies, right?) to prompt you on dates and details. This step saves everyone precious time during the appointment and spares you the frustration of recalling every detail for every question.

Don't let this multiple quizzing frustrate you. There's a method to the madness of three different people asking you the same question — usually some form of "Why have you come to see the doctor?" They know that the second or third time a patient answers that question, he may provide additional information without even realizing it.

Many doctors send a questionnaire to help patients gather essential information about themselves and their medical histories. Even if you don't receive such a document, be prepared for your doctor's questions by writing down the following information and taking it with you to your initial exam:

- Patient's legal (full) name and maiden name
- Date of birth
- Birthplace
- Parents' names with dates and causes of death
- Current prescribed (Rx) medications, dosing routine, and purpose (example: diazide, 10mg 1 x day for hypertension); list each Rx separately
- Current over-the-counter (OTC) medications taken regularly, including vitamins, supplements, and such (example: calcium + D, 600 mg 2 x day); list each separately
- Any medications (Rx or OTC) taken over the past year but not currently taken
- Known allergies or adverse reactions to medications or common medical equipment (example: latex gloves)
- Other physicians seen regularly (example: allergist, cardiologist) — name, address, telephone
- Current health problems and dates of onset
- Dates and circumstances of past illnesses or medical events (example: fractured rib, heart attack, accident)
- Dates and reasons for hospitalizations
- Dates and reasons for surgeries
- Recent changes in physical health
- Recent changes in mental or emotional health
- Current situations that may contribute to health changes (consider family, work, and other factors)

Stepping through your initial exam

Okay, you have everything in order and today's the appointment. Take someone with you. If you think you have PD (and it turns out that your doctor agrees), you'll need that extra set of ears to hear what you're bound to miss after you hear that you may have a chronic and progressive condition. Most likely, this will be your care partner if the diagnosis turns out to be PD. The role of this person is to take notes and listen during the appointment and then help you digest and decipher that discussion after the appointment.

Much of what happens at the doctor's office is already familiar to you: the wait (complete with dog-eared selections of last year's magazines); the weigh-in, blood pressure and updating of your medical history; the second wait (this time in the exam room). Use this time to go over the information and questions you've prepared. The doctor's going to ask why you think you have PD, and you need to be prepared to offer specifics (your symptoms, when and how often they occur, when they began, what seems to relieve them, and so on). If you've made a list, you're ready and can just review it.

The doctor may be giving you extra time for your appointment, but that's not the same as endless time. You need to use the time you have wisely by coming to the appointment as well prepared as possible. For more tips on knowing what to expect from a diagnostic appointment and getting the most from that appointment, see "Working with Your Neurologist to Determine Whether This Is PD" section later in this chapter.

Leaving with the answers you need

You'll probably have a gazillion questions by the end of the initial appointment, and you're just as likely not to be able to think of a single one. So once again, be prepared. Prepare a list of questions in advance and use that list. You may even want to hand a copy to your doctor.

If you've brought another person with you to listen and take notes, this is the time she may want to speak up and ask questions also. You can use the following sets of questions as a guide during the appointment. But feel free to add your own.

If the diagnosis seems pretty clear from the start

Although your PCP may believe the diagnosis is clear, he most likely will deliver the news as *possibly* or *likely* Parkinson's and recommend you see a neurologist (a specialist in disorders of the central nervous system). Your PCP may talk in lingo that's unfamiliar to you (*parkinsonism, bradykinesia, postural instability,* and such). Don't be afraid to ask for a clear, layperson's explanation by asking the following questions:

- What is the diagnosis — in plain English?
- What is the prognosis (how quickly will the condition progress)?
- How will the diagnosis be confirmed?
- Does this diagnosis require me to see a specialist?
- Can you recommend a specialist and help set an appointment for me?
- In the meantime, what should I do?

If the doctor orders tests

Even if your doctor believes the diagnosis is fairly clear, she may want to rule out other possibilities. For example, some of the medications you've been taking may be interacting in a way that produces a slight shaking (tremor) in your hand. Or, maybe your primary symptom seems to be depression and apathy; the doctor may want to refer you to a psychologist for evaluation. If she recommends these or other tests, ask the following questions:

 ✔ What are the tests and why are you ordering them?

 ✔ What is the procedure for each test?

 ✔ How quickly will you have the results?

 ✔ What will be the next steps after you have the test results?

If the PCP recommends treatment

Especially if you live in a small community or rural area, your PCP may be the only name in town for treating a wide variety of complex conditions. Even if you live in a larger community that has several specialists including neurologists, your doctor may be aware that your economic situation and lack of adequate insurance may keep you from seeking these services. In any case, if your PCP does not recommend seeking a specialist as a next step but does recommend a plan of treatment, ask the following questions:

 ✔ What is the treatment?

 ✔ Why are you choosing this treatment option?

 ✔ What are the risks or possible down sides of taking these medicines or following the recommended therapies?

 ✔ What is the cost and will this be covered by my insurance?

 ✔ What are the benefits?

 ✔ How quickly should the treatment work?

 ✔ How will you monitor and follow up on the treatment plan?

 ✔ What are the alternatives to this treatment plan?

If It Looks Like PD. . . Connecting with a Neurologist

The initial suspicions of you and your PCP will likely lead to an appointment with a neurologist who can administer further tests to confirm the diagnosis. (If your PCP has already diagnosed PD, then your neurologist helps manage your care.) The following sections suggest how to find a specialist in your area and how to know whether you'll make a good team.

Locating an experienced and qualified neurologist

If possible, look for a neurologist who specializes in movement disorders (like Parkinson's). If you're very fortunate, you live in or near a community that has a Morris K. Udall Parkinson's Disease Research Center of Excellence program. These programs — often in a medical university or institution — are involved in clinical research specifically for the benefit of PD patients. (See the "Morris K. Udall Parkinson's Disease Research Centers of Excellence" sidebar for more information.)

This section suggests resources for finding a neurologist who can help you deal with your PD — now and down the road.

Surfing the Web

The Internet can be a huge help to locate a doctor. Several sites locate physicians by specialty as well as by location, and the sites provide important information about a doctor's training, expertise, possible ethical or treatment violations, and so on. Try an online search with the phrase *neurologists finding*.

You can also get information by checking with the local or regional chapter of a national PD organization. (See the next section and Appendix B for the national organization's info.) Ask whether your area has a local PD support group. If it does, ask for the name and contact information of the group's facilitator. When you call the facilitator, ask whether any members of the group have been treated by neurologists that you're considering. If possible, contact those patients (preferably including patients who have changed doctors) and ask about their experiences with those doctors.

Checking with the local chapter of PD groups

The following organizations have chapters and support groups in communities across the country. You can call them to get names of neurologists in your area.

- ✔ National Parkinson's Foundation (NPF): 800-327-4545
- ✔ American Parkinson's Disease Association (APDA): 800-223-2732
- ✔ Parkinson's Action Network (PAN): 800-850-4726

If you live in a small community, you may have to connect with the group in a larger community nearby (or even at the state level), but the information from these experienced groups is invaluable as you look for a neurologist that's right for you.

Asking your family doctor

Your PCP may be an internist or, if you live in a small community or rural area with limited access to medical care, he may be a general practitioner. For some women, an Obstetrician/Gynecologist (OB/GYN) is their PCP. Whatever your doctor's focus, he's probably aware of local leading doctors in various specialties.

A key question to ask your PCP is: Which specialist do you recommend for working in tandem with you (the PCP) and me to manage my overall health and PD? This question is important for many reasons, but mainly because it is enormously important that your neurologist be consulted before any other doctor prescribes medications or treatment that may adversely affect your PD medication routine or worsen your symptoms.

When your town has no neurologists

Speaking of small communities, what are your options if the closest neurologist is some distance away? First, consider that you're not going to see this specialist weekly or even monthly after the diagnosis is confirmed and you begin routine treatment. Second, assuming the neurologist and your PCP are willing to work together, you have the emergency back-up of your PCP if you need immediate attention.

Don't be tempted to just let your PCP manage your PD for the sake of convenience. At the very least, you want to have your neurologist reevaluate your treatment and status two to four times a year depending on how much change you experience between visits. If you have questions between appointments, try the phone and e-mail. But, taking a day every two to three months to see the neurologist — the specialist in treating your PD — is time well spent. You're worth every minute of it!

Evaluating your neurologist

First things first. You can't expect a neurologist to cure you because a cure for PD doesn't exist — yet. But you can and should expect a professional partnership. You and your neurologist (as well as other team members that we introduce in Chapter 6) will work together to manage your PD symptoms and maintain your physical, mental, and emotional health to the highest possible levels during the years ahead.

You're looking for a specialist who seems curious about *your* Parkinson's:

✔ How it's affecting you now

✔ How you can manage those symptoms best

✔ How to postpone onset of new or worsening symptoms for as long as possible

---

Morris K. Udall Parkinson's Disease Research Centers of Excellence

Morris K. Udall served in the United States Congress for 30 years and was well-respected by colleagues on both sides of the aisle. He also lived with Parkinson's disease from his diagnosis in 1979 until his death in 1998, serving in the House of Representatives until 1991. In 1997, Congress passed the Morris K. Udall Parkinson's Disease Research Act, and President Clinton signed it into law in 1998. This legislation contributed to the establishment of 12 Parkinson's research centers funded by the National Institute of Neurological Disorders and Stroke (NINDS), a division of the National Institutes of Health (NIH). As a result, the legislation cast a national spotlight on the need for collaborative, coordinated research efforts for new treatments and a cure for PD.

The 12 centers are:

✔ Brigham and Women's Hospital, Boston, MA

✔ Columbia University, New York, NY

✔ Duke University, Durham, NC

✔ Harvard University (McLean Hospital), Belmont, MA

✔ Johns Hopkins University, Baltimore, MD

✔ Massachusetts General Hospital (Massachusetts Institute of Technology), Boston, MA

✔ Mayo Clinic, Jacksonville, FL

✔ Northwestern University, Evanston, IL

✔ University of California Los Angeles (UCLA), Los Angeles, CA

✔ University of Kentucky Medical Center, Lexington, KY

✔ University of Virginia, Charlottesville, VA

✔ University of Pittsburgh, Pittsburgh, PA

The 1997 legislation was a good start, but more work is needed. In 2005, Congressman Lane Evans of Illinois, who also has PD, introduced H.R. 3550, a bill to amend and further the work of the original legislation. The new bill would require NIH to hold a conference to review the progress of the work at these Centers for Excellence every two years and produce a strategic plan (including a budget, expected results, actual spending, and actual results) and a report to Congress. H.R. 3550 was referred to a subcommittee in August of 2005. As of this writing, that was the last action on the bill. The Parkinson's Action Network (PAN) maintains a watch on this bill and other legislation critical to the fight. The Web site is www.parkinsonsaction.org.

Along with expertise, you're looking for a certain quality of empathy — a chemistry between the two of you. (See more discussion on this relationship in the next section.) You don't want a godlike figure that makes decisions *for* you rather than *with* you. After all, who has to live with this PD? Not the neurologist.

Preparing for that first visit

Use the following checklist as you prepare for meeting the neurologist:

- ✔ When you make the appointment, ask for the first or last appointment of the day. This choice should assure additional time for questions.

- ✔ Make sure your PCP has sent copies of your records to the neurologist's office. Assuming that it was your PCP who referred you to the specialist, you may think that the records are transferred automatically. Guess again. You need to stay on top of this transfer and follow up with both offices to make sure the transfer actually takes place.

- ✔ Take a copy of your personal medical history and the results of any recent lab work with you. (Refer back to the section "Preparing for your initial exam" earlier in this chapter for more about the history.)

- ✔ Be sure to update that history to include your medications with the strength and dosage routine (or pack up the actual meds in a plastic bag — seriously!). Also list any vitamins, supplements, or other OTC meds you take on a regular basis.

- ✔ A few days prior to the appointment, call the office to confirm the appointment and ask whether they've received your records. If they haven't, follow up with your PCP. You may need to pick up copies of the records and take them with you to the appointment.

- ✔ Arrive half an hour before your scheduled appointment so you can complete their paperwork without cutting into your time with the doctor.

Interviewing the good doctor

Everyone wants the best neurologist out there. But, because of PD's chronic and progressive nature, you also need a neurologist who's a good fit for you and your care partner. Start with the basic nuts and bolts. The following list contains the most essential factors you need consider:

- ✔ Of course the neurologist has a medical degree, but is he *board-certified* (has he completed and passed nationally recognized exams to test his expertise)? If he has special training in *movement disorders* (PD is one), count yourself ahead of the game.

- ✔ What professional organizations and societies does he belong to?

✔ How many people with Parkinson's (PWP) are currently under his care?

✔ How long has the doctor been treating PWP? (If the good doctor is a good *older* doctor, how long does he anticipate practicing?) If the doctor is relatively young, check background and experience. Has this person worked with more experienced PD specialists?

✔ Who are the partners in his practice, and what are their backgrounds? No partners? Where does he send patients when he's unavailable?

✔ What days and hours does he see patients? (If the doctor is well known and sought after but has really limited office hours, that situation may send up a red flag for getting appointments when you need them.)

✔ Are the office hours and location convenient for you? If not, is that a deal breaker for you? Keep in mind that in the early stages of your PD (see Chapter 3) you'll probably see your neurologist infrequently, perhaps every six to eight weeks. If the distance and schedule still seem inconvenient, you can look elsewhere, but please try not to sacrifice experience and skill for convenience.

✔ If the doctor orders lab work, does his office provide the service? If not, is the office part of a hospital-physician complex where labs are easily available? If the answer is "No" to both questions, you'll most likely go to your area hospital or walk-in clinic for the lab work.

✔ What's the cost of an office visit?

✔ If you need to consult with him by phone, does he charge you for it?

✔ Does he accept your insurance? If you're on Medicare, does he *accept assignment* (charge only what Medicare assigns as the cost)? See Chapter 20 for more help on those sticky insurance questions.

Reviewing your first impressions

Okay, the neurologist passes your basic tests. Now for the tough part: How well will the two of you work together? First impressions can say a great deal, so pay attention to details like the following:

✔ Does the doctor seem rushed or distracted when she meets you?

✔ Does she listen and ask questions that draw out additional information, or does she cut you off making pronouncements rather than recommendations?

✔ What is her treatment philosophy on PD? Medication right away? Medication only after symptoms start to interfere with life routines? What about the use of new or proven surgical procedures?

The right answer, of course, includes a reminder that all patients progress differently and under varying circumstances, so the treatment regimen varies person to person.

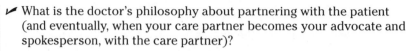

✔ What is the doctor's philosophy about partnering with the patient (and eventually, when your care partner becomes your advocate and spokesperson, with the care partner)?

✔ Is there chemistry (we're not talking magic here, just good vibes)? Do you feel an intangible connection — where you can rely on this doctor's partnership to explore ways to manage symptoms and maintain functionality as long as possible?

Moving forward if it's a good fit

Finally, if this doctor seems a good fit, you have just a few more questions to ask him:

✔ How does the doctor prefer that you prepare for an appointment? For example, does he want you to e-mail questions or concerns in advance, or can you bring written questions to the appointment? Can you bring a tape recorder to tape the conversation so you can listen to it again?

✔ What is his preferred way of communicating with you between appointments: by phone or e-mail; through his nurse or physician assistant? (If you're to contact the nurse or physician assistant, be sure you meet this person and get direct contact information.)

✔ What hospital does the doctor use for treating patients?

And what if, after all of this, the doctor just isn't for you? No chemistry. Of course, you can move on and start the whole process with another doctor. On the other hand, if this doctor is considered the best in your area, perhaps you should give the relationship a chance. After all, the two of you are relative strangers. How well did you click with other professionals in your life on the first appointment? Keep in mind that this is first and foremost a professional relationship; you will rely on this expert to plot the course you'll navigate through the challenges of PD. This doctor may not be especially interested in seeing pictures of your first grandchild, but if the treatment plan he puts together clearly focuses on your individual journey through PD and helps you enjoy that grandchild for years to come, do you really need anything more?

Working with Your Neurologist to Determine Whether This Is PD

Neurologists use a variety of methods to make a definitive diagnosis of PD:

✔ The physical examination

✔ An assessment of your function through mental and performance testing

✔ Sophisticated imaging equipment that permits a look inside your brain

Despite all these methods, your doctor may still need to rule out other explanations for your symptoms before she's prepared to state, without question, that you have PD.

This section takes you through the usual steps of that first visit.

Navigating the clinical exam

No single diagnostic test (like doctors have for measuring blood pressure or cholesterol levels) can confirm a clinical diagnosis of Parkinson's disease. So your neurologist's skill of observation and his experience in diagnosing and treating PWP is key. Your initial appointment will probably include the following three levels of examination:

History taking

The first level of examination is a discussion of your complete medical history. The printed copy you provide (see "Compiling your medical history" earlier in this chapter for help with this step) can help, but you'll probably hear some questions two or three times in this first appointment. Be a *patient* patient (pun intended). A good neurologist asks these questions not only to review your symptoms but also to rule out less-typical types of parkinsonism or other neurological conditions, which sometimes entail radically different management. (See "Parkinsonism, But Not PD" later in this chapter.)

Physical exam

After recording your medical history, the doctor performs a physical examination that may include such standards as:

✔ Measuring your blood pressure (while you're lying down and then again standing up)

✔ Checking your pulses, heartbeat, lungs, and abdomen

The point of such routine observations is to make sure your symptoms aren't due to problems in other parts of your body.

Neurological exam

The final level is the neurological examination, which is largely a process of observation. The neurologist tests your coordination and balance while observing you walk, stand, sit, turn, extend your arms and hands, and so on.

This exam may also include any of the following tasks:

- ✔ Opening and closing your fists or tapping your fingers several times
- ✔ Touching the doctor's finger and then your nose with your index finger (it looks silly but can give the neurologist a wealth of information)
- ✔ Recovering your balance after the doctor pulls you gently from behind your shoulders as you stand with your eyes open or closed
- ✔ Answering several simple questions from the doctor to test your attention and memory
- ✔ Drawing a figure on a piece of paper and then duplicating it

Don't be surprised by the apparent simplicity of these questions and tests; they are all part of a standardized exam!

After the neurologist has completed the initial interview, the physical exam and neurological observations, he (or an assistant) may use standard screening tools to further confirm the diagnosis or the stage or severity of your PD. This next section covers those tools.

Establishing the severity and staging the progression of your PD

Your neurologist may use a variety of tools for establishing your PD's progression through the various stages or levels. (See Chapter 3 for more about these stages.) The rating scales in the next section are useful in setting a benchmark for the doctor. Neuroimaging tools are also helpful in tracking progression and ruling out other possibilities for symptoms you may experience.

Rating scales and neuroimaging tests are tools available to your doctor to assist in establishing the progression of your PDC. They aren't used in confirming the diagnosis.

Rating scales

In any major disorder like PD, neurologists may use standardized rating scales to measure symptoms and stage the disease. (For a refresher on *staging*, flip over to Chapter 3.) These instruments are helpful in determining how advanced your symptoms are and how best to address them. The scales also form the basis for a more extensive medical history if a patient needs to change doctors in the future. In addition, clinical researchers frequently use these scales to monitor the effects of new and experimental therapies on patients. (See Chapter 14, where we discuss the trials more completely.)

✔ **Hoehn and Yahr Rating Scale:** This diagnostic tool stages the level of a person's PD by using broad measures of disability. This scale was originally devised by Melvin Yahr and Margaret Hoehn following a detailed study of the natural progression of PD in the late 1960s. They observed five general stages in PD, ranging from Stage 1 (unilateral disease, limited to one side of the body) to Stage 5 (wheelchair bound or bedridden unless aided). However, as we mention often in this book, PD doesn't progress in neat, little, predictable stages. Therefore, the more complex (and more informative) Unified Parkinson Disease Rating Scale (see the next section) usually accompanies and complements this tool.

✔ **Unified Parkinson Disease Rating Scale (UPDRS):** The UPDRS focuses on several facets of PD's disability, such as its effects on daily activities, motor skills, and mental capacity (including behavior and mood). It consists of a painless interview and a focused neurological exam, with a score for each item from 0 (normal) to 4 (severe). Therefore, the higher the UPDRS score, the greater the disability from PD.

The UPDRS — when administered correctly — is "an exquisitely sensitive test for detecting early PD," according to a Parkinson's Disease Foundation article. It may be the best tool for the neurologist to assess symptom levels and design treatment plans. The UPDRS is currently under revision by the Movement Disorders Society and will be soon updated to better reflect the multifaceted reality of PD disability.

✔ **Schwab and England Activities of Daily Living:** This tool rates a person's ability to perform the normal routine activities of daily living using a percentage rating. The patient usually rates himself with the help of set definitions presented by the doctor.

For example, people who consider themselves to be completely independent and functional qualify for a 100 percent rating. They can perform all activities without difficulty. In contrast, a person who takes three to four times the normal time to perform a task (such as dressing) has a 70 percent independence rating. And a person who can manage only a few chores from time to time (and always with great effort) has a 30 percent rating.

Neuroimaging

A thorough neurological exam and the proper administration of the UPDRS is usually enough to diagnose a new case of PD. However, neuroimaging techniques now permit neurologists to pinpoint the diagnosis of PD and follow its progression by observing the affected nerve cells.

Two recently developed imaging techniques, positron-emission tomography and single photon emission computed tomography, can confirm the diagnosis of PD and distinguish PD from other Parkinson-like disorders. (See "Parkinsonism, But Not PD" later in this chapter for more discussion on other disorders.) Both scans use low levels of radioactive materials and pose little, if any, risk for the patient. I describe both of these scans in the following:

✔ The *positron-emission tomography* (PET) scan uses a radioactive form of *levodopa* (the drug that enhances dopamine production in the brain), which is injected intravenously into the patient, to highlight the loss of normal *dopamine* cells (the neurons primarily affected by PD) in the brain. As dopamine cells uptake levodopa, a reduced signal from labeled (radioactive) levodopa is usually found in PD.

✔ The *single photon emission computed tomography* (SPECT) scan is another imaging technique able to measure metabolic and physiological functions of specific areas of the brain. When using radioactive markers able to link to dopamine cells, SPECT scans can measure the progressive loss of these neurons caused by PD.

A couple of factors limit the use of neuroimaging: cost and availability. At this writing, some insurance companies consider such scans experimental and as a result, don't cover any of the costs. In addition, the equipment and expertise for performing and interpreting the scans aren't widely available.

Ruling out the red herrings: What else can it be?

What else looks like PD? That answer may depend on your *presenting* symptoms (the information you tell the doctor) or on other facts that the doctor gathers through interviewing and examining you.

For example:

✔ If you don't present with any of the *TRAP* symptoms (check out Chapter 3 for a quick review of these) but you talk about a loss of energy, the doctor may want to explore that symptom more. After further questioning, your doctor may see that depression plays a role in your loss of energy. If so, is the depression associated with PD, or is it related to some other life-changing event, such as the death of a loved one or the loss of a job?

✔ Even if a hand tremor was your reason for seeing a neurologist, is the tremor confined to one hand or both? Does it stop after the hand is engaged in activity, or does the tremor continue?

Don't try to second-guess your symptoms. Is it PD? Maybe. Is it something else — something easier to treat and cure? Possibly. Either way, you need to know. Why postpone treating a curable condition simply because you think it may be more serious? And if it does turn out to be PD, then you want to get a jump on managing symptoms as early as possible — when you have the greatest opportunity to maintain independence and flexibility.

Parkinsonism, But Not PD

If it walks like a duck and quacks like a duck, it's a duck, right? So if it looks like PD and acts likes PD, then it's PD, right? Not always.

The same symptoms that indicate PD can also indicate other conditions, thus *parkinsonism* is a generic term referring to slowness and mobility problems that look like PD. Parkinsonism is a feature in several conditions that have different (and perhaps known) causes, but those conditions don't progress like PD. As a result, years may go by before the differences between PD and the other disorder are apparent; the PD diagnosis may then be reversed.

Taking antiparkinsonian medications (such as levodopa) may be the first indicator that parkinsonism isn't actually PD. By definition, PD promptly responds to this medication, which improves its symptoms in a consistent way, at least for a few years. But, in parkinsonism, improvement is often erratic or nonexistent from the beginning. In fact, your neurologist will always closely monitor your response to treatment in order to rule out the possibility that your condition is a disorder other than PD.

Two categories of non-PD disorders are:

- ✔ **Parkinson's Plus syndromes:** This group of neurodegenerative disorders has parkinsonian features, such as *bradykinesia* (slowness), *rigidity* (stiffness), *tremor* (shaking), and *gait disturbances* (balance). See Chapter 3 for more about these PD symptoms. However, they are also associated with other complex neurological symptoms that reflect problems in brain areas other than the *dopaminergic system* (the network of neurons able to make and release the neurotransmitter *dopamine*). These conditions progress more rapidly than PD and don't respond as well (or at all) to antiparkinsonian medications. The most common Parkinson's Plus syndromes are *Multiple System Atrophy* (MSA), *Progressive Supranuclear Palsy* (PSP), *Cortico-Basal Ganglionic Degeneration* (CBGD), and *Lewy Body Dementia* (LBD).

- ✔ **Secondary parkinsonisms:** The symptoms of these disorders relate to well-defined lesions in the brain from strokes, tumors, infections, traumas, or certain drugs. Like Parkinson's Plus syndromes, these syndromes are usually less responsive to levodopa. However, if the primary cause of parkinsonism is controlled, these symptoms tend to be less progressive.

In addition to Parkinson's plus and secondary parkinsonisms, *Essential Tremor* (ET) is another source of possible confusion. As the most common movement disorder — as much as 20 times more common than PD — ET's only symptom is a tremor that affects the hands (only while they're moving) but may also affect the head or voice. ET can run in families and is usually benign and non-disabling. The much-admired actress, Katherine Hepburn, may have suffered from ET — not PD.

This Is Your Life — Getting a Second (or Even Third) Opinion

Whatever the diagnosis, if you have concerns, questions, or doubts, then you have every reason to get a second or even a third opinion. After all, you know your body and its symptoms better than anyone else. So if you live within a reasonable distance of a Udall Center (see the sidebar "Morris K. Udall Parkinson's Disease Research Centers of Excellence" earlier in this chapter) or a medical center with a reputation for excellent PD care and research, see whether you can get an appointment and check out what those folks say. Even if you have to travel some distance, the information will be worth the trip.

Another reason to seek a second or third opinion is to find a neurologist you have chemistry with. The doctor who delivered the initial diagnosis may be a fine neurologist with great credentials and experience, but maybe the two of you had no connection and you don't see a partnership with her. With PD, you don't want to be switching from one doctor to another. So, find a doctor that you can build a real partnership with now — one with a proactive and optimistic philosophy about meeting the challenges of living with PD.

The danger lies in seeking one opinion after another just because you didn't like the first (or second or third) answer — even though, in your heart-of-hearts, you're sure it's true. That's called *denial*. Because you may not want to face the future, you keep running after more opinions, hoping some day some doctor will say you don't have PD.

After a doctor has confirmed the diagnosis (and perhaps another doctor has reconfirmed it), you need to accept it and prepare yourself and your family for the journey. Maybe you've already made significant progress by finding a neurologist that you and your PCP can partner with to maintain and manage your health for the long term.

Chapter 5

You've Been Diagnosed — Now What?

. . . .

In This Chapter

▶ Facing your fears about Parkinson's disease

▶ Establishing your long-term vision and short-term goals

▶ Caring for the future: Advice for your partner

. . . .

*O*kay, it's official — you have Parkinson's disease (PD). In these first days following that blow, no doubt your emotions are rocketing. And like a pinball, they're bouncing moment to moment and hour to hour around those Five Stages of Grief that Elisabeth Kubler-Ross introduced:

✔ Can't be (denial)

✔ Shouldn't be (anger)

✔ Don't let it be (bargaining)

✔ Why me? (depression)

✔ IS! (acceptance or at least realization)

A sixth stage to consider in facing a diagnosis of PD is *hope*. You can find some measure of control as you continue toward the future you had already planned — one that did *not* include living with a chronic and progressive illness.

And that's the purpose of this chapter — to help you move beyond those first jumbled emotions of diagnosis toward a clearly focused, take-charge attitude of this disease. In this chapter we first talk you through the emotional steps and then guide you toward healthy goals and plans for coming to grips with PD. We also address your care partner, the one who plans to walk that walk with you, and offer advice for these early months after the diagnosis.

Sorting Out Your Emotions

Depending on your past awareness or experiences with PD, either you have some idea of how your life is going to change or you have no idea at all. In either case, your imagination can get carried away with all the what-ifs.

Stop! This is a new challenge, but it's not so different from other challenges that have taken your life in unexpected directions. Every day people face unplanned events that change the course they thought they were on — job losses, break-ups in relationships, unplanned moves to different locations, the loss of a loved one, hurricanes, and floods. Life happens.

Take a breath. Any challenges that you faced (and survived) in the past (like raising your children, building your career, caring for aging parents, and such) gave you key building blocks and tools to face this new challenge.

Now, give yourself time to:

- ✔ Understand that a PD diagnosis is not a death sentence. You have a life to live and choices to make about how you'll face each day, probably for years and even decades to come.
- ✔ Believe that past experiences have given you the tools you need to cope with PD.
- ✔ Accept the difference between what you can and can't control. Focus on what you can.
- ✔ Connect with people who are positive and upbeat.
- ✔ Banish negative self-talk ("I can't," or "I won't," and such), and turn the negative to a positive ("I can" and "I will").
- ✔ Embrace the joys in your life — your partner, children, friends, work or avocation, love of music, art, sports, and so on.
- ✔ Help yourself by helping other people — volunteer, get involved, make a difference.
- ✔ Recognize the opportunities you have to educate others, advocate for change (and a cure), make new friends, and know your deeper self.

Basically you have two choices: Define your life as a person with Parkinson's (PWP) or live that life to the fullest — the same as if you'd never been diagnosed with PD.

Dodging denial and meeting your diagnosis head on

When you get the confirmed diagnosis, you and your family — especially your partner — need time to digest the news and react. And the first reaction for one or both of you may be denial. Your partner may become overprotective and treat you as if you're gravely ill. Financial concerns may pop up; your partner may wonder about the costs and sacrifices. Underneath your partner may first feel cheated out of the life you had planned and then angry at such a selfish thought when you're facing a debilitating illness. (For more help in dealing with such difficult feelings, see Chapter 22.)

Neither you nor your partner may admit any of these feelings initially. Big mistake. Your fastest route to coping is to work through such feelings together by openly communicating your fears and concerns and then working through possible solutions to each. Following the guidelines set forth in the remainder of this chapter can help.

Denial can take two forms. First, many people who receive the diagnosis of PD — or any other serious illness — soon realize that the early symptoms have been there. Perhaps you dismissed those early warning signs for weeks or even months because you were afraid or didn't want other people to know you had some troublesome symptoms.

The second form of denial comes after you've received the diagnosis. Now the facts are out there. You're human, and no doubt the actual news that you have PD has come as a real blow. *Initially* refusing to believe this is happening is your mind's way of giving you time to gather the necessary strength to go forward.

However, *sustaining* that denial takes an enormous amount of energy — energy that can be much more valuable in facing the actual challenge. Refusing to acknowledge the truth means you're forcing yourself to keep a secret from other people and yourself.

In spite of your denial, deep inside you know this diagnosis is real. You may even be surprised to realize you have a slight feeling of relief because the enemy has a name, and now you can begin to fight it. You can't go back and not have PD. But you can decide how best to move forward.

Allowing yourself to get angry

Anger is an understandable reaction to news like this. The question is: Who's on the receiving end of that anger? The world in general? Your friends and family who've never taken care of themselves like you always have? Your significant other (who you fear — in your current, warped state of mind — may leave you)? God? How about yourself?

Go ahead — rant, rave, and howl at the moon. A little healthy anger is good for you, and certainly you deserve to indulge that anger — within reason. Try these tips for giving anger your best shot:

- ✔ Keep the focus on the object of your anger — having PD. It's easier than you may suspect to broaden that focus until suddenly everything and everyone makes you mad.

- ✔ Start figuring out ways you're going to get back at this enemy that's attacked your perfectly good life (the same way you'd think of ways to get back at the boss who passed you over for that promotion). For example, you can say to your Parkinson's, "I'll show you that I can still lead my life in spite of the challenges you throw my way!"

- ✔ Set limits. When you're overwhelmed by your fury at the unfairness of this diagnosis, set a kitchen timer for 10 minutes. When the bell dings, you're done — at least for today.

- ✔ Find the humor — black though it may be — in this unexpected and unwanted situation and defuse your anger with that humor.

Anger (like denial and a bunch of other normal reactions to news of a chronic, progressive illness) is non-productive *unless* it leads you to fight back. Permit yourself some time to work your way through this news. (For some people, this will be a matter of days; for others it's a couple of weeks.) If the feelings continue longer than that, you need to get some help to resolve the anger. Throughout the course of your PD, you're going to be upset and angry from time to time. Your goal is not to dwell in that anger but to transform its energy into determination to regain control and move forward.

Admitting you're scared

Chances are good that you still don't have a handle on the full impact of this diagnosis. Getting your head around the concept of a lifelong, progressive illness is a pretty tall order, especially in the beginning. It's enough to scare the bejeebers out of anyone! You have so many questions and fears. How do you deal with them?

There's no shame in admitting you're scared. The title song from the musical *Cabaret* says, "Start by admitting from cradle to grave, it isn't that long a stay." In other words, life is what we get — no promises and no guarantees. The unknown can be intriguing, exhilarating, or frightening. And certainly, when that unknown is PD, you may find yourself even feeding that fear through your responses to it.

Instead of further terrifying yourself by reading every case study, article, or book you can get your hands on about PD, place limits on how much information you need and can handle — especially at the beginning. Instead of smiling politely as some well-meaning clerk or neighbor relates his horror story about a fifth-cousin-twice-removed who had PD back in the dark ages, thank him for his concern and leave. Instead of allowing other people to educate you based on hearsay, observations from afar, and an article they read about former Attorney General Janet Reno, educate yourself.

Using the reputable and frequently updated resources listed in Appendix B, you can gather the information you need to become the true expert on what is and isn't possible with PD. Then, when people start telling you about your condition and how to manage your life, quietly but firmly correct them. Trust us; nothing silences a know-it-all like someone who really does know. And nothing helps you get a handle on that gut-wrenching fear like educating yourself on the realities, possibilities, and opportunities for expanding your life — of living with PD.

Getting to acceptance

No one is denying that you need to work through a whole range of emotions, but you can't stay locked in those emotional prisons. When you move through them, you free yourself to fully live your days.

You have a chronic and progressive illness, but

- ✔ You have years ahead of you.
- ✔ You're still productive.
- ✔ You have time to pursue dreams and goals.
- ✔ You can live life on your terms if you accommodate PD as *part* of that life, not *all* of it.

How to go about that? Start with these key steps:

- ✔ Get the best treatment you can after you have the diagnosis. Part III of this book is all about treatment options, some that you may find surprisingly easy to incorporate into your life.
- ✔ Deal with the emotional roller coaster of living with a chronic progressive illness. Chapters 13 and 22 offer tips on facing the depression, anxiety, and other difficult feelings that are part and parcel of living with any chronic progressive conditions.

✔ Manage your inevitable lifestyle changes and social adjustments with family and friends (and theirs with you). Check out Chapter 7 for tips on who, how, and when to tell about your PD; then look at Chapter 15 for more in-depth advice on maintaining key relationships.

✔ Protect your unique sense of self-worth and identity. Well, we could just remind you to read this whole book because our key message in every chapter is that you can live with this condition. In fact, you can have a full and satisfying life —it just won't be the life you thought you were going to have (but isn't that true for most people?).

Sometimes acceptance comes most easily when you turn your attention to the people who love you and have heard your diagnosis. They're wrestling with high anxiety too. Of course, their first concern is for you, but a part of that concern is PD's effect on their relationship with you. How will their lives change with yours? When you acknowledge their fears (as well as your own) and explore that with them, you create an environment of "we're in this thing together" that goes a long way toward sustaining everyone when times get tough. (Tips for ways you can best communicate with other people are in Chapters 7 and 15.)

By taking the lead in figuring out how to live with PD, in many ways you become a mentor. You're the person others look to and trust to show the best way to face this life-changing situation. For many of us, actor Christopher Reeve and his wife, Dana, were the poster couple for finding grace in the face of unspeakable adversity. Think about it: If you built your career as *Superman* and ended up unable to move much less leap over tall buildings, wouldn't you be tempted to feel sorry for yourself? Instead Christopher Reeve found the will and the courage to use his adversity to inspire and motivate people and make a real difference in the world.

No one expects you to become a national icon now that you have PD. But you can become that mentor for people closest to you. Through your attitude and approach, you can set the tone for the way others interact with you and incorporate PD into the relationship.

Taking charge and moving forward

Prepare but don't project needs to be your mantra. The temptation to look ahead and worry about the future can be overwhelming. Our advice: Fight that instinct! Given a diagnosis of a chronic and progressive disease that has no cure, a person's natural tendency is to try and foretell the future. Major mistake!

With PD, every patient's journey is unique, so projecting what may happen can only increase your anxiety. You and your care partner can go crazy, racing around and trying to cover all your possible challenges even before they develop.

The point is that you have a disease that will require — like most health conditions — changes to your lifestyle. For example,

✔ What will you do if you can no longer manage the stairs in your current home, but the bedrooms (and the main bathroom) are all upstairs?

In Chapter 21, we explore many options for staying in your current residence in spite of obstacles such as this. For example, you may have a room on the first floor that you can adapt as a bedroom; maybe you can convert a half-bath into a full bathroom (with the addition of a shower); or your stairway may be wide enough to accommodate an electric chair lift.

✔ As your ability to move decreases, how will you handle an emergency such as getting out of the house in the event of a fire?

Even if you didn't have PD, common sense should move every family to have an emergency plan in place. So sit down with the family and figure this one out — for you and everyone else in the household. One solution is to talk to people at your local fire and police department and get their suggestions.

Our guess is that throughout your life (and certainly as an adult) you've planned for the possibility of unexpected changes or events. And even though those plans may come in a year or not at all, you've still considered the options and are prepared to act.

Taking Action

Think of PD as a 400-pound lineman constantly in your face. He's there when you wake up and when you go to sleep. He gets in your way, blocking you when you try to work or play and when your friends come around. Sometimes he's well-behaved, maybe even sitting on the sidelines for a while. But mostly he's charging, blocking, and even tackling to keep you from doing what you want.

How do you get around this lineman? The answer is that sometimes you won't. But other times — most of the time —you can find new and innovative ways to live life on your terms. Managing a chronic illness means you need to give up control over some parts of your life and take control in new ways. Some of those new controls are:

✔ Educating yourself and your family about your PD

✔ Developing a long-range strategy for managing your PD

✔ Turning negatives into positives through creative problem-solving

✔ Being a real team player — with your healthcare team (see Chapter 6), your care partners, and other PWP

Arming yourself with good information

The key to gathering information is making sure it's trustworthy and evidence-based. The Agency for Healthcare and Research (an agency within the Department of Health and Human Services) recommends these resources:

✔ **healthfinder** (www.healthfinder.gov) is sponsored by the U.S. Department of Health and Human Services. The site includes links to government agencies, clearinghouses, non-profit groups, and universities.

✔ **Health Information Resource Database** (www.health.gov/nhic/ #Referrals or 800-336-4797) is sponsored by the National Health Information Center. This site offers information on more than 1000 organizations and government agencies that provide health information on request.

✔ **MEDLINEplus** (www.nlm.nih.gov/medlineplus) is sponsored by the National Institutes of Health (NIH). The site has extensive information from NIH and other trusted resources on more than 650 diseases and conditions.

✔ **Non-profit organizations** such as the National Parkinson's Foundation and The Michael J. Fox Foundation focus specifically on PD. For a complete list and contact information, see Appendix B.

In addition, try checking with medical libraries in your area (but keep in mind that this information is for physicians, medical students, and researchers — the reading can get fairly technical).

Ignore information from

✔ Product advertisements that

• Make extraordinary claims, such as *scientific breakthrough* or *secret formula*.

• Claim to work for a number of different conditions.

- Claim the product is available from only one source or for a limited time.

✔ Well-meaning friends who have

- Heard of some therapy but can't recall the source.

- Had a relative who tried *x-treatment*. It worked for that person, so it's bound to work for you!

✔ Well-meaning strangers who, in their zeal to show sympathy for your condition, rattle off several ideas about treatment.

Jotting down the questions you have

Chances are good that you were pretty numb as you sat in the doctor's office and received the news. (See Chapter 4, where we cover the initial visit with the neurologist.) But now you realize you have all sorts of questions. Or perhaps you asked questions at the time and your doctor offered information, but you really didn't take it in.

Schedule a second appointment (if you haven't already) and let your doctor (or the nurse) know that you want to be able to ask questions and discuss issues that have come to mind since the diagnosis. At that appointment, bring your list of questions (as well as your care partner for that second set of ears) and be ready to take notes. The following questions are a sampling of some concerns you may want to cover.

✔ What's the technical name of my condition, and what does that mean in plain English?

✔ What's the *prognosis,* my outlook for the future?

✔ How soon do I need to make a decision about treatment?

✔ Will I need additional tests? If so, what kind and when?

✔ What are my treatment options, and what are the pros and cons of those treatment options?

✔ What changes will I need to make in my daily life?

✔ What resources and organizations do you recommend for support and information?

✔ What resources can your office provide (books, pamphlets, audio or videotapes, and such) that I can review right away?

✔ And, the question uppermost in your mind: Am I going to die from this?

Establishing realistic and attainable goals

If PD is to be part of your life but not your entire life, then you need a game plan. Fact: If you don't have a plan for dealing with PD, then it will dominate every facet of your life. This section takes you through specific steps toward making and living that plan.

In the world of business, executive teams meet regularly. Their purpose? To plan for the future success of their business. Their process usually follows a three-step course:

1. **Establish a long-term vision.**

2. **Set short-term goals toward achieving that vision.**

3. **Identify and prioritize tasks necessary to attain those goals.** (This is known as the *Plan of Action,* or POA.)

To apply these three steps to PD, the first step (the vision) is already established: to live a productive and satisfying life for as long as possible in spite of PD.

The second step (setting goals) requires you to set aside sentimentality. As much as people wish otherwise, PD (as of this writing) has no cure. So, a goal of being cured is neither realistic nor attainable. As you consider your real goals, remember the following principles:

- ✔ Keep them simple.
- ✔ Keep them practical.
- ✔ Keep them specific.

The third step is the POA. Did you ever see a milk stool, the three-legged variety farmers sat on to milk cows? That three-legged approach is the way you need to think about your POA over the long term because living with PD is not only a physical challenge; it's also a mental and emotional one. And, just like the milk stool, if one leg is missing, the plan will topple.

The following sections provide examples of three goals and their POAs that support a long-term vision for PD.

Goal 1: Maintain maximum physical function

PD has no magic pill. So, after confirming your diagnosis, your neurologist will probably have a number of recommendations that may include management of symptoms with proven medications, physical and occupational therapy, and perhaps a program for diet and exercise.

Although medications and traditional medical interventions may help minimize your symptoms, you enhance your opportunity to achieve your long-term vision when you maintain your best physical condition. On the other hand, if you ignore the doctor's prescription for changes in your lifestyle (such as adjustments to your diet and activity routines or a specific timetable for taking your medications), you compromise your overall vision. (See Chapter 9 for more about the importance of sticking to your medication schedule and Chapter 12 for a full discussion of exercise and nutrition.)

No one has all of the symptoms. Although PD is a chronic, progressive condition, its path varies tremendously from one person to the next. You are unique — as a person and as a PWP. You and your medical team need to keep that in mind as together you select those options (medications, therapies, and lifestyle changes) that have the greatest effect on maintaining your physical function for as long as possible.

Goal 2: Keep your mind sharp

You're certainly going to have a lot on your mind in the days and weeks to come as you and your medical team put together a viable plan for managing your PD symptoms. And you're going to hear a lot of new words — words that PD specialists, PWPs, and their care partners throw around as easily as *apple* or *orange*.

You can refuse to follow that technical PD jargon (and everything else about this intruder), or you can become an expert, someone who actively seeks out background information about PD, understands and uses the technical lingo, and keeps up with the research and new treatment options.

This advice doesn't mean PD has to become your life's work. You have more important (and fun!) ways to spend your time. But remember: Knowledge is power, and seeking out that knowledge exercises your brain. Get started using the resources listed in Appendix B. Getting a grip on PD (what it is and isn't) is a good place to start — but don't stop there.

What are your interests and how did you challenge your mind before you had PD? Are you a sports enthusiast who enjoys statistics and box scores? Do you enjoy brainteasers, like crossword puzzles, jigsaw puzzles, or word games? Do you love good music, art, and theater?

Continuing to engage your mind in enjoyable ways is as important to your POA as pushing yourself physically. Don't turn your back on the intellectual life you enjoyed before PD.

Goal 3: Embrace the power of emotional and spiritual well-being

Going through a range of emotions post-diagnosis is normal. But anxiety and depression can be viable symptoms of PD as well as viable responses to its diagnosis. Your doctor needs to know if you're experiencing persistent (longer than a couple of weeks) sadness or apathy. (See Chapter 14 for a full discussion of the effects of anxiety and depression in PD.)

Although your neurologist or primary care physician (in consultation with each other) can prescribe medication and professional counseling to help you through these negative emotions, you can also be proactive by

- Acknowledging that these persistent negative feelings are abnormal.
- Finding a support group where you can discuss feelings with other people who

    Perhaps have similar emotions.

    Recognize these emotions as part of the adaptive process in dealing with PD.

- Accepting the support of family and friends as you come to terms with PD and its effects on all your lives.

In concert with your medical team, you can address physical, mental, and even emotional needs as part of your POA. However, one facet of your care plan only you can develop is a plan for your spiritual health. This facet goes beyond faith and religious rituals, although those resources certainly help.

Spiritual health means going inside yourself and coming to terms with your illness day by day. For some PWP, coping comes through challenging activities: participating in sports, continuing to pursue a career, traveling, and so on. If these challenges help you find inner peace and comfort, great!

Other PWP may find spiritual healing in quieter pursuits: a walk in the park or along the beach; music; reading; sitting quietly in a secluded, deserted place. These activities are also excellent choices for maintaining spiritual health.

Take care that your solitude doesn't become a regular hiding place to wallow over your losses. Be aware that seclusion can sometimes lead to depression.

Living your life to the fullest

You can perform a lot of actions to fight PD and its effects. But thousands of PWP believe that a huge part of fighting PD is to approach it as only a piece of their lives. The point is this: Those facets of your life that defined you before you were diagnosed are still there — at least for the most part. If you were a parent before, you still are and your child (children) needs you as much as before. If you had a career that you enjoyed (even loved), don't allow PD to become your new, full-time occupation. If you enjoyed sports, music, and other leisure activities, get creative about finding new ways to enjoy those pastimes. In short, LIVE!

The road will be challenging, but as actor and PD advocate, Michael J. Fox, wrote in his biography, *Lucky Man,* "If you were to rush into this room right now and announce that you had struck a deal — with God, Allah, Buddha, Christ, Krishna, Bill Gates, whomever — in which the ten years since my diagnosis could be magically taken away, traded in for the person I was before, I would, without a moment's hesitation, tell you to take a hike."

Next steps

Getting information you can trust so you can form the questions to ask so you can establish some clear goals for managing this condition — pretty tall order! Consider these three concrete steps that you can take right now to get started:

1. **Go online and bookmark the sites listed in Appendix B if you have access to a computer.**

   These national organizations are your best resource for the latest updates on treatments as well as tips for managing your PD symptoms. Get into the habit of regularly checking in on the sites you find most useful. If the site offers an e-list, sign up.

2. **Call the toll-free numbers for the PD organizations if you don't have access to a computer.**

   Ask them to send you their printed materials and add you to the mailing list for new materials in the future.

3. **Keep reading.**

Before you turn to the next chapter, take a moment to read through the following with your family — especially the person who is most likely to be your primary care partner. Even though these sections (scattered throughout this book) are labeled *for the care partner,* try to read them together. The information applies to both of you because you have a responsibility to acknowledge that your care partner has a life beyond helping you manage your PD. (You may also want to check out Chapter 24 for more tips about how to give and receive care and support.)

A Word for the PD Care Partner

In many chronic, progressive illnesses (for example, Alzheimer's disease), family members must increasingly take charge. With PD, however, the PWP can be in charge most of the way. As the care partner, you may want to take over, especially as tasks become more difficult and decisions take longer for your partner to process. But resist that urge. Partnering-in-care is not doing *for* — it's doing *with*.

But where does that leave you as you face your own fears and anxieties about living with someone who has a chronic, progressive condition that won't go away but will color your lives for years to come? Go back and reread this chapter. Everything we suggest for the PWP applies to you as well:

✔ Sort through your emotions; deal with the anger, the fear, and the realities of how life is going to change (see also Chapter 22).

✔ Adopt a take charge/move forward/don't look back outlook and start preparing for eventualities that may occur down the road. (You may especially want to read Chapters 20 and 21 about housing options and financial and legal matters.)

✔ Be proactive. Educate yourself; go to doctor and therapy appointments with the PWP and take notes; become a combination of cheerleader and coach as your loved one faces new challenges.

✔ Set goals that allow you to maintain a life and identity beyond your role as care partner.

The best support you can offer over the long term is to be a fierce advocate for your loved one's autonomy and independence. The next best way to show support is to take care of yourself and see that your needs are also met. By working together — in partnership — the two of you can take something that could have destroyed you and turn it into a life-experience that enriches you in ways you cannot yet imagine.

Chapter 6

Drafting Your Healthcare Team and a Game Plan

. . . .

. . . .

Knowledge may be power, but with today's constant bombardment of information, you need a team of experts that can answer questions and address unexpected situations with the most-advanced procedures.

People with Parkinson's (PWP), like people with other chronic-care needs, must rely on the expertise of several different professionals throughout the course of their illness. In this chapter, professionals and their roles in managing your Parkinson's symptoms are defined. You also take a look at how best to handle hospitalizations, emergency room visits, and other unexpected medical predicaments and complications that are possible for PWP. Last, but not least, your care partner gets ideas for building his own team.

Introducing Your Teammates

Each member of your professional Parkinson's disease (PD) team has special talents and expertise that can help you manage symptoms and maintain normal function and quality of life, often for years following the initial diagnosis. In this section, you discover a list of professionals and their roles in your care, and then you uncover your role in helping these pros perform at their very best.

Lining up the doctors

At least two doctors will help set the course for your care after your PD diagnosis. In addition, you may have other specialists (or you may add them at a later date) if you have other chronic conditions, such as arthritis, hypertension, and the like. The more doctors you have, the more vital it becomes for one doctor (most likely your primary care physician) to take the role of quarterback to oversee and coordinate the plan to meet all your health needs.

Your primary care physician

Your *primary care physician* (PCP) may be a general practitioner (GP) who focuses on family medicine or that person may be an internist who treats adults only. You've probably been seeing this doctor for some time and have built a trust and style of communication that works for both of you. Now that you have PD, you need to talk with your PCP about two things: his willingness to consult and communicate with your neurologist (who'll take the lead on treating your PD symptoms), and how your PD treatment can integrate with your overall healthcare plan.

Your neurologist

Chances are good that your PCP referred you to a neurologist to confirm the PD diagnosis. If so, these two professionals may already have a good working relationship. However, if you went for a second (or even third) opinion and chose another neurologist to oversee your PD care, be sure that these two doctors meet and show a clear willingness to work together. It's also helpful if your PCP and neurologist are on staff at the same hospital in case you need hospitalization or emergency treatment down the road. (For tips on locating and choosing a neurologist, see Chapter 4.)

Other specialists

In the event you need to consult with other specialists (a cardiologist, urologist, or the like) for new medical situations that arise, these physicians must work closely with your PCP and neurologist so they're all communicating from the same play book (to continue the sports analogy). Think of these doctors as coming off the bench. When they get into the game, they need to get up to speed on your game plan and their specific roles.

Before you keep an appointment with a specialist ask your PCP (and neurologist, if appropriate) to send the specialist(s) a copy of your most recent records. After your visit with one of these doctors, ask that a copy of the office visit report be sent to your PCP with a copy sent to you at the same time. With this exchange of information between doctors — and by assembling your own file of reports — you enhance the likelihood that everyone is on the same page, working from the same information.

Calling up the therapists

Because PD is a movement disorder that affects your ability to perform basic movements, your physical, occupational, and (possibly) speech therapists are very important. These professionals offer proven methods to enhance and prolong your control of symptoms, and improve your overall sense of well-being. Their services may or may not be covered by insurance unless your doctor's prescription notes them as *medically necessary* to treat your PD.

Physical therapist

A *physical therapist* (PT) can teach you how to build muscle strength, increase flexibility, and improve coordination and balance to prevent falls and serious fractures. Techniques may include exercise programs (standard as well as alternatives, like yoga), heat and cold packs, and water therapy (exercises in water).

Your PT can design a program of exercises specific to your individual symptoms and abilities to preserve and even increase your muscle strength and flexibility.

Although exercise doesn't appear to slow the progression of PD, recent studies indicate that exercise may help prevent the orthopedic muscular and skeletal effects of *akinesia* (slowed or impaired ability to move) and lessen *rigidity* (stiff muscles). Exercise helps you maintain balance and prevent falls.

Your PT can't work miracles. If you only exercise when you go to a session with your PT, you're not likely to see ongoing or long-term benefits. When the physical therapy sessions end (or when the time between sessions stretches to two weeks or more), you need to pursue your own regular program of stretching, strengthening, and aerobic exercises if you want the physical therapy to be successful in the long run. See Chapter 12 for a suggested program of stretches and exercises.

Occupational therapist

Essentially, the *occupational therapist* (OT) helps preserve your sense of independence and self-confidence by showing you new ways of performing simple and routine tasks (known in the medical profession as *activities of daily living* or *ADLs*) that may have become difficult for you. One significant benefit of working with an OT is simply knowing that you can preserve your control (with alternative techniques) when the loss of control seems a foregone conclusion. For example, she may teach you new techniques (such as a *cueing* or a *reminder system*) and provide assistive devices (such as a special cane) that help you perform certain movements and tasks.

For more information on ways to adapt to your changing symptoms, check out the information in Part III on living with PD.

Speech therapist

Not every PWP needs speech therapy, but if you're experiencing a softened vocal tone, unintentional mispronunciations, or wrong word choices, a speech therapist can help. These professionals can also help if you ever develop swallowing or other throat muscle problems that can come with PD.

If a trained speech therapist isn't available in your area, consider trying a program especially for PWP called the Lee Silverman Voice Treatment or LSVT. For more information about the LSVT Foundation, its programs, and links to other PD groups, see www.lsvt.org.

Drafting other team players

As a PWP, you have your front-line defense consisting of your PCP, your neurologist, and trained movement and speech therapists. But, have you considered the number of other professionals that can help you to manage your symptoms and continue living a normal life as long as possible? Be sure that you include the following care professionals and experts when you're assembling the team.

Pharmacist

Your pharmacist is in the business of knowing medications and their interactions. She knows your current medications, their potential side effects, and the possible impact of any new medication that your PCP or neurologist may prescribe. And, because this is her area of expertise, she's your best resource for answering your questions after you've carefully read the printed information on your prescriptions. (For more information about prescription medicines, be sure to check out Chapter 9.)

Your job? Pick one pharmacy (or chain that shares information among all branches) to fill all your prescriptions and stick with them. Then be sure the pharmacist knows which over-the-counter (OTC) medicines you're taking or considering taking.

Psychologist or counselor

Anxiety and depression are part and parcel of having PD, and they're perfectly normal reactions to hearing a diagnosis of a chronic, progressive condition. A trained and licensed counselor can be a key member of your professional care team. Whether you see this person on a regular basis for *talk therapy sessions* (see Chapter 13 for more on this topic) or just now and then for some emotional unburdening, go ahead and identify this counselor shortly after your diagnosis is confirmed.

Support groups

Throughout this book we tout the benefits of joining a support group — for you and your care partner. You may reject this idea in the early stages. "I don't want to sit around talking to a bunch of strangers or listening to them complain about their PD. I've got my own problems." Wrong! Well, sort of. You definitely have your own problems. But, here's the point you're missing: A support group can help you find ways to cope with those problems.

Many types of support groups are around for PWP and their care partners. Some groups take a broader advocacy approach, while other groups focus more on their members. All support groups should have a trained professional that leads or facilitates the discussions (someone with experience and credentials). For more information, see Chapter 13 or to locate a group in your area go to www.apdaparkinson.org.

Legal and financial advisors

Your PD may eventually affect your ability to make key decisions about finances and legal matters, about the future of your family, and about your own future. Although this problem may never arise, working with an expert as early as possible after your diagnosis to put key documents and plans in order is just smart planning — whether you have PD or not. (For a full discussion of the legal and financial matters that need attention, see Chapter 20.)

Given the complexities of PD costs, drafting an insurance advisor for your team is a wise maneuver. This person can guide you and your care partner through the multitude of questions related to disability (short and long term), Medicare, Medicaid, Health Management Organizations (HMOs), Preferred Physician Organizations (PPOs), Health Savings Accounts (HSAs), and any other alphabet-soup plans that will undoubtedly surface in the future.

Spiritual advisor

Taking a holistic approach — caring for yourself physically, mentally, and spiritually — can give you a jump on managing your PD symptoms. Many people focus on the physical and mental but figure the spiritual will take care of itself. Remember: Your spiritual well being has just as many levels as your physical and mental health. If you have a spiritual mentor that you can tap to join your professional care team, do so early on. This person may be your clergy, someone who's mentored you through other passages, a practitioner of alternative or complementary medicine, or even the counselor that's mentioned in the "Psychologist or counselor" section of this chapter.

Making the cut

Drafting a team of experts in your battle against PD has benefits well beyond the expertise of each member. When you choose them carefully and treat them with respect, you find these men and women will go to great lengths for you. They even become some of your most enthusiastic cheerleaders, offering support and encouragement, humor, and affection as you confront the challenges of living with PD.

How do you evaluate each member of the team? The criteria are pretty standard — regardless of the profession:

- ✔ Does this person have the right stuff — the appropriate credentials and experience — to handle the job?

- ✔ Is it a good fit — are you comfortable with this person? Can you talk about anything or ask the silliest question without feeling intimidated?

- ✔ Does this person really listen? Is he open to ideas that aren't his own?

- ✔ Does this person give you the time you need — especially when your PD may slow your movements, thinking, and ability to put thoughts into words?

- ✔ Is this person willing to admit limits to her knowledge and expertise and refer you to someone more qualified to handle a specific issue?

- ✔ Will this person be there when you need him?

Working with Your Team to Manage the Unexpected

Stuff happens, and worst-case scenarios happen unexpectedly. Maybe you fall or burn yourself while preparing dinner and end up in the emergency room. Or, despite all precautions, you experience an adverse drug interaction that requires a stay in the hospital. Nonmedical emergencies — a fire, a weather event (such as a severe storm or tornado) — can also crop up. Our advice throughout this book is this: Have a plan in the event something unexpected happens. This doesn't mean you're assuming the worst. You just want to be ready — or as ready as possible.

Establishing an emergency plan

Be prepared — the motto of the Boy Scouts of America is just as useful for PWP and their care partners. You or your care partner may never need to dial 911, but what if . . . ? Why not think in the relative calm of your normal routine and prepare for that possible unexpected event? These next sections provide specific recommendations to help you prepare and then deal with a variety of emergencies.

The home front

Start your emergency plan with home safety by reviewing the tips for accident-proofing your home in Chapter 21. Then consider what to do in case of a medical emergency, such as an allergic reaction or a dislocated shoulder or some other emergency beyond your control — a fire, a flood, a blackout. Who do you call? Where do you go? What do you do?

Your home is unique, just like you, so the best way to prepare for a safety emergency is to contact your local fire department. It may have a program where a firefighter comes out, assesses your home for fire safety, and then offers pointers for handling emergencies. Another resource that offers a checklist for creating your own evacuation plan is available through the American Red Cross at www.redcross.org.

Personal records

Take advantage of the following tips that put you ahead of the panic if a medical or safety emergency does arise:

- ✔ Gather this vital information:
    - • A list of all prescription and OTC medications and a list of any allergies and chronic health conditions you have besides your PD
    - • Insurance or Medicare numbers
    - • Your medical history
    - • Names and contact numbers of your doctors and for an emergency contact person, like your significant other, for example
- ✔ Date all this information and update it regularly, especially when you add or discontinue meds.
- ✔ Make sure you and your care partner have copies of this info at all times in your wallet or purse and in you car(s).
- ✔ Let key others (your employer, a trusted neighbor who may respond to an emergency) know where to find the information should you be unable to direct them.

✔ Prepare a folder specifically for the emergency room. (People administering care don't have time to read old records.) Include the following pieces of information in the folder:

- All information listed in the previous section, "Personal records."

- A copy of your *advance directive* (a living will and a medical power of attorney), even if the hospital and your doctor already have it on file. If you don't want the medical staff to provide certain interventions or extraordinary measures to save your life, you must provide that information. (See Chapter 20 for more info on these and other legal issues.)

✔ Prepare a fireproof box with copies of key documents: insurance and Social Security cards; bank and credit card account numbers; wills, powers of attorney (financial and medical), and photos of valuables in case of a fire or weather catastrophe (such as a tornado or hurricane).

✔ Post critical emergency contact numbers near your home phone. Those numbers include local hospital emergency room, fire department, police department, utility company (for power outages), doctors, pharmacist (in the event of an adverse drug reaction), and a relative or friend to contact.

Easy access

You may never need emergency intervention, but you're better off to be prepared with information that an emergency team can readily access. Take the following measures to prevent glitches when seconds count.

✔ Distribute duplicate house keys to trusted friends and neighbors.

✔ Be sure your care partner can access financial funds any time you may not be able to take financial actions such as writing checks to pay bills or transferring funds from savings to checking accounts as needed.

✔ If you live alone, get a medical alert system, which enables you to call for help if you're unable to get to a telephone. (Yup, we're talking about that classic TV commercial — "Help! I've fallen and can't get up!")

Decision time

In an emergency, don't waste time worrying whether you should call for help. Risking a little embarrassment rather than your life is always the wise move.

However, if you do need to call for an ambulance or go to the emergency room, be realistic about your expectations. Keep in mind that the United States has nearly 40 million people with no health insurance; for these folks, the ER doctor is likely their doctor of choice.

Note: The Centers for Disease Control estimates the average waiting time in the ER (if you're not critically injured or ill) is three hours; in cold and flu season the wait can be much longer.

Because of possible delays, you need to

✔ Speak up if you're experiencing symptoms such as extreme pain, trouble breathing, dizziness, and other signs of distress.

✔ Tell every ER person who examines or assists you that you have PD (and any other chronic conditions such as diabetes or hypertension) even though someone has taken your history and you know these facts are on your patient information sheet.

✔ Be proactive. Make sure that the people who treat you are aware of your medications and allergies.

If your situation is serious but not life threatening, call your doctor or the nearest urgent-care or walk-in clinic for faster response and care. And if your doctor does advise you to get to the ER, he can speed up your process by calling the hospital and telling the ER staff that you're on the way.

The hospital stay and its aftermath

If you need to be admitted to the hospital, the cause isn't likely to be your PD. The more likely reasons will be a serious injury (such as a hip fracture or head trauma from a fall) or another heath condition (such as heart problems or diabetes). Regardless, be prepared with the necessary information (see the previous section for suggestions) to make the stay less stressful for everyone.

Leave valuables (checkbook, credit cards, jewelry, and the like) at home. If you must bring them because of an emergency and the haste in leaving for the hospital, hand them off to a trusted family member or friend as soon as possible. Or ask a staff member whether the hospital has a safe place to keep the valuables until you can make arrangements for them.

The same suggestions outlined for an emergency (see the previous section "Establishing an emergency plan") apply for a hospital stay. But, because you'll likely be in the hospital for days rather than hours, you must monitor the orders for your PD medications. The attending physician and the staff may not realize the importance of your PD meds' strict dosing and timing. For example, your neurologist's orders for medication at 8 a.m., noon, 4 p.m., and 8 p.m. may be interpreted by the hospital staff as four times a day over a 24-hour period, or 8 a.m., 2 p.m., 8 p.m., and 2 a.m.

I'm not fooling around and I'm not drunk — I have Parkinson's disease

To offset any misunderstandings that may occur during your hospital stay, consider packing a copy of the following note in your bag and showing it to the staff. In spite of its lighthearted tone, the note provides critical information about your care.

To whom it may concern:

First of all, let me say how much I appreciate everything you'll be doing to care for me while I'm here. My care partner and I understand that you have other patients to attend to besides me. In return I ask that you understand some things about me:

✔ You may have noticed that I'm moving pretty slowly and I probably couldn't walk a straight line if my life depended on it. Am I intoxicated? Nope. I've got this thing called Parkinson's disease.

✔ Other times you may notice that I seem to be doing just fine — doing normal stuff like brushing my teeth, washing my face, walking around on my own — and then my call bell will light up, and I'll be asking you to please come help me get to the bathroom. What gives? I have Parkinson's, and the medications I take to control it have these *on-off* cycles. One minute I can perform routine things, and the next I need all the help I can get.

✔ Speaking of meds, I really need for you — and everyone involved in treating me while I'm here — to know that certain medications commonly used in hospital settings can really mess with my PD symptoms. Please check with my neurologist, Dr. _____ at _____, before ordering or administering any new medication — especially antinausea or antipsychotic meds.

✔ And finally, as long as the subject of antipsychotic is on the table, please be aware that my Parkinson's may cause me to experience confusion, disorientation, and even some interesting misperceptions about where I am and what you're doing. I may also start to hallucinate — fortunately these *visions* I experience are usually benign and silent, so no voices are suggesting that I do you bodily harm. Again please check with Dr. _____ before administering any meds.

That's pretty much it in a nutshell. Having PD and being in the hospital can be a challenge for both of us, but hopefully now that you understand, we'll both have an easier time of it. Thanks for understanding and thanks for your care and concern.

Sincerely,

(Put your name here)

Sometimes your PD meds need to be suspended so new medications for the condition that landed you in the hospital can work. Again, be vigilant about your care. Have your care partner alert your neurologist (or the doctor managing your PD care) as soon as you know you're going to the hospital and insist that the hospital on-call physician (or any doctor who orders the suspension of your PD meds) consults with your neurologist before ordering *any* changes in medication.

Any time that your medications are being administered *for* you (as in a hospital setting) instead of you taking them yourself, be sure that you or your care partner carefully examine the pills you get. If any of the meds look different from those you take at home, question it. Also, since hospital staff is responsible for administering medications to a number of patients with diverse conditions, there may be a delay in your getting your PD meds on time. If necessary, have your neurologist contact the attending physician at the hospital to discuss the correct medication regimen. Also, make sure the attending staff knows which medications may be *contraindicated* (harmful) for PWP. (Copy the list of red-flag medications provided on the Cheat Sheet at the front of this book and ask the admitting doctor to add it to your file.)

In addition to monitoring your medications, you may have another battle to wage: The hospital staff, even though they're medical professionals, may have limited or no experience with PD and may misinterpret your PD symptoms — on-off cycles, dykinesias, confusion from the stress of a hospital environment, and the like. For example, if a nursing assistant sees you up and mobile at 2:00 and comes back at 3:00 because you want assistance getting to the bathroom, he may think you're just looking for extra attention. For one good idea for heading off any staff resentment or misunderstanding, see the nearby sidebar, "I'm not fooling around and I'm not drunk — I have Parkinson's disease."

More tips for managing the unexpected

Emergencies arise for all kinds of people. But because you have PD, such crises may carry the extra elements of stress and panic. You and your care partner may want to consider taking a basic first-aid course through your local Red Cross or YMCA to better prepare yourselves for unlikely emergencies, such as bleeding, choking, medication reaction, falls, and so on.

If you need to call 911, be prepared to give the following information:

- ✔ Phone number you're calling from
- ✔ Address and directions to help the ambulance get there quickly
- ✔ Description of the person's condition (breathing? conscious?)
- ✔ Your name

In addition, follow these steps:

1. **Don't hang up until the emergency operator tells you to.**

2. **Be sure you unlock the door and turn on outside lights.**

   Even if it's not night, the lit porch light makes locating the right house easier.

3. If possible, have another family member or neighbor wait outside to direct the emergency personnel.

4. Stay close so you can provide answers to key questions, but let the emergency personnel do their jobs.

5. Gather the information you've prepared (see the earlier section "Establishing an emergency plan") and get ready to go.

Consider having only cordless phones so you can move around the house (unlocking doors and turning on lights) while you're talking on the phone with the doctor or emergency operator.

A Word for the PD Care Partner

This book has a number of chapters that you may want to read and heed. This is one of them. Putting together a network of professionals that you and the PWP can call upon as issues crop up will make life easier for both of you.

Within this group of professionals, you need to find your own experts — three people you can turn to with your concerns of managing and coping:

- **Primary care physician:** You may have the same general practitioner or internist as the PWP. As long as this physician attends to *your* needs and concerns when you're the patient, that's fine. However, you may want to consider a PCP who isn't involved in your PWP's care. This is your decision, but remember: You need someone to focus on maintaining your physical health and well being.

- **Counselor or therapist:** Being a partner in care can be extremely stressful, especially as the needs escalate. But you'll be better prepared to cope with the unexpected twists and turns along the way if you take time now to connect with a professional who counsels care partners. Don't be stubborn about this. You are at risk for episodes of anxiety, panic, and depression as much as the PWP.

- **Support group and spiritual advisor:** Okay, so we cheated and lumped two into one. But your spiritual health is a vital piece of your ability to partner in care. A support group can provide a safe place to talk about (and let go of) those bad feelings you may be wrestling with (see Chapter 22 for more on this topic). And it has folks who can laugh and share some of the black humor that comes with being a care partner — they all know, understand, and feel your pain. As for a spiritual advisor, you know yourself best. Your clergyperson, a trusted mentor, your counselor or therapist, and your support-group leader are all good candidates to fill this role.

Chapter 7

Choosing How and When to Share Your News

. . . .

In This Chapter

▶ Setting a course with your care partner

▶ Keeping the story straight: How to share the news with your family

▶ Sharing with your inner circle: That's what friends are for

▶ Determining who else needs to know

▶ Taking the high road: People who overreact and folks who poke their noses in your business

. . . .

iving with Parkinson's disease (PD) can go well beyond the person diagnosed with PD. Day in and year out, the disease also affects the people who live with, work with, care about, and love the person with PD (PWP). It affects generations — children, grandchildren, and even aging parents (in the case of young onset PD, see Chapter 8), who may be facing their own health challenges.

Everyone has concentric circles of personal contacts. In the closest circles, we have our immediate family (spouse, partner, kids, parents) and perhaps a couple of truly best friends. Next comes a little wider circle — friends we socialize with, extended family, and perhaps a couple of professionals, like our doctor or clergyperson. Further removed from the core of our lives is another group — our employer and co-workers, acquaintances, and neighbors. Deciding when and how to tell each person or group about your diagnosis is an individual decision, one that you have to base on the dynamics of your relationships and your comfort level in sharing this kind of news. But first . . .

Before You Start Spreading the News

Even if you initially share your diagnosis with very few people, you need to plan how you want these people to react — both immediately and in the future.

Establishing your ground rules

Start by determining your ground rules and the level of support you want. The following categories identify some of the more common PWP stances:

- Some PWP are fighters: They go on immediate offense, take charge, and fight this enemy with every ounce of strength and all the resources they can muster.

- Other PWP take a flight (or more defensive) position: In some ways they choose to ignore the whole situation. Flight folks use their energy and resources to assure everyone (and most of all themselves) that nothing has really changed — life goes on.

- A third group of PWP falls somewhere in the middle, combining facets of fight and flight: Although they want life to continue as normally as possible, they realize they have to fight back to keep their PD's progression at bay.

Whichever group you're in, you need to think about your ground rules for living with PD. What kind of meaningful care and support can the groups of people in your life offer as you face life with PD? Those who care about you — family members, friends, neighbors, co-workers — naturally want to help. In many cases, they're not sure how to offer that support. You need to explain the ground rules and indicate what will — and won't — be helpful.

Preparing to state your needs

Think through now — alone, or preferably with your care partner (the person who will most likely be with you for the whole journey) — how other people can help. Initially you may need people to listen, to distract you when necessary, and to give you the gift of normalcy just by being themselves.

As your needs become more specific and as you accept the hands-on help of others, you also discover three really important outcomes:

✔ You empower people by allowing them to contribute something truly meaningful to you.

✔ You ease some of the responsibility that may have fallen on your care partner's shoulders.

✔ You prevent yourself from becoming isolated, and you actually increase your ability to take control of situations as they arise.

Accepting help is not a sign of weakness; in fact, it's a sign of strength. Acceptance shows you haven't surrendered to the challenges of PD. And when you can't fight the battle alone, you still win because you have people willing to step up to the fight for you.

Meeting the challenge with good humor

We can't say this too often: An upbeat, optimistic attitude is one of your most effective weapons against PD. And right next to it is the ability to laugh — with others, at yourself, and especially at your PD. We're talking black humor here, folks.

Bill of Rights for people with Parkinson's

Declarations of individual rights are nothing new. Perhaps you've noticed *rights* lists posted when you visit a hospital or care facility. But we think it's important that you — the person with PD — know your own inalienable rights. Feel free to edit and add your own ideas to the following list. Then bookmark it and reread it regularly.

I have the right

✔ To take care of and make decisions for myself for as long as I am capable and to expect my care partners to respect my wishes, should the time come when they speak for me

✔ To seek help from others as I recognize limits to my own endurance and strength

✔ To maintain those facets of my life that were part of my identity before my PD diagnosis for as long as possible — even if each task takes three times as long

✔ To occasionally (and humanly) get angry, be depressed, and work my way through other difficult feelings

✔ To reject any attempt by others (either consciously or unconsciously) to limit my independence because it'll make life easier for them

✔ To expect and receive consideration, respect, encouragement, affection, and forgiveness as long as I offer these same qualities in return

✔ To take joy and pride in my accomplishments — regardless of how small — and the courage it takes to achieve them

✔ To speak out and demand that new resources and eventually a cure be found — if not for me, then for those who follow

For example, a diet-center leader famous for her wonderful sense of humor inspired her feeling-sorry-for-themselves clients with the story of her father, a large, barrel-chested man who had always been bigger than life. Then he got cancer and started fading away — literally. One day toward the very end, when he was but a shadow of his former robust self, he said to his daughter, "You know I want to be cremated." She nodded in agreement. "Well," he added, "if I keep dwindling away like this, I think you'll be able to do the job in the microwave!" His daughter was first stunned and then burst into laughter. That's black humor, folks – and it works because it helps you keep your perspective as you face the sometimes tough days of living with PD.

Breaking the News to Your Care Partner

Chances are your care partner was with you when the diagnosis of PD was confirmed. If you learned the news together, then the telling part is done. But the two of you still need to spend some time working your way through the questions of how this diagnosis is going to affect your lives — individually and together.

If your primary care partner is not your significant other (perhaps she's a sibling or an adult child who works, has a family of her own, and lives in another community), give yourself a day or so to digest the diagnosis and think about how you prefer to break the news.

When you're ready (don't wait too long; a day or week at most), try to have the conversation in person and allow enough time to work through the discussion. If you can't talk in person, choose a time when this person isn't distracted by other activities and have the discussion by phone. When you deliver the news, reassure this person that the diagnosis is not life-threatening and you have no need for immediate action. Then set a time when the two of you can discuss your present needs, your needs down the road, and her willingness and capability for fulfilling those needs.

If you have to deliver the initial news by phone, urge your care partner to check out some of the Web sites in Appendix B. Or call the folks at the National Parkinson Foundation at 800-327-4545 and ask them to send copies of their excellent (and free) booklet, *Parkinson's Disease: Caring and Coping* to both of you. (In fact, while you're at it, ask for copies of the entire series of booklets.)

During this sit-down conversation with your care partner, allow enough time to:

> ✔ Share immediate emotional reactions — even if you've had a couple of days or a week since you and your care partner heard the news.
>
> ✔ Be prepared for different responses. One of you may react with denial and the other with anger. (Before this discussion, you may both benefit by reading the section on personality differences in Chapter 5.)
>
> ✔ Set down in writing a list of steps to take. Include a tentative timeline for each one based on the tips we offer in the next section.

Resist the urge (by you or your care partner) to leap ahead and take dramatic and life-changing actions such as putting your home up for sale and moving in with your daughter or assuming that you need to quit your job. You have time. You are years — and perhaps decades — from needing to make these lifestyle changes because of your PD.

Telling Your Family

When and how you deliver the news to your immediate and extended family is an individual choice that's influenced by

> ✔ The status of individual family relationships.
>
> ✔ Your personal feelings about how soon you want even close relatives to know.

When you're ready to talk to family members, the easiest way may be a family gathering (if geography allows) where you tell all the adult members at once. Everyone can hear the same version, and details won't get distorted through repetition. However, because families are so spread out in today's world, a family meeting may not be possible. In that case, consider arranging a conference call. Again, the goal is to deliver the news to all the adults at the same time.

If you have children, find a place and time to share your news with them before that larger meeting, especially if your PD is of the young-onset variety and your children are still living at home. Your children will make this journey with you; they deserve to have the same time and privacy to digest this news as your care partner had.

Give adults the facts

When you deliver the news to the adults in your immediate and extended family, stick to the basics:

✔ What PD is

✔ Whether others in the family are at risk

✔ How PD is treated

✔ What your prognosis is

Some family members may have suspected a serious illness of some kind; others may be completely shocked at the news and take it hard. In either case, a good first step is to educate and inform.

PD associations offer a number of basic educational and informational materials for fundamental questions about PD. These excellent materials are listed in Appendix B. Handing out this printed information at a family meeting (or e-mailing it if your family lives elsewhere) gives them a reference for questions after the initial shock wears off. By selecting the same material for everyone, you lessen the chances of that information becoming distorted.

Set a positive tone

After you share the facts of PD with adult family members, consider setting the tone for your emerging new relationships. For example, you can add, "There's a lot I don't know, but I do know I can live a relatively normal life in spite of my symptoms. The tough part is figuring out how to live it without people feeling sorry for me or treating me differently." With that simple statement you've laid out the ground rules:

✔ You have PD, but you're still you.

✔ Most important, you want other people to continue treating you the same. (Okay, so Cousin Fred can let you win a few more poker games and your mother may finally call someone else to get the cat out of the tree each week.)

✔ How much you say beyond that — symptoms, research, no present cures and such — is strictly up to you and your assessment of how much information this group can handle at the first telling.

When that question of "What can I do to help?" comes up, perhaps the best answer is to make these three points:

✔ Help me by being yourself and finding ways to continue our relationship as normally and fully as before.

✔ Help me make sure my care partner maintains a life outside of mine.

✔ Help me most of all by understanding that I'm still the same person inside. Don't let my PD symptoms scare you or make you treat me any differently.

Don't sugarcoat the situation for kids

Today's children are bombarded with information from every possible angle. Put another way, this generation is far savvier at a far younger age than most adults can imagine. On some level, even very young children can understand that something has changed in their environment. Don't underestimate their capacity for feeling stress and tension, especially when they can sense the undercurrent in the household but no one's talking with them about it.

✔ Teenagers can usually handle the same information you give the adults. If your teen is especially sensitive or perhaps struggling with other emotional challenges (the break-up of a relationship or not making the sports team, for example), you may want to have the conversation with that teen separately so you can focus on reassuring and comforting her.

✔ With younger children (or grandchildren), keep details as simple as possible. A terrific resource for telling young children (under age 12) about PD is the book entitled *I'll Hold Your Hand So You Won't Fall: A Child's Guide to Parkinson's Disease* by Rasheda Ali and her father, Muhammad Ali.

✔ In some cases, children in their middle years (ages 9 to 12) are mature enough to be included with the adults in the general family meeting. But just because they seem to understand and accept the news, don't assume that they don't have concerns or a gazillion questions about how your lives are going to change.

✔ If the child is your grandchild, decide with the parents the best way to deliver the news.

Regardless of the ages (or seeming maturity) of the children, never forget that they're children; they haven't lived long enough to pile up the life experiences and tools for coping that an adult has. Check in with your children and grandchildren often through positive techniques such as:

✔ Seeking their help with innovative ways you can cope with certain limits to normal tasks (like dressing) when your PD symptoms hinder you

✔ Continuing to pursue activities the two of you have always enjoyed — even if you have to find ways to adapt, such as getting a recumbent bicycle instead of riding your old one

✔ Providing the opportunity (place and time) for them to raise questions and concerns about what your PD means for the future

Giving Close Friends the News

Soon after you break the news to your family, consider how and when to tell your closest friends. Again several issues are at play here, including the fact that friends may have already noticed your symptoms and discussed their concerns with each other. They may not have brought their concern to you directly because they didn't want to intrude.

How and when you choose to tell this group depends in part on the nature of the group. In other words if your close friends are also close with each other, then inviting everyone over to your house and telling them all at the same time may be best. The advantage is that everyone hears the same words (although they may process them differently) at the same time directly from you. In addition, they can see your response to the diagnosis — hopefully upbeat and optimistic — at the same time. And they can all hear the ground rules for how you want them to respond to your diagnosis.

In cases where you have close friends who are not close with each other or friends who live in other places, you may want to tell each individually. If so, try to do it face to face (or at least by phone — not e-mail) so the person can see and hear how you're handling the diagnosis.

Consider providing the same helpful information (fact sheet and list of Web sites) that we identify in the two previous sections so your friends can pursue questions that may occur after you tell them.

Friendships can be critical to your overall sense of control and well-being when you're living with PD. Unfortunately, a lot of PWP make the mistake when they get the diagnosis of pulling away from their friends or denying their need for that support (tangible support like cutting the lawn or intangible support like just being there to listen).

When PWPs (or their care partners) react as if the support is an insult or a statement of the PWP's incapacity, they make matters worse. This reaction can have a snowball effect because the friend who wanted to help feels rejected (even embarrassed) at apparently adding to your stress. Before you know it, those treasured friendships (along with the normalcy and pleasure they brought your life) have disappeared.

As soon as you and your care partner are ready to go public with your news to friends, take control and set the tone by doing the following:

✔ State your needs regarding your approach to PD. For example, tell them you understand that they may want to rush in and start helping you (preparing meals, handling the household and yard chores, and such), but the best support they can offer is to help you maintain as normal a life (and relationship) as possible for as long as possible.

> ✔ Appreciate any offer of support and help (even if you shudder to think that they believe you need that help).
>
> ✔ Be prepared to suggest alternate ways they can be a part of your network of support and caring.

Another way to think of outside help is to consider your care partner and his soon-to-be-filled-to-capacity schedule. By maintaining a normal routine with friends and associates, you give your care partner a break to pursue life aside from PD.

When you respond to your friends' invitations to activities you enjoyed before PD with "I can't . . .," they may stop offering and gradually get on with their own lives. Instead, try an attitude of "I'd love to [play cards, bike, meet you at the coffeehouse]. Help me figure out how we can make that happen." Then you can brainstorm options together.

As Lance Armstrong (the seven-time Tour de France winner and cancer survivor) has said, "C'mon, man. *Everything's* an option."

Widening the Circle: Informing Others

On the outer fringes of those concentric circles we describe at the beginning of this chapter are those people who play a role in your life but not a vital or intimate one (neighbors, community group associates, professionals you rely upon, and so on). Breaking the news to this last circle of contacts (with the possible exception of your boss and co-workers; see Chapter 16 for the specifics on that special group) is not a responsibility that you need to feel compelled to do right away — or ever. Basically, your condition's really none of their business.

On the other hand, don't underestimate the unexpected support and management resources that may come from one of these people. For example, your barber or beautician may offer to make a house call as your symptoms change. Or your neighbor may be happy to be on call for emergencies when you're alone and your partner's at work.

When the timing seems right during the first months following your diagnosis, let these people know you have PD. Only you can decide how much information they need or what kind of support and response they may provide. But, as with anyone you tell, be prepared to set the tone for their response, to correct misinformation they may have about PD, and to appreciate their concern and support however they express it.

Handling Sticky Conversations

Having said that, we need to get real here. Some people (and they may be in your closest circles) are more hindrance than help when they hear you have PD. One type simply can't handle bad news of any sort, so you end up spending a lot of time and energy comforting and emotionally supporting their (mostly unfounded) fears and anxieties. Another type believes they have all the answers even though they have zero real knowledge about PD. They, too, can use up your resources of energy and good humor as you try and educate them to the realities of living with PD. Consider these tips for handling those sticky situations:

✔ For people who simply can't cope with difficult news, consider being prepared with a specific request. You can ask, for example, "You're such an avid biker, would you be willing to bike with me once a week? My doctor tells me that exercise, especially now in the early stages, is really important, but I'd rather not go out alone."

If this person is a close friend or family member, you may want to speak with him separately and acknowledge his obvious fears and anxieties. Then let him know that he can be most helpful by trying to remain upbeat and positive — at least in your presence.

If all else fails, allow such people an initial period of mourning over your news. Then insist that they get over it or else you'll have to limit your contact with them. This is not about these people. You're the one with PD and, bluntly stated, you just don't need other people bringing you down.

✔ For the well-meaning folks (even strangers!) who see your tremor or some other PD symptom and start telling you the story of their uncle's wife's brother who also had PD, you need a different tactic. No doubt such people mean well, but they'll never be part of your care team. This empathy and advice (or showing off!) is about them, not you.

Don't allow unwanted advice or comments to upset you. Of the two of you, *you* are the expert at PD. Acknowledge their effort to help, and then walk away.

Chapter 8

Special Advice for Those with Young Onset Parkinson's Disease

*W*hen it comes to Parkinson's disease (PD), no one's more famous than the popular actor Michael J. Fox. The twinkle in his eye and his legendary self-deprecating humor — even about life with PD — make him less the celebrity and more the national support-group leader for millions of people with Parkinson's (PWP) and their care partners.

In a 2006 interview in *AARP, The Magazine,* Fox reported that as many as 40 percent of the 60,000 new PD cases each year involve someone younger than age 50. This figure alone blows holes in the myth that only old people get PD. The fact that Fox was first diagnosed in his 30s shines an even brighter light on the growing numbers of young and active people who face this challenge.

The cause of *young onset Parkinson's disease (YOPD)* is as debatable as the cause of traditional onset PD (see Chapter 2). But what isn't debatable is the fact that it hits people in their prime, plays havoc with their established roles (spouse, parent, adult child of aging parents), derails rising careers, and overrides plans for the future.

In this chapter we take a look at the specific issues facing people diagnosed with YOPD. When the information is the same for any PWP, we refer you to other chapters in the book. But if you're 30, 40, 50, or not yet 60 and have PD, this chapter's for you.

Comparing YOPD to Traditional Onset PD

The term *onset age* means when symptoms first appear — not when a diagnosis is made. If the onset age is earlier than age 50, the diagnosis is usually YOPD. (In very rare cases, PD symptoms appear before a person reaches the age of 21; the term *juvenile Parkinson's* distinguishes it from traditional or YOPD.)

Two excellent resources for information specially aimed at people with YOPD are Young Onset Parkinson's Association (YOPA) at www.yopa.org and The Michael J. Fox Foundation at www.michaeljfox.org, where you can sign up to receive regular *Fox Flash* e-mail bulletins. These periodic updates cover upcoming foundation activities and provide valuable tips and information for PWP and their care partners.

How they're the same

PD is chronic, progressive, and (at least at this writing) incurable regardless of your age and when you get it. On the positive side, it's possible to live for many years — in some cases a regular lifespan — in spite of having PD. It's possible to continue to work, to raise a family, to see children marry and have children of their own, and to enjoy many of the same activities you enjoyed before being diagnosed.

How they differ

YOPD and traditional onset PD differ in three basic ways:

- People with YOPD are less likely to experience the dementia (memory problems) or balance problems that affect people whose PD begins when they're older. Part of the reason for the difference is that older people are more likely to have multiple conditions (such as Alzheimer's, a series of small strokes, or adverse medication interaction) that affect memory and balance.

- People with YOPD may experience a condition known as *dystonia* (unusual muscle cramping, aches, or abnormal movement in a particular area of the body such as a foot or shoulder). For reasons that still aren't clear, older patients seldom experience dystonia but tend to have *tremor* (shaking), a symptom that's less common for a person with YOPD.

Although dystonia is well recognized as the possible first symptom of YOPD, your diagnosis may be delayed if your doctor isn't familiar with such PD symptoms in younger patients. According to the Young Onset Parkinson's Association, the number of people with YOPD may be significantly under-reported for the very reason that many people experience early symptoms for years before they get to a doctor who considers PD as a possible diagnosis.

✔ In general, people with YOPD appear to respond well to antiparkinsonian medications, yet side effects (such as *dyskinesia* — uncontrollable movements) may affect them more quickly than older PWP.

In an article for the American Parkinson's Disease Association, Lawrence I. Golbe notes that people with YOPD experience two specific medication-related problems more than older PWP: early wearing-off of the medication benefits and on-off fluctuations (when PD meds lose their effectiveness so symptoms reappear before the next dose is due).

Many people with YOPD (and their doctors) elect to postpone treatment with antiparkinsonian meds as long as possible to avoid some of these escalated symptoms and side effects. *Note:* Research shows no clear evidence that early withholding of therapy has long-term benefits.

Faster or slower? What's the prognosis?

The jury's still out on the pace of progression for people with YOPD. However, more advanced therapies may eventually postpone the progression of symptoms for a longer time — perhaps adding years to the person's relatively normal life.

PD — regardless of the age of onset — affects each individual differently. As with any health issue, your physical and mental health at the onset of PD (and your fight to maintain that well being through a balanced diet and regular exercise program) can have an enormous effect on the prognosis. Nothing is carved in stone regarding the progression of symptoms — no matter how old or young you are when they start.

Facing the Special Challenges of YOPD

If you have YOPD, the most difficult challenge may be the very fact that you're young. You had planned a life packed with many goals, and one of them was *not* living with a chronic and progressive condition!

Most people in their young adult years tend to see themselves as invincible. They may take steps to ensure financial security for their family and themselves in the unlikely event that something bad happens, but they really don't consider it a possibility.

But, now it appears that the *unlikely* event has happened: You've been diagnosed with YOPD. And it's standing directly in the way of the life you've planned. At first you can see no way around it. But you know better. You know something this scary, this bleak can enrich your life in many ways.

Stop for a moment and consider other times when you faced what seemed like an impossible challenge. How did you respond to that challenge? Maybe it was a basketball game when your team was down by a point with only seconds to go and you were at the line for two free throws. Maybe it was a far more serious situation like financial difficulties or the possibility of losing your job. Maybe it was when you needed and wanted to prove yourself to someone you admired and respected. Whatever the challenge, you took some mental steps early on to face the threat or achieve what you wanted.

In this section we give you the mental steps to help you get through this diagnosis and come out on top — again.

Getting an accurate diagnosis

The diagnosis of YOPD is based on the same cardinal signs used to diagnose PD at any age:

- ✔ Tremor at rest (trembling when body part is not engaged in activity)
- ✔ Rigidity (muscle and joint stiffness)
- ✔ Bradykinesia (slowed or impaired ability to move)
- ✔ Postural instability (impaired balance)

Cases of YOPD tend to present less often with tremor and more often with bradykinesia, rigidity, and abnormal muscle cramps (dystonia) that frequently affect one foot.

When a person develops PD at a young age, the doctor must make sure that the patient doesn't have another disorder that can mimic parkinsonism (see also Chapter 4). Your doctor should always check for two rare diseases in particular: *Wilson's disease* (which requires a different treatment) and *Dopa-responsive dystonia* (DRD), which has a prognosis very different from PD.

The genetic element (see Chapter 2) seems to be more prevalent in YOPD than older PD patients. In some cases, the doctor may order a test for *Parkin* mutation, which is more frequent in YOPD. If you agree to have this DNA test, be sure you ask to see a certified genetic consultant in order to discuss all the implications (emotional and practical) of this test for you and your family.

Handling the diagnosis: A positive attitude is the best offense

Get ready for a ride on the emotional roller coaster after you get the diagnosis. Your initial reaction may range from disbelief to denial to anger to all of the above and then some. Your mind may rocket from image to image — will you see your kids grow up, graduate, and marry? Will you be able to work and support yourself and your family? What about the dreams you had of traveling, starting your own business, running that marathon? What about those words *no cure*?

Give yourself some time to mourn the fact that your life does not — for the moment — seem to be headed in the direction you had hoped. And then get on with it. This is the life you've been given. Everyone has to deal with challenges and tough choices at some point in life. PD is yours.

Because you're under 50 (even under 40), you have young onset PD, which has no cure — yet. However,

- ✔ Researchers have already developed proven techniques and therapies for managing and treating symptoms.

- ✔ You can maintain function and a relatively normal lifestyle over a period of years and — in your case — possibly decades.

- ✔ You will not die from Parkinson's disease

- ✔ Much of the life you imagined is still within your reach. The odds are very good that you'll

  - • See your children grow up, graduate, marry — and have children.

  - • Continue working for years to come and even realize the dream of starting a second career.

  - • Travel. Why not? (The marathon may be a little trickier.)

  - • Get very good at finding ways to adapt PD to goals that are really important to you.

And the best defense is a good offense

Okay, so you've taken time to digest the diagnosis and you have the attitude thing going. Now what? Take a look at the following sections to keep moving in the right direction.

Brain power

You initial response may be to run to the library or computer and look at every statistic you can find on YOPD. What were the odds that you'd get PD? What's the likely prognosis in years? What percentage of PWP your age are able to keep working, see their children grow up, have sex?

Mark Twain said there are three kinds of lies — lies, damned lies, and statistics. You can choose to believe the statistics and project them onto the rest of your life or you can refuse to be a statistic. You can determine that you're unique and that you'll custom design (with your care team — see Chapter 6) your PD management for you — and only you. But the immediate challenge is to get to work educating yourself (and your family and friends) about this diagnosis.

You've already taken a positive step by reading this book! It's chock-full of chapters offering information for anyone living with PD — young or not-so-young. After you've read it (and, of course, shared it with people close to you!), keep it handy. As you make this journey with PD, use this book as a guide to the resources you'll need along the way.

Carpe diem: Seize the day!

The overriding emotion you may feel early on is a sense that you've totally lost control of your life. But you can only lose control if you surrender to it — if you choose to hand it over to someone else and simply follow other people's orders. There's a better approach to PD for you and your care partner — one that gives you the best chance of living the life you planned before the diagnosis.

Take charge of this thing — the same way you'd attack any other unlikely event (like losing your job or your home being damaged by fire). Life can hand you bigger problems than PD — really! Unlike people facing a terminal illness, you have time and a reminder to be proactive and do what matters most now, not some day.

Without going all the way to Pollyanna-mode, consider the advantages of a can-do and optimistic outlook:

✔ The very fact that time becomes more precious can instill the determination not to waste an hour or a day.

✔ Close relationships can be strengthened — marriages, parent-child connections (yours as a parent and yours as the child of aging parents).

✔ Genuine and dedicated friends will stick; hangers-on will not (and you may be surprised at who's who in the bunch).

✔ New people — interesting and stimulating, understanding and fun — come into your life.

✔ There's nothing like a progressive illness to make you get off your butt, take that trip, write that novel, or go back to school.

✔ You now have the opportunity to work with other people to make a real difference in the lives of millions. How many people do you know who can say that?

✔ In some ways you're getting a fresh start — the chance to change you. Suddenly you understand in a very real way that life *is* finite.

Staying on track in your career

A question that's bound to be at the top of your mind is whether or not you can continue working. On so many levels, your ability to pursue a career, run a business, or maintain financial security is integral to living the life you envisioned. Be sure to read Chapter 16 for a full discussion of PD in the workplace.

One of the key messages you want to send to your employer, co-workers, and yourself is that the prognosis of YOPD is good. With proper management of PD symptoms through exercise, diet, and medications, your career can be good to go for years to come. When your neurologist, physical therapist, and nutritionist fully understand your job's requirements, they can structure your care plan (and timing of meds when you begin taking them) to provide optimal function when you need it most.

Before you sit down with your employer to discuss your diagnosis and its possible effects on your work, plan ahead by

✔ Exploring options such as flexible hours or telecommuting. If your employer makes such options available to other employees (like new parents or regular part-timers), then you're not asking for special consideration.

✔ Thinking through the demands of your specific job and how to handle them. Anticipate the questions (and doubts) your employer may have about your ability to continue.

If you think it's necessary, ask your neurologist to prepare a letter that explains the status of your PD in relation to your work.

Stress can pack a double whammy when it comes to maintaining your job and career because stress comes with the territory in many (make that *most*) jobs and can do a real number on your YOPD symptoms. Take a look at Chapter 16 for ways to manage stressful situations in the workplace — this is a huge step toward successfully maintaining your position for years to come.

Dealing with PD's impact on relationships

Now that you have PD, your diagnosis can become the two-ton gorilla in the room, sitting squarely between you and other people — if you let it. When you fear that your lover, child, best friend, or co-worker can't see you because PD's in the way, then take the initiative. Make sure these people remember that you're still you! By addressing PD issues that may affect your most important relationships, you can remove that gorilla from the room.

Your role as a spouse or significant other

The roles you and your partner have settled into may undergo quite a make-over as your PD progresses. Fortunately, this progression usually occurs over a period of years with ample time to adjust. But that delay doesn't mean you can't or shouldn't prepare for necessary changes. In other words, begin communicating now. Communication and patience are your best resources for adapting later to these inevitable changes. These are some examples:

- If your tremor worsens and you've been chief handyperson for the household, how's that going to work out? Talk about ways that you can manage the task with more time, or use this opportunity to teach a child how to wield a hammer.

- If small, cramped handwriting is an early symptom of your PD and you're the lead check writer and bookkeeper, can that continue indefinitely? Maybe you can pay bills online or install software to print out checks that you only need to sign.

- If you've been the family's gourmet cook but now you take hours longer to turn out one of your signature meals, then you (and those around you) need to practice patience by allowing for the extra time you need. Then again, you may consider graciously (and willingly) accepting some help.

Don't rush into changes before they're necessary. Do take time to plan with your partner the ways that you can adjust certain tasks or roles before you give them up.

As your symptoms progress and your medication timing switches unexpectedly into on-off mode, your spouse or significant other may find it tough to believe you're suddenly struggling with a task that you managed fine just a minute earlier. Be honest about what's going on. Acknowledge that it looks like you don't want to do this task, but — for now — you really can't. Communication and patience are paramount here!

Another common concern when you have YOPD is the question of intimacy. Okay, to put it bluntly — you're wondering about its impact on your ability to perform sexually. The answer: If you experience a change in your sexual desire, performance, or pleasure, a host of underlying causes are possible. Some of the more common ones are:

- ✔ Side effects of medications

- ✔ Effects of certain cardiovascular conditions (high blood pressure, circulatory problems, reduced blood flow, heart disease and such)

- ✔ Impact of other conditions such as urinary incontinence, menopause for women, or prostate problems for men

- ✔ Effects of depression, stress, or anxiety

- ✔ Symptoms common to PD (tremor, stiffness, on-off episodes, dyskinesias and such) that can affect movement (not to mention the mood!)

PD may cause sexual dysfunction, but this symptom usually occurs several years into the progression of the disease, and other symptoms (including those listed above) can play a role. Don't simply assume that a change in your desire for intimacy or ability to make love is a normal part of PD. Solutions are available, so talk to your doctor and look at Chapter 19 for more information on sexual dysfunction.

Intimacy means more than the act of making love. Think about the progression of your relationship. Maybe it began with flirting and progressed to the sheer romance of the courtship before you two decided you were in this for the long haul. Maybe you surprised your partner with an unexpected romantic gesture — flowers for no reason, holding hands at the movies, the funny card, or handwritten note. Rekindle those little moments that led to falling in love and the commitment of a long-term (or even lifetime) relationship.

Maintain a sense of humor. Surely even at your healthiest you had those moments — embarrassing, silly, laugh-out-loud times when it all went haywire at a critical moment. Plan to roll with them. Shared laughter can be incredibly sexy.

Your role as a parent

How life may change for you and your kids will depend on their ages when you're diagnosed. If they're very young, you can keep the news simple and guide your children as they grow up and your symptoms progress. By the time they reach their middle or high school years, living with a parent who has PD will seem so normal that it'll be their friends' parents who seem different.

If your children are older (middle or high school) when you're diagnosed, communication may be more difficult. At this age your children are dealing with a lot already. They're trying to locate their own sense of identity among their peers and within the family unit, they're trying to live up to adult expectations, and they're facing ever-escalating pressure to make the right choices. No wonder they shut down sometimes!

Now you come along and deliver the news that you have PD — a disease they may have heard about but one that they may have some real misinformation on. Depending on their age and your relationship, your children may or may not ask questions, but don't assume that they have none. On the other hand, dole out information carefully. You may hear "TMI!" (too much information) from your teen when you start throwing around terms like *bradykinesia, substantia nigra,* and such.

If you have teens or middle-schoolers, you may want to ask for help in researching information. They're undoubtedly proficient on the computer. Give them a focused PD topic to research and ask them to share it with the family. For example, put them to work locating and bookmarking the best PD Web sites for the family. What organizations can they find? What are the strengths of each site? By proactively including your children in a management plan for your PD, you take away a lot of their fear and distress that can come from being left out of key discussions and decisions.

Your role as a friend

If you're fortunate enough to have a network of close friends — even if that network is only two or three people — you have a fabulous resource for coping with your PD. Friends can listen when you really don't want to burden your spouse or significant other. And they can take your focus off PD to get you back on the track of living the life you'd planned. Friends can make you laugh and let you cry. They can push, shove, and irritate you until you'll do anything to get them off your case. They can admire your courage, wonder at your ability to contain this beast, and celebrate each passage — just as they did when you didn't have PD, and just as you've done for them.

Friendship is a two-way street. Your friends can only be there if you let them, and they'll be there for the long term only if you let them know you'll do the same for them. For more ideas on PD and friendships, see Chapter 15.

Your role as a co-worker/employee/employer

By some estimates, up to one-third of PWP (at any age) are actively employed. As the news of your diagnosis spreads at work, your co-workers will probably take one of two positions: Some will immediately come forward, express their concern, and ask what they can do to help; others will pull back, take a let's-see-how-this-goes position.

As with all your relationships, this one is yours to manage. Frankly, your best bet is to let people know that you have PD (after you've told your employer). Otherwise the rumor mill is going to be the messenger. Consider sitting down with members of your department (with your supervisor's approval) to give them some brief, basic facts about YOPD. You can then ask these co-workers to use these facts to squelch rumors they may be hearing.

If you're the employer (or department head), be aware of immediate employee concerns for you *and* for themselves. What does your PD mean for the future of the business and their job security? Again carefully prepare by anticipating questions and concerns (from good employees seeking other positions or ambitious staffers eyeing your position) for you and your business.

Whatever your job, you need to realistically assess (and reassess regularly and frequently) your ability to handle the job. Your greatest barrier will be stress, and the greatest stress comes when people around you clearly question your ability to do the job. For ways you can address this problem and the related challenges of PD in the workplace, see Chapter 16.

Your role in the community

Over time your PD becomes more and more difficult to disguise. Even if you can manage the outward symptoms like a tremor or impaired movement, the stress of trying to keep it a secret can drain you. But why expend so much energy to keep people in the dark when they may become unexpected sources for support and outright help?

Maintaining (or instigating) community relationships isn't just about the personal returns. When you volunteer at your child's school or join in for a charity walk or bike event, you're making a better world for others — and that's empowering. You're not this poor PWP; you're someone who chooses to take advantage of an opportunity to make a real difference for yourself and the community around you.

Speaking of community action, the Parkinson community — national, regional and local — is well organized and a great place to get involved. By taking an active role in advocating for more research dollars, better therapies, and eventually a cure, you empower yourself and other PWP. Not a marcher or the outspoken sort? Not a problem. Check out www.parkinsonaction.org or any of the national organizations listed in the appendix of this book for ways you can get involved behind the scenes.

The Dollars and Cents of YOPD Financial Planning

Definition of *terrifying*: The experience of a person in the prime of life getting news that he has a chronic and progressively debilitating illness. Although people with YOPD can hope for a cure in their lifetime, basing their financial futures on such a pipedream is, unfortunately, unrealistic.

Realistically you'll live with PD for many years to come, years that may include getting married, raising a family, sending kids off to college, securing the future for your partner, caring for aging parents — a host of emotional and financial challenges. Our suggestion? Regardless of your economic status, take your partner and get to a financial planner *now* (see Chapter 21 for tips on choosing one) to help you plan for the future.

If you're in debt now, you need a plan to manage that debt and end it as quickly as possible. If you have plans for major financial commitments (such as buying a car or home or sending your child to college), you need to ask yourself whether such plans are still viable.

Financial planning is one of those tasks where preparing for the worst scenario is the wisest move. You may ask, "But what if I never need to put the plans in action?" The best answer is a different, more challenging question: What if you *do* need to?

If you haven't already done so, take time to ask the big questions:

- ✔ What are my current health insurance plan's benefits?
- ✔ What hospitalization, disability benefits, and programs may be available through my work?
- ✔ What are the benefits and limitations of the COBRA program if I have to stop working?
- ✔ What long-term care insurance program can I (or my partner) benefit from?
- ✔ Am I eligible for that program?

Connecting with other YOPDers

"I have plenty of friends," you say, "so I don't need to connect." Oh, but you do. You have a condition that usually strikes people decades older than you. You have a chronic, progressive condition that's going to impact every facet of your life. On top of that, you have this life — of work and relationships and social events and community functions and. . . . So, you're going to have times over the coming months and years when the very person you need to talk with is someone who understands what it means to have YOPD, someone who's been there, who's still there — someone who can tell you to knock it off, stop wasting precious time, and get on with your life when you start feeling sorry for yourself.

So where can you find these people? If you're really fortunate, a YOPD support group is close enough for you to conveniently attend meetings. If it isn't, then check with the facilitator of any PD support group that meets in your area to see how many of the participants have YOPD. If that fails, ask your neurologist whether she treats other YOPD patients. If she does, perhaps names and contact information can be exchanged.

Your best resource may be the Internet. One established organization specifically for YOPDers is Movers and Shakers at www. pdadvocates.org The Parkinson Action Network at www.parkinsonsaction. org is another great place to connect with PWP of all ages. The National Parkinson Foundation at www.parkinson.org sponsors an annual conference for YOPDers and their families. In addition, chat rooms and other sites offer people with YOPD a chance to connect — even in the wee hours of the morning. Two such sites are www.braintalk.org and www. plwp.org.

The point is that you (and your care partner) can connect with others your age that understand and have experienced or are experiencing many of the same frustrations you are. Your friends and family members may be terrific — supportive and concerned — but how can they possibly understand the full impact of YOPD? Not even your neurologist can fully appreciate what it means to have PD in the prime of your life.

Connecting with YOPDers isn't about giving up on friendships that have sustained you (and that still sustain you). But connecting with other YOPDers can lessen your sense of isolation and provide you with resources and news to manage your symptoms in a variety of situations. Another person with YOPD may not become your new best friend — but then again, don't rule out the possibility.

If you have no insurance, talk to your financial planner immediately about options that may be available in your state or through federal programs. If the financial planner can't answer your questions or provide information in a timely manner, find another planner!

In addition to your financial planning, take the following measures to help your medical providers:

> ✔ Establish a *durable* power of attorney for healthcare decisions as well as financial decisions.
>
> ✔ Write a living will or advance directive; make sure you distribute copies to every doctor who treats you and carry a copy with you in case you need to go to the hospital or emergency room.
>
> ✔ Be sure that the people you appoint to speak for you know what you want them to say and do!

For a more detailed discussion of legal and financial concerns that need your attention sooner rather than later, turn to Chapter 20.

A Word for the PD Care Partner

When you discover that someone you love has a condition that takes that person's functions and abilities, your instinct may be to go into full caregiver-mode and take charge. Please resist that urge! The person you love is exactly the same person that he was before the diagnosis. PD doesn't change a person overnight. In fact, the changes are gradual enough for the two of you to take the time to adapt, prepare, and plan.

But you don't want to run away either. Throughout this book we talk about the fight-or-flight response to tough situations. If you're a person who takes flight (backs away and finds reasons to become disengaged), then you need to reassess that instinct. The person you love and are devoted to needs you — your support and understanding — in the early going, and she may eventually need more of you as her spokesperson and advocate.

If you're a fighter (a person who takes charge or refuses to lose), you may need to dial it down a notch or two. Although you're the care partner, the operative word is *partner*. You're not in charge; you don't have YOPD. Contribute and discuss options — yes. Coax and encourage — absolutely. Defend your right to a life beyond your partner's PD — positively. But in the final analysis, the person with PD has the right (as well as the ability) to decide how she wants to face this challenge. It's called *patient autonomy* and it's the very foundation of medical ethics.

Part III
Crafting a Treatment Plan Just for You

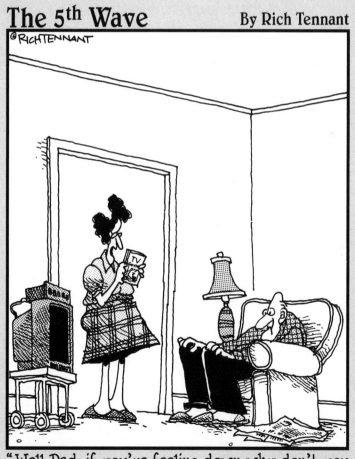

The 5th Wave   By Rich Tennant

"Well Dad, if you're feeling down why don't you watch some TV. Let's see, there's 'Silent Killers', 'When Puppies Attack', and 'War of the Worlds.'"

In this part . . .

You can explore the variety of options available to treat your PD and help manage symptoms. These include medications and surgery as well as complementary and alternative medical treatments. Our chapter on diet and exercise includes an illustrated program of stretching and strengthening exercises that you can take to your doctor or physical therapist for review. Finally we have a chapter on clinical trials where we discuss the pros and cons of participating in such projects and what you need to know before you make a commitment.

Chapter 9

Managing PD Symptoms with Prescription Medicines

*Y*our Parkinson's disease (PD) diagnosis will include treatment options for managing your symptoms. If you have no symptoms of functional disability at the time of your diagnosis (in other words, if the PD isn't interfering with your ability to live your normal life), then your doctor will most likely prescribe programs like exercise and nutrition counseling, a support group, and, of course, regular visits to his office to monitor symptoms and any signs of progression.

As your symptoms begin to affect your work, social, and routine activities, your doctor will likely add *pharmacologic* therapy (prescription medications) to the treatment plan. In this chapter, we look at the most common medications for managing symptoms, some that have been around for decades and others that are relatively new to the scene. We also pass along some suggestions for staying on top of your medication regimen.

Because PD has no cure at this time and there is no means of preventing its progression, the treatment goal is to manage the symptoms, postpone their progression, and minimize the onset of new symptoms for as long as possible.

Managing Motor Symptoms with Proven Prescription Medication

In managing your symptoms, your doctor may prescribe a variety of medications to help prolong your current level of function. The medication may be available only as a brand-name drug (meaning it's still under patent protection), or it may be available in the generic form (meaning the patent has expired). Brand drugs are usually newer, more expensive, and possibly more beneficial than generics.

All medications for PD have one goal: to restore brain concentration of dopamine to near-normal levels. To achieve this goal, your doctor may prescribe one or more pills with different mechanisms of action (similar to different foods that we routinely use to restore sugar levels in our body, such as pasta, fruit, and sweets). The number of pills doesn't necessarily correlate to the gravity of the disease!

Almost 40 years after its introduction, the combination of *levodopa* and *carbidopa* (usually prescribed under the brand name *Sinemet*) is still the preferred treatment for most people with Parkinson's (PWP). The following sections cover the components of this medication and the role each one plays.

L-dopa — The gold standard

The most effective prescription medication to date for controlling PD symptoms is *levodopa* (often abbreviated to *L-dopa*), which brain cells use to produce more *dopamine*, the neurotransmitter that PD reduces. Producing more dopamine permits relief for PD symptoms such as stiffness, tremor (shaking), facial mask, cramped handwriting, slow movement, and impaired gait (walking).

Historically, L-dopa was administered alone, which caused a whole list of side effects including nausea, loss of appetite, vomiting, lowered blood pressure (leading to dizziness and possible falls), and rapid heart rate. Because these side effects were so significant, researchers almost dropped L-dopa from the regimen before they discovered the advantages of prescribing it with its now-conventional partner, *carbidopa*. Coupled with carbidopa, L-dopa can almost completely control PD symptoms for a *honeymoon* period of two to eight years.

Unfortunately, 50 percent of PWP develop motor complications after 5 years of levodopa therapy; virtually all of them experience a decline in the benefit of levodopa after 10 to 15 years of therapy.

Carbidopa — L-dopa's companion

Any time the treatment seems worse than the condition, researchers look for ways to make the treatment more palatable for the patient. Carbidopa's main purpose is to offset the serious and uncomfortable side effects of levodopa without causing side effects of its own. In addition, carbidopa

- Allows your system to absorb the essential vitamin B_6
- Lessens the amount of levodopa you need to control symptoms

When your symptoms do require medication, the prescription will probably be a low dose of carbidopa/levodopa. The prescription includes two numbers — usually 25/100. The first number refers to the amount of carbidopa and the second is the amount of levodopa. Your doctor monitors your symptoms on this low dose (usually taken at regular intervals three to four times a day). If you experience side effects, he can double the amount of carbidopa in your prescription. As the symptoms of PD progress, your doctor may increase the dosage and shorten the periods between doses.

Two other formulations for this medication are:

- The controlled-release (CR) form of Sinemet, which prolongs the effect of levodopa
- The orally disintegrating tablet (ODT) form of carbidopa/levodopa (brand name *Parcopa*)

  With ODT delivery systems, you place the tablet on your tongue and it melts (like a mint) in a matter of seconds without water.

Entacapone — Another bodyguard for L-dopa

Recently a new class of drugs, *catechol-O-methyl transferase* inhibitors (*COMT-I*), has been added to PD therapy. COMT-I blocks the enzyme 3-O-methyldopa and allows even more levodopa to reach the brain. (Imagine levodopa with two body guards — carbidopa and *entacapone* or *tolcapone* (see the following paragraph) — to shelter it from dangerous enzymes on its journey toward the brain.) Other advantages of adding COMT-I to L-dopa are

- Longer duration of the L-dopa effectiveness
- Potential for reducing the dosage of carbidopa/levodopa
- The possibility of managing *off* times more effectively (See "Tracking the on-off fluctuations of your meds" later in this chapter.)

Entacapone (brand name *Stalevo*) is a new L-dopa therapy that combines the COMPT-I with carbidopa/levodopa. This three-in-one combination makes dosing easier because you take one pill, not two. Another COMT-I, *tolcapone* (brand name *Tasmar*), is available but has some limitations associated with liver toxicity.

Other effective prescription medicines

Your doctor may prescribe other medications in addition to your carbidopa/ levodopa to better manage your symptoms. We cover the most common classes of these companion drugs in the following sections.

Dopamine agonists (DA)

Unlike levodopa, which is transformed into dopamine, *dopamine agonists (DA)* imitate the characteristics of dopamine. Your doctor may recommend that you try a DA before prescribing Sinemet as a first-line treatment in order to delay the complications associated with the use of levodopa over the long haul. (See the previous section "L-dopa — the gold standard" for more about Sinemet.) DAs have been in use for two decades with proven effectiveness in treating PD symptoms. But their use may be limited by troubling side effects, such as daytime sleepiness, low blood pressure, edema (swollen feet), vivid dreams, and, on occasion, hallucinations.

Four dopamine agonists are available. Older generation drugs (bromocriptine and pergolide) are rarely used because of possible cardiac side effects. But newer generations of DAs (including *pramipexole* and *ropinirole*) offer effective management of symptoms with relatively fewer side effects.

Of the four DA medications available, studies haven't proven one to be more effective than another. Therefore, if you have an unfavorable response to one DA, ask your doctor about trying a different one to see whether it's more successful.

Monoamine oxidase inhibitors (MAOI)

This class of drugs works by interacting with *monoamines,* chemicals in the brain that transmit messages between nerve cells. Of the three monoamines (dopamine, serotonin, and norepinephrine), dopamine is the focus for PWP because it controls messages related to movement.

Although MAOI has two subtypes (Type A and Type B), only MAOI-B is used to treat PD. Its fundamental task is to inhibit the *oxidation* (burning) of dopamine, which clears the dopamine from the *synaptic space* (the tiny space between brain cells where chemical messages are exchanged). As a consequence, more dopamine is available and PD symptoms improve. Interestingly, MAOI-B may provide an additional benefit by acting as a kind of neuroprotector (see Chapter 2), possibly slowing the progression of PD and delaying the need for carbidopa/levodopa therapy.

The original drug from this group is *selegiline,* which doctors still prescribe for the early stages of PD because it provides some control of PD symptoms. A new formula of orally disintegrating selegiline *(Zelapar)* has recently been introduced with a lower incidence of side effects and a once-a-day dosing schedule. The most recent drug in this class to receive FDA approval is *rasagiline* (brand name *Azilect*), also taken once a day for the treatment of early PD. For PWP in the moderate to advanced stages, a combination of selegiline and L-dopa can improve symptoms.

The downside to MAOIs is their potentially serious effect on blood pressure, especially when the patient is taking other medicines that also affect blood pressure. Take these precautions to avoid serious problems:

✔ Be sure all doctors know you're on this medication and always check with your pharmacist before using:

- Over-the-counter (OTC) products such as cold-cough remedies (especially those including *dextromethorphan*) and diet supplements

- Prescription medicines such as antidepressants that increase serotonin levels

✔ If you're scheduled for surgery, be sure the anesthesiologist knows you're taking rasagiline because anesthesia combined with the MAOIs can cause a dangerous drop in blood pressure.

✔ Be aware that MAOIs can cause abnormalities of blood pressure known as *tyramine* (or *cheese effect)* when the patient is eating aged cheese or drinking red wine.

Consult your doctor if you have additional questions about the serious side effects of MAOIs.

Transdermal patch — A new delivery system

In most cases, prescribed medications come in a tablet or capsule form. But researchers are working on other ways to get the drug into your system with improved effectiveness, fewer side effects, and a shorter waiting period before the drug takes effect.

As one example of such research, at this writing the Food and Drug Administration (FDA) is in the process of reviewing a *transdermal* (skin) patch for the delivery of rotigotine, a dopamine agonist. You apply the patch to your skin (back, shoulder, or abdomen) once a day. The advantage of the patch is its consistent delivery of medication throughout the day. Consistent delivery of the dopamine agonist helps smooth out the amount of medicine you receive unlike the peaks and valleys that occur when taking tablets or capsules multiple times each day. This new method may improve symptom control and reduce side effects. Patches for the delivery of levodopa are also under study.

Amantadine

Amantadine is another older medication that doctors occasionally prescribe in early stages of PD because it can provide some benefit before levodopa is needed. Exactly how amantadine helps relieve symptoms isn't clear. In fact, it was originally (and continues to be) a treatment for the flu, but scientists serendipitously stumbled on its potential PD benefits. Most recently doctors have noted amantadine's benefits in managing *dyskinesia* (the writhing, twisting of the body) that may occur after long-term levodopa therapy.

Keeping the names straight

Your doctor has a growing arsenal of medications with which to treat your PD symptoms. Table 9-1 provides a handy reference for their generic and brand names.

Table 9-1	Generic and Brand Names of Common PD medications	
Class of Drug	*Generic Name*	*Brand Name*
Carbidopa/Levodopa		
	Carbidopa/levodopa	Sinemet
	Carbidopa/levodopa controlled-release	Sinemet CR
	Carbidopa/levodopa/entacapone	Stalevo
	Carbidopa/levodopa orally disintegrating tablet (ODT)	Parcopa
Dopamine Agonists (DA)		
	Bromocriptine	Parlodel
	Pergolide	Permax
	Pramipexole	Mirapex
	Ropinirole	Requip
	Rotigotine (transdermal system)	Neupro
COMT Inhibitors		
	Entacapone	Comtan
	Tolcapone	Tasmar

Class of Drug	Generic Name	Brand Name
MAO-B Inhibitors		
	Selegiline	Eldepryl
	Selegiline ODT	Zelapar
	Rasagiline	Azilect
Others	Amantadine	Symmetrel

Treating Non-Motor PD Symptoms

PWP must deal with a whole range of symptoms — only some of which involve movement. In the chapters that follow, we discuss in detail the PD symptoms of depression and anxiety and symptoms that may occur as your PD progresses. (See Chapters 13 and 19.) However, if any of the following non-motor symptoms become disruptive to your routine and life, talk to your doctor about medications that may be helpful:

- ✔ **Dizziness or changes in blood pressure when you stand after lying down or sitting:** Report this to your doctor! Treatment may include changes in habits (such as increasing fluid intake or wearing support stockings) or a change in medications.

- ✔ **Increased saliva or swallowing problems:** Again, your doctor needs to know about this because it may be a side effect of a medication or it may be the progression of your PD. Either way, don't ignore it!

- ✔ **Sleep disturbances:** The disease itself and some of your antiparkinsonian meds can cause sleep disturbance. Ask your doctor whether a sleep aid may be helpful. In some cases where sleep disturbances are especially troublesome, a more specific sleep study may be indicated.

- ✔ **Pain, cramping, or dyskinesia:** These symptoms are often worse at night or bedtime. A change in your evening dose of Sinemet (higher or lower) may solve the problem, or ask your doctor whether anti-inflammatories (such as ibuprofen), muscle relaxants, or dopamine agonists may help.

- ✔ **Nausea, stomach upset, constipation, and heartburn:** These symptoms may be part and parcel of your medication routine. Talk to your doctor about when, how often, and to what degree of discomfort these symptoms occur.

- ✔ **Urinary frequency or urgency:** Conditions other than your PD (such as prostate hypertrophy) may be at play here. Talk to your doctor if you experience any change in urinary habits, especially if you experience pain or any sort of discharge with urinating.

If you're seeing another doctor or taking medication for high blood pressure or another chronic condition, be sure your neurologist and all doctors consult with each other before prescribing new meds for you.

Using Your Medication Safely and Effectively

As a person with PD, you need to pay close attention to your medication timing and dosing. You also need to be aware of changes in performance and function (mental or physical), especially if such changes seem to relate to your medication routine. In short, you need to

- ✔ Take an active role in monitoring your medications and the results you get (or don't get) from them.
- ✔ Inform your doctor and pharmacist of any side effects, new symptoms, or worsening of current symptoms.

This section covers the important ways you can work with your doctors and pharmacist to maintain a healthy regimen with your meds. We also pass along some advice for keeping track of your meds and their effectiveness with your PD symptoms.

Partnering with your doctor and pharmacist

Work with your neurologist to review *all* your medications from time to time. Be sure to include any OTC products you take regularly. And remember to pay special attention to any dosing changes or new prescription meds another doctor may have ordered.

When your neurologist and other doctors write a new prescription for you, ask the following questions:

- ✔ Why are you prescribing this medication at this time?
- ✔ What results should I expect after I begin taking this medication?
- ✔ How soon should I expect positive results?
- ✔ How should I take the medication — timing, dosing, with (or without) food and so on?
- ✔ What side effects might I experience?

Keeping the costs of meds under control

If the cost of your medications is overwhelming, you may be eligible to receive some of your prescription medications for a reduced cost or even for free. The American Parkinson Disease Association (APDA) partners with a coalition of health providers, pharmaceutical companies, patient advocacy groups, and other organizations to help you get the medicine you need. Call 888-477-2669 or go online to `www.pparx.org` for full details on eligibility. You can also check with your state Office on Aging or go to `www.benefitscheckup.org` or `www.needymeds.com` for more information.

✔ What side effects should I notify my doctor about immediately?

✔ What side effects would require me to get to an emergency room or call 911?

✔ What does the medication cost?

✔ Can I get the same benefits a less expensive way?

> For example, Stalevo is convenient but can be expensive. Taking Sinemet and Comtan separately may save money.

✔ Are any interactions possible between the new medication and other prescription or OTC meds that I'm already taking?

When you get the medication the first time, be sure the pharmacist prints out and reviews the prescribing information sheet with you. (If you don't have a regular pharmacist, ask your neurologist to recommend pharmacies in your area that she respects and communicates well with.)

Before you leave the pharmacy:

✔ **Ask questions if anything on the information sheet raises a red flag for you.** For example, if a side effect of the new med is low blood pressure and you're taking medication to manage high blood pressure, how will the new drug affect it?

✔ **Check the label to be sure you can read it and that you have received the right medication according to your doctor's instructions.** If a substitution has been made (a generic for the brand your doctor prescribed, for example), ask the pharmacist to call the doctor to be sure the switch is okay.

✔ **Open the package and look at the medicine, especially if it's a refill**. If the pill or tablet doesn't look like the med you've been taking, immediately bring that question to your pharmacist's attention.

Mixing prescription and OTC medications

Pick up any magazine these days and you'll likely find an article touting the advantages of some herbal supplement or vitamin. Or maybe a friend recommends some OTC product for your heartburn, headache, or cold symptoms. The question is: How will these commonly used products interact with your prescription meds — especially your antiparkinsonian meds?

Anyone who takes a prescription medication to manage or treat a chronic illness needs to vigilantly read labels on all OTC as well as prescription products for potential interactions. Call the primary care physician or neurologist and talk to the pharmacist before taking the meds to let these professionals help you decide if this med is right for you.

Common signs of potentially dangerous drug interaction include accelerated or slower heart rate, diarrhea or constipation, heartburn, nausea or cramping, fever, skin rashes or unusual bruising, dizziness, confusion, loss of appetite, or abnormal fatigue. If you experience any such side effects, contact your doctor. If side effects are severe — or a doctor is unavailable — call 911 or get to an emergency room.

Note: Ask your doctor whether grapefruit juice can have an effect on your medications. Studies have shown that grapefruit juice can interfere with the liver's ability to break down some medicines — especially prescription drugs.

Balancing the benefits of medications against their potential side effects is delicate. In partnership with your doctor, determine what combination works best for your lifestyle and quality of life. The goal is to keep you *in* control — as opposed to *under* the control — of your meds and your PD.

Setting up a routine for managing your meds

Being human, we have a tendency to ignore or bend the rules, especially when it comes to faithfully following a medication regimen. We skip doses, miss the timing by a couple of hours, cut the dose to save money, and even share prescription meds with other people (because it did so much good for us).

With PD, taking medicine and taking it in the prescribed and timely manner is critical. And, because you probably take more than one medication for PD (not to mention the meds you may take for other conditions such as high blood pressure), timing is indeed everything.

As your PD progresses, you may experience memory problems, so it's enormously important that you figure out now how you're going to remember to take your meds. This section offers suggestions for both organizing your medication regimen and remembering it.

Three keys to avoid problems with your medications:

✔ Make sure one (and only one) doctor (your neurologist is the best choice) oversees all your medications, including OTC vitamins, supplements, or herbal remedies.

✔ Choose one pharmacy (or one pharmacy chain that maintains your records regardless of where you are) to fill all your prescriptions.

✔ Take a list — if not the actual meds — to every doctor's appointment (including dentists, podiatrists, and so on) and to the hospital or emergency room if you need to go there.

Hospitals use several medications to combat nausea following anesthetic that are *contraindicated* (or *not to be used*) for PWP. These drugs not only worsen PD symptoms but can actually produce Parkinson-like symptoms in people with no diagnosis of PD. For a complete list of these drugs, see the Cheat Sheet in front of the book.

You also need to get organized at home — where you most likely take your meds. You've probably seen or even used those plastic pill-containers that organize meds by day (or even by dose throughout the day). Some of these containers come with a beeper that signals the time for a dose. Other varieties have large sections to accommodate several pills or larger pills.

Consult with your pharmacist on the best choice in medication organizers for your purposes. Think about your daily activities:

✔ Are you home all the time?

If you are, then one large, multi-sectioned container may be a good choice.

✔ Are you at work when one dose comes due?

Then a smaller pocket container or one with the reminder alarm is a good choice for that dose.

Establish a regular time (the same time and day every week) for loading the meds into the proper container. Then place the container(s) in the most obvious place to remind you. (For example, you may want your morning and bedtime meds next to your toothbrush.)

Tracking the on-off fluctuations of your meds

As if multiple motor, cognitive, and other symptoms of PD aren't enough, the common PD medications can also affect the course of the disease. Read any PD article or get into a discussion with any PD patient or care partner, and sooner or later you hear the terms *wearing off* and *on-off*.

The *wearing-off* effect may appear when the PWP has been on the same dosage for some time. Over time, the positive effect of the med simply wears off before the next dose. In that window between the end-of-dose benefit and the delivery of the next dose, the PWP may experience heightened symptoms of PD, such as tremors, difficulties with balance and coordination, and so on. Such incidents commonly occur after a relatively long *honeymoon*, when the antiparkinsonian meds effectively control the symptoms. The usual solution is to shorten the time between doses, increase the dose, and/or add other meds.

The *on-off* phenomenon (which is fairly unique to PD) refers to the PWP's ability to perform common physical activities one minute and then be totally incapable the next minute, all within the same dosing cycle. Another way of looking at this phenomenon is that the wearing off effect loses its predictability so PD symptoms emerge without warning. Some PWP actually refer to the sensation as someone flipping a switch. Usually this effect occurs when the PD is in the advanced stages.

We recommend that you track your on-off fluctuations after they begin by noting the following and reporting your findings to your doctor:

- ✔ The time the meds start wearing off in relation to your next scheduled dose of medicine.
- ✔ The exact symptoms that reappear.
- ✔ The frequency of the off-period. Is it every dose or just now and then? If it's now and then, is there a recurring pattern?

Finally, *dyskinesia* (involuntary movements) is another treatment-related symptom that may become apparent as the disease progresses. Movements may range from dance-like to irregular and jerky motions, and they usually occur when the medication dose is at its height.

For friends and family, this seemingly random ability of the PWP to act normal one minute and need help the next minute may appear calculated, to gather sympathy or manipulate other people. But the cause is simply not known. Recent theories link the continued loss of dopamine-producing cells and years of drug therapy as a possible cause. Both the PWP as well as family and friends must understand that this on-off effect isn't within the PWP's control, isn't a deliberate attempt to gain sympathy, and may not respond to a change in the medication routine.

Chapter 10

When Surgery Is an Option

As Parkinson's disease (PD) progresses, medications often lose their effectiveness; sometimes they cause, rather than alleviate, problems for the patient. In these instances, surgery may bring much-needed relief and even restore some level of normalcy to the patient's functions and life for many years. In this chapter, we explore current surgical procedures and raise the important questions for you to ask before deciding to proceed.

Deciding Whether You're a Candidate for Surgery

First things first: Of the many people with Parkinson's (PWP), which ones are more likely candidates for surgery? The following questions are a general guide to help you understand your chances for a successful outcome from surgery.

- ✔ Have you successfully used antiparkinsonian medications (primarily L-dopa therapy) for several years?

- ✔ In spite of an optimal medication regimen, are you experiencing increasing freezing episodes (sudden difficulty in moving), on-off fluctuations (shortened time between response to meds and time for next dose), and dyskinesia (twisting motion — a major side effect of taking the antiparkinsonian meds)?

- ✔ Is your tremor so severe that medication can't control it?

Of course, your age, past medical history, and general health are always considerations before deciding to undergo surgery, but you're more likely to benefit from surgery if you answered "Yes" to all of the above questions.

Note: Unfortunately, PWP whose main issues involve cognitive loss, impaired balance that doesn't respond to L-dopa, poor speech (*dysarthria*), or swallowing problems (*dysphagia*) are less likely to be helped by surgery.

Even if you appear to be a prime candidate, you have a great deal to consider before deciding whether surgery's right for you. Most importantly, remember that you may experience relief — even significant relief — of some symptoms, but your PD will progress. In particular, symptoms that surgery can't address (such as autonomic dysfunction or cognitive decline) may still be a factor in the progression of your PD.

On the other hand, if certain symptoms (like tremor, bradykinesia, dyskinesia, rigidity, and on-off fluctuations) have begun to rule your life, surgery may buy you some much-needed relief and time to enjoy a higher quality of life. This isn't a decision you or your doctor should make lightly.

Weighing Your Surgical Options

At this writing, surgical options for treating PD are virtually limited to *deep brain stimulation* or DBS (see section below). But scientists continue to seek new procedures that may prove more effective in controlling symptoms or stopping them altogether, allowing the patient to remain symptom-free for a period of time. (See the sidebar "Stem Cell Research: The Controversy" later in this chapter.)

Deep brain stimulation (DBS)

The new standard for surgical treatment is a process called deep brain stimulation. Since the FDA approved DBS in 2002, over 25,000 PWP have had the procedure. In addition, DBS can effectively treat other neurological conditions such as essential tremor and dystonia (See Chapter 4 for more information.) Follow-up studies have shown consistent benefits for up to five years. However given the relatively recent introduction of DBS to PD therapy, the long-term safety and effectiveness of this procedure is still being studied.

According to a 2004 report from the University of Florida Movement Disorders Center, of 174 PWP referred to the center as candidates for DBS, only eight met the criteria that indicated they could benefit from the procedure. Proper screening by a medical team experienced in DBS is essential.

During the DBS procedure, a specially trained surgeon implants a *neurostimulator* (a battery-operated device similar to a pacemaker) to send electrical stimulation to those areas of the brain that control movement. The procedure follows these steps:

1. The surgeon drills a small hole in the skull and then inserts an electrode (called a lead), positioning it in a targeted area of the brain.

2. The surgeon then inserts an implantable neurostimulator (sometimes called a pulse generator or IPG), or battery pack, under the skin in the area of your collarbone.

3. In a procedure that takes place two to four weeks after the implant of the lead, a thin, insulated wire (called the extension) connects the battery pack to the lead.

4. Your neurostimulator is then programmed to send signals appropriate to your individual condition and symptoms. (Several sessions may be necessary to get the programming right for you.)

Advantages of DBS include:

✔ The possibility to tune the device at any time in order to maximize benefits and minimize side effects

✔ A significant reduction in the amount of medication you need

✔ Significant relief from the troublesome side effects (such as dyskinesia) of those medicines

✔ The possibility of reversing the procedure in the future if a new, more promising procedure becomes available

Downsides of DBS include the following:

✔ This is still brain surgery with potentially severe — though rare when DBS experts perform the surgery — complications, including the potential for brain hemorrhage (bleeding).

✔ DBS isn't intended to stop the progression of your PD, although long-term studies are needed to clarify the long-term benefits of DBS.

✔ Two significant factors you must consider are cost and proximity to the center where the procedure is performed.

Find out in advance whether your insurance covers the cost of DBS. Also make plans for making the trips to and from the DBS center for follow-up visits.

Lesion procedures

Procedures such as *pallidotomy* and *thalamotomy* were the earliest surgical procedures to relieve PD symptoms.

- ✔ Pallidotomy destroys (or *lesions*) the *globus pallidus* (a part of the brain that becomes overactive in PD) in an effort to restore movement control.
- ✔ Thalamotomy is a similar surgery aimed at controlling tremor by surgically destroying a selected portion of the brain's thalamus.

Despite some encouraging results in the 1980s and 1990s, doctors recommend these lesion surgeries much less frequently today because benefits tend to regress after five years. In addition, serious side effects (such as difficulty in speaking, poor balance, and cognitive dysfunction) are possible, especially if the surgery is on both sides of the brain. Unlike DBS, these procedures are not reversible and will probably prevent the patient from taking advantage of more effective surgeries in the future.

However, for a small number of patients, this procedure may be more appropriate. Candidates include patients with poor access to programming and continued follow up after DBS, patients with higher risk of infections from a foreign body, and patients that — for one reason or another — can't have a stimulator.

Gamma knife surgery

Gamma knife surgery is an alternative technique for pallidotomies and thalamotomies in PWPs. Not a knife at all, the gamma knife is actually a machine that uses powerful, focused beams of radiation to precisely target the specific area of the brain. The procedure is usually on an outpatient basis, takes under an hour, and uses only local anesthetic. According to a study from Emory University in Atlanta, although lasting benefits in some patients have been reported, gamma knife surgery may have a higher complication rate than has previously been indicated due to delayed onset and under-reporting of changes.

Looking to the future: Surgical possibilities

Scientists are working on improvements to DBS, focusing on such details as a smaller and longer-lasting battery pack or a battery pack in the electrode so everything operates as one unit in the scalp. Another possibility is providing branch leads in the stimulator that network to various parts of the brain that control movements.

Stem cell research: The controversy

Until scientists can prevent the loss of or repair damage to dopamine-producing brain cells, PD will continue to be a chronic and progressive disease. This is where the controversial topic of stem cell research comes into play. Actor Christopher Reeve was an outspoken and tireless advocate for stem cell research, believing it was the only hope for people with brain or spinal injuries. Other spokespeople in favor of stem cell research include former first lady Nancy Reagan for Alzheimer's disease, Mary Tyler Moore for juvenile diabetes, and of course, Michael J. Fox for PD.

The debate is not only scientific but ethical. Scientists have ample evidence that cell transplantation may be the key to curing or preventively treating millions of people suffering from various conditions. In a nutshell, stem cell research focuses on transplanting renewable cells to replace lost or damaged cells due to problems such as chronic and progressive conditions, brain or spinal injuries, and the like. However, as researchers begin using human subjects to test the cell-transplant models already proven in animals, the need for a renewable supply of stem cells from human fetuses creates a heated debate.

Opponents' primary argument is that these cells are part of a viable fetus; therefore taking them is the same as aborting a human life. Further, they argue that scientists have no real evidence that cell transplants will work, especially in diseases like PD, where the root cause is unknown. People in favor of stem cell research argue that stem cell research isn't limited to finding cures; it focuses on the larger arena of understanding, preventing, and treating disease more effectively.

Scott Stern, associate professor of management and strategy at Northwestern University's Kellogg School of Management sums it up this way: "To stop stem cell research now because there are no immediate applications would be like stopping work on transistors in 1947 when their main application was considered as a potential hearing aid."

For more information on the stem cell debate, go to www.parkinsonaction.org or www.michaeljfox.org.

Beyond DBS, researchers hope to prevent, stop, or even reverse the death of dopamine-producing cells through advances in gene therapy and cell regeneration. (See the sidebar in this section, "Stem cell research: The controversy.")

Undergoing Deep Brain Stimulation

Brain surgery is pretty scary, but it certainly places a whole new light on managing PD's symptoms and living a full and functional life for as long as possible. Keep in mind that this surgery is elective — it's *your* call, not the doctor's.

Note: Because DBS has virtually replaced all previous types of surgeries to treat PD, we focus on it in the remaining pages of this chapter.

Asking the right questions before DBS

Regardless of what your doctor tells you, this decision is yours to make. So take time to educate yourself (and your family), and consider this surgery from all points of view.

Before making a decision, take advantage of the following suggestions:

- ✔ Read the literature your doctor offers, and educate yourself fully about the procedure, the benefits, and the risks. Get written information about possible complications and risks. A primary question to ask is, "Can DBS make my PD worse?"

- ✔ Meet with your neurologist and the neurosurgeon. As with any potential surgery, ask questions and expect definitive answers about the risks and worst case scenario. (For example, less than 5 percent of patients will experience serious complications, such as stroke or bleeding, from DBS surgery, but a slightly higher percentage may develop an infection at the implantation sites.)

- ✔ Ask the neurosurgeon what percentage of his total practice are DBS procedures. Also ask whether the surgeon has ever been sued for malpractice related to a DBS procedure and how many procedures he has performed.

- ✔ Ask the neurosurgeon who will follow up with you after the implant. Does he collaborate with an experienced programmer and movement-disorder specialist to manage the settings on your neurostimulator? Is he part of an established DBS program or does he work on his own?

- ✔ Ask your neurologist (or your support-group facilitator) to introduce you to two other patients who have had the procedure — at least one of whom is a few years postsurgery. Talk to those patients about their experiences before, during, and after the surgery.

If you decide to go forward after weighing all the pros and cons of surgery, read on so you and your family know what to expect.

Passing the presurgical tests

Before your procedure can be scheduled, you need to pass several presurgical tests. These tests are fairly standardized and usually include a general medical examination to be sure you're healthy enough to endure the stresses of surgery; neuropsychological testing to be sure you don't have dementia and are emotionally and mentally prepared; brain imaging tests (such as an MRI or CT scan); and the usual blood tests, electrocardiogram, chest X-ray, and such.

Ironing out the details

After successful preliminary testing, the next step is scheduling the procedure. DBS is never an emergency, so the surgery date should be based on the surgeon's schedule and availability but also on your (and your family's) convenience.

Before the doctors get to work on your brain, cover the following two issues:

- ✔ Everyone involved in the surgery and postsurgical care needs to be aware of your medications (for PD and anything else). Be sure a clear plan is in place for managing all your medications (including those for other conditions, such as high blood pressure or diabetes) during post-surgical care and throughout your recovery.

  See the Cheat Sheet inside the front cover for a list of common post-surgery drugs that can be a real problem for PWP in the postsurgical recovery period.

- ✔ Make sure your family knows when and where they can expect to see the doctor following surgery.

Knowing what to expect during and after surgery

Okay, everyone's in place and ready to go. The day of surgery isn't too pleasant, but then surgery's rarely a walk in the park.

For three to six hours, you'll be under local (or possibly no) anesthetic, off your medication, aware of your surroundings and the doctors, and experiencing the full range of your PD symptoms. The good news is that you'll be so integrally involved in the procedure — answering questions from the surgeon and other people as they work — that you'll probably be less aware of the discomfort than you imagine. (Prior to surgery, your doctor can provide printed information and a full description of the procedure).

Because DBS requires precise work, your head will be in a helmet-like contraption that attaches to your skull and the operating table to ensure that your head remains still throughout the procedure. (Sounds like something out of a sci-fi or horror movie, but in most cases, the only complaint is a post-surgery headache.)

The steps necessary to implant the neurostimulator are precise and demanding. Fortunately modern technology has special brain-imaging equipment that permits your surgeon to calculate the precise coordinates of the targeted area deep in the brain. In addition, most centers proceed to *map* your brain activity by recording the electrical activity of different groups of cells encountered during the journey from the surface to the depth of the brain. In fact, every area of the brain has a distinctive electrical *language*, which allows the surgeon to match the initial coordinates with the proper area activity. (Someone has compared this process to a tourist traveling blindfolded through Europe trying to identify his position based on the local language.)

After the lead is in place (see the previous section "Weighing Your Surgical Options" for more about this process), your surgeon may implant the battery and extension wire at the same time or wait up to a week before connecting the system.

Compared to implanting the electrode, connecting the system is child's play:

1. While you're under general anesthesia, your surgeon makes a small incision near your collarbone and inserts the implantable pulse generator (IPG) in a pocket formed under the skin.

2. Next, he runs a small wire from the IPG under the skin up your neck and behind your ear to connect the IPG to the DBS lead in your scalp.

3. Finally, your surgeon closes the incision with stitches or staples.

Hospitalization for DBS surgery is usually two to three days. For more complicated surgeries (when postsurgery confusion, infections, or other complications occur), the stay may be longer. In most cases, however, recovery is a matter of resting for a number of reasons: to get past the emotional and physical exhaustion that can be a part of any surgery; to rest after the possible slight headache (because of the helmet apparatus); and, in some cases, to reduce the mild confusion. Most DBS patients are able to leave the hospital the morning following the procedure.

Most routine postoperative conditions clear up after the first day. The stitches or staples in your scalp will be removed by your doctor a week or so after your discharge. The IPG (battery pack), which is usually implanted two to four weeks later, will be visible as a slight bump in your chest (especially if you're slender), but you don't feel the wires or apparatus as they work.

Programming DBS into Your Life

Surgery of any type takes a lot out of you. There's stress and anxiety from anticipating the procedure, exhaustion from the procedure itself, and suspense and concern about whether it worked, whether it was worth the trouble. This section helps you anticipate your life after your DBS surgery.

Changes you can expect

Following DBS surgery, your neurologist determines the best time to begin reducing your medication. But first, your neurostimulator must be programmed. This process may take one long session (*initial programming session*) and several outpatient visits, because just as you have unique responses to medication, you may have unique responses to the stimulator.

You may not realize the benefits of DBS for weeks or even months, although most people experience some effects the same day the unit is programmed. Tremors and dyskinesias are usually the first symptoms to respond. Be patient as your doctor works with you to balance the settings on your stimulator with your medication regimen.

During this sometimes-exasperating process, you may have some temporary discomfort, such as minor shocks or muscle spasms. These symptoms are related to adjusting and programming the neurostimulator and should be brief. Before you leave the office after a programming/adjustment session, your doctor may want you to wait an hour or so, just to be sure you're okay with the new settings.

Warning signs you need to heed

Although you may experience some discomfort and unusual symptoms as your neurostimulator is programmed, let your doctor know whether you experience any of the following symptoms after implantation or between programming sessions:

- ✔ Shocks or tingling sensations
- ✔ Numbness or spasms, especially in the face or hands
- ✔ Impaired balance or dizziness
- ✔ Slurred speech

 ✔ Blurred or double vision

 ✔ Depression

 ✔ Dykinesia-like movement

As you go about your normal routine, take these precautions:

 ✔ Ask for a hand-check when you go through security while traveling. If the electromagnetic field of the security equipment causes your stimulator to shut down, you can turn it back on with a handheld remote. Not to worry: Airport security personnel are accustomed to travelers who have implants such as a defibrillator or pacemaker.

 ✔ If you play sports, carefully rethink any high-level contact sports like basketball. Repeated direct blows to the implant or connections can cause harm or the need for replacement.

 ✔ At home, try to stay away from microwave ovens (while they're in use) and be aware of the magnetic strip that keeps the refrigerator door shut. Swiping it near your chest may inadvertently turn off your neurostimulator.

 ✔ Check with your neurologist before any doctor orders imaging tests such as an MRI or CT scan for you. The test may be perfectly safe for you, but it doesn't hurt to be sure.

 ✔ Other common warnings are provided in the patient-information manual you receive. Review them in detail with your treating physician or programming nurse.

Chapter 11

Considering Complementary and Alternative Medicine Therapies

....

....

Medication and surgical procedures are only two of the options for treatment of your Parkinson's disease (PD) symptoms. Increasingly the healthcare profession is embracing the benefits of some complementary and alternative medical treatments.

This chapter helps you understand the differences between complementary and alternative therapies so you can sort through the various options and weigh the potential benefits of each. It also helps put you in touch with reputable practitioners if you decide to expand your treatment plan.

Don't underestimate the importance of diet and exercise to your success in managing your PD symptoms. These topics are so vital that they get their own discussion (see Chapter 12). In this chapter, though, we look at therapies you may have heard of but never considered as viable complements or alternatives to the conventional plan you expect your doctor to recommend.

What's in a Name? CAM Therapies Defined

Techniques, medicines, and therapies that take a holistic (mind, body, and spirit) and unconventional approach to the treatment of disease are often called *complementary* or *alternative medicine* (CAM) therapy.

Alternative medicine usually refers to approaches (yoga, T'ai Chi, acupuncture, special herbal remedies, diets, and the like) that aren't standard in Western society but are quite common in Eastern societies.

Complementary therapies, on the other hand, include techniques and approaches (physical, occupational, and speech therapy; modifications to diet; regular exercise, and such) that are more familiar to Western societies.

Alternative treatments often *replace* more conventional treatments, and complementary therapies *augment* conventional methods.

Although alternative and complementary treatments may work in tandem with more traditional medical treatment, they usually haven't passed (or even been required to pass) the rigorous, scientific, evidence-based tests that conventional medicines and treatments must navigate for the Food and Drug Administration's (FDA) approval.

However, in 1998 the National Institutes of Health (NIH) established the National Center for Complementary and Alternative Medicine (NCCAM) because of

✔ The growing popularity of alternative and complementary therapies.

✔ The need for establishing standards for practitioners.

✔ The need for a respected resource for validating information and conducting research on their benefits.

NCCAM focuses on four key areas:

✔ Research

✔ Training and career development for researchers working on projects related to alternative or complementary treatments

✔ Public outreach and education

✔ Integration of CAM treatments with conventional medicine

You can find information about specific therapies on the NCCAM Web site www.nccam.nih.gov or by calling (888) 644-6226.

Before you consider any alternative or complementary therapy, talk with your neurologist and make sure the therapy is from a licensed, certified practitioner. (See the section "Finding the Best Practitioner" later in this chapter for tips on determining the right practitioners.)

The following section explores the major categories of CAM treatments available today.

Debunking the myths about treating PD

PD treatment has a number of urban myths that surface from time to time about what does and doesn't work. Often these falsehoods are from credible sources (such as members of your support group or even articles in respected, usually trustworthy publications). The Internet is another prime source for such rumors. For these reasons, remember to seek and confirm information by asking questions of your doctor or other trusted healthcare professionals (such as your pharmacist). And use only reliable PD information resources, such as those listed in Appendix B.

The following are some of the more prevalent myths floating around:

✔ Levodopa is toxic. (Actually it's been working for PWP for over 40 years.)

✔ Levodopa will stop working after a while. (No, but symptoms may escalate, causing you to need stronger, more frequent dosing.)

✔ You die from PD. (How you're going to die is as much a mystery now as it was before you were diagnosed — could be a car accident, lightening, a heart attack, and so on.)

✔ You're definitely going to be in a wheelchair. (Keep in mind that PD is unique to every person. Your chances of being in a wheelchair are probably higher than some PWPs and far lower than others'.)

✔ You're definitely going to be demented — a vegetable. (PD has no definites. As for being a vegetable? Just focus on eating vegetables and stop predicting the future.)

✔ My children will have PD. (Go back and read Chapter 3 — right now.)

✔ You can't eat proteins while taking levodopa. (Ah, the protein myth — see the section "The protein factor" later in this chapter. Meanwhile, eat your protein.)

✔ Surgery doesn't work for PD. (Right, it may not work for some people, but it does work in combination with prescription medications for many others, and you may be one of them.)

✔ You can cure PD with alternative therapies such as glutathione and nicotinamide adenine dinucleotide, NADH. (We've said it before and we'll say it again — PD doesn't have a cure yet.)

✔ And our personal favorite: You can cure PD with foot massage. (We're not even going to comment on that one.)

As you can see, each myth has a little bit of truth. Remember, somewhere along the way you were told: If something sounds too good to be true, it's probably not true. So when someone tries to sell you the snake-oil-of-a-cure, or a concoction that reverses symptoms, or a plan that halts PD's progression, just walk away. Your best weapons against this web of half-truths? Be informed, keep up with new research, and ask questions.

Introducing Your Options

The concept of any therapy other than traditional medical methods (medications and surgery) may be new to you. And one of the beauties of reading up on these various CAM options before you talk to your doctor about them is that you can do so in the privacy of your own home.

In this section, we introduce you to several of the more prevalent therapies. Before taking any action, though, be sure you discuss with your neurologist the potential of such therapies for helping your PD symptoms. (Then again, maybe your neurologist has suggested one or more of these techniques, and you're reading this section because you [wisely] want to get a better idea of just what you're in for.)

East treats West: Acupuncture and other traditional Chinese medicine

For centuries Western medical experts considered Eastern medical techniques to be experimental at best and quackery at worst. But much of that attitude has changed dramatically in the last decade. Traditional Chinese Medicine (TCM) is founded on the concept of *qi* (or *chi*), when the person's natural flow of energy is in balance. This system includes forms (such as exercise, herbal remedies, acupuncture, and massage) that work with identified energy points in the body.

Perhaps the most familiar TCM is acupuncture. This therapy usually requires a series of appointments by a trained and licensed therapist who inserts sterile needles (about the size of a human hair) into a part of the body believed to affect the area needing treatment. Although acupuncture has not been shown to relieve PD symptoms, it may help persons with Parkinson's (PWP) who experience cramping, stiffness, pain, or sleep disturbances.

In 1997, the NIH noted the increased use of acupuncture by a growing number of physicians and other medical professionals in the United States for relief or prevention of pain.

Ohhh! Ahhh! Experiencing body-based CAM therapies

Treatments that manipulate or move various parts of the body (such as muscles and joints) are considered body-based CAM therapies. Major examples of this category are chiropractic and osteopathic therapy and body massages.

Chiropractic and osteopathic therapy

Chiropractors focus on the structure of the body as it relates to the function, preservation, or restoration of various parts. *Note:* In chiropractic literature you may find some poorly defined theories that relate PD to previous head and neck traumas, which then suggest neck manipulations to treat (and cure!) the disease. Given that these assumptions are criticized even within the chiropractic profession, the role of chiropractic therapy in PD is unknown at this time.

Osteopathic medicine is a more-conventional medical system based on the principle that all the body's systems work together. When one system is affected, then other systems are likely to be affected as well. The hands-on techniques of some osteopaths to manipulate various body parts are considered a CAM therapy.

Massage

Many people associate massages with a ritzy spa or salon. But many medical professionals view regular massage therapy by a trained and certified therapist an important complement to conventional medical care. Massage can help relieve some of the stiffness and muscle contractions common in PD by

✔ Increasing blood supply to the muscles.

✔ Increasing range of motion.

✔ Stretching the muscles for greater flexibility.

The bonus to these physical benefits is the mental payoff: reduced stress and anxiety. You and your care partner may find that regular sessions with a massage therapist are a great way to relieve stress, build a sense of well being and calm, and improve circulation.

Massage is also a good form of relaxation. Under the right circumstances, it offers an environment conducive to meditation and centering. See the next section, "Exploring mind and body options to relieve tension, stress, and anxiety," for more about these benefits. You can also check out *Massage For Dummies* by Steve Capellini and Michel Van Welden (Wiley) for more info.

Therapeutic massage and other CAM therapies may be covered by your insurance if your doctor prescribes them as medically necessary.

Exploring mind and body options to relieve tension, stress, and anxiety

Mind and body therapies rely on the mind's ability to influence physical function and symptoms. They include meditation, creative outlets (as in music, art, or dance), and so on.

Employing relaxation and meditation techniques

Living with a chronic and progressive illness takes a lot out of you. Combine that reality with life's thousand other pressures (like work, relationships, financial security, crime, the weather, and such) and you have a prescription for stress. So when you have PD, finding ways to eliminate tension from your mind and body makes especially good sense.

You can have planned relaxation without going anywhere, hiring anyone, or paying any money. It's a simple matter of finding a quiet place to focus totally on *you* for at least 15 minutes twice a day. At the end of that time, close your eyes, hum a mantra, or sit cross-legged on a pillow — it's totally up to you.

Start by being aware of your *physical* tensions. Slowly and softly breathe in and out as you relax each muscle group one at a time: forehead, neck, shoulders, arms, hands, fingers, torso, hips, thighs, calves, ankles, feet, and finally toes. As you become more aware of your body relaxing, you have a better idea of where you tend to store that stress and tension (for example in the neck and shoulders, the fingers, or perhaps the jaw). Soon you'll be able to consciously relax those areas beyond your planned relaxation sessions.

Another tool is meditation, which you can use when your tension is not only physical but also mental and emotional. It can take many forms; consider the mantra-chanting practice of Zen meditation or the visualization techniques that follow recorded prompts to imagine (visualize) a calm, peaceful setting.

If you've never tried meditation, the Mayo Clinic recommends these tips to help you get started:

- ✔ Select a form of meditation that fits your lifestyle and daily routine and works with your fundamental beliefs.

- ✔ Set aside the time. If 15 minutes twice a day seems too much, start with 5 minutes and work your way up to longer sessions.

- ✔ Forgive your slips. If your mind wanders, recognize it. Then come back to your focus on relaxing and calming your mind, body, and spirit.

- ✔ Experiment until you find the timing and method that works best for you.

In combination with relaxation, meditation can reduce stress for mind and body. But, like all complementary and alternative practices, meditation should supplement — not replace — your doctor's traditional therapies.

Getting in touch with your creative side

Quilting. Woodworking. Gardening. Knitting. Playing an instrument. Dancing — by yourself or in a group. Writing poetry or stories. Journaling. Everyone has a creative side. And, as one sage said, "If something is worth doing, it's worth doing badly." You may not be Picasso or Mozart but you can find pleasure in creating something unique. Who knew that such pleasure could be good therapy as well?

At the 2006 World Parkinson Congress in Washington DC, one of the most popular areas was a wonderful art exhibition by dozens of PWP. To supplement the display, there were delightful performances by musicians, poets, storytellers, and others. Some of the work was good enough to be in a fine gallery or shop, but the real beauty was in the obvious joy and delight of the artist in creating it. To see examples of the exhibit, go to www.pdcreativity.org.

Take these steps to get your creative side in gear:

- ✔ Find a new or return to a former hobby, art, or craft that appeals to you. Establish a regular time to pursue it — an hour every evening or once or twice a week if time is tight.

- ✔ Consider taking lessons at a local art center, community center, or shop. You can enjoy the dual therapy of creativity plus socialization.

Letting those creative juices flow isn't about being good. It's about finding pleasure, escape, and relief from the daily grind of managing your PD symptoms. Just say "Ahhh!"

Staying active via alternative exercise

Postural instability (the loss or impairment of your natural ability to hold yourself upright and maintain balance) can be a major problem for PWP. The greatest danger, of course, is falling. But a close second is the fear of falling that causes you to overcompensate for these off-balance positions, further jeopardizing your stability. One of the benefits of regular physical activity is realizing that alignment, stability, and balance are vital to our overall well being and independence.

For PWP, Eastern exercise programs may be as beneficial, if not more so, than the traditional, strenuous Western types. Eastern exercise therapies tend to be performed slowly and focus on stretching motions that can enhance flexibility. These Eastern methods aren't for everyone, but if you haven't been off the couch and gotten real exercise in a while, you may want to consider this variation.

Check with your doctor before beginning any exercise program — conventional or alternative.

T'ai Chi

This ancient, low-impact Chinese exercise combines measured breathing with slow, dance-like movements that develop flexibility, enhance cardiovascular well being, and improve balance. Although books and instructional visual aids are available, the best way to get started is by working with a trained professional to understand the proper moves and breathing combinations. Check with your local community center, senior center, or health club for classes in your area. *T'ai Chi For Dummies* by Therese Iknoian (Wiley) can provide a solid introduction.

Yoga

Another exercise program that incorporates stretching and balancing exercises in a slow, rhythmic pattern of movement is yoga. Forget the painful-looking, pretzel-like positions you may have seen on television or in movies. Yoga — properly done — combines stretching with breathing and meditation to achieve a greater sense of physical, mental, and spiritual balance.

As with T'ai Chi, yoga classes have levels from beginner to advanced and different styles of teaching. For example, some instructors focus more on the physical movement; others distribute the focus between the physical, breathing, and mind exercises.

If possible, find an instructor who can and will modify the traditional yoga positions and movements to accommodate your limitations. For example, if getting up and down from a mat is difficult, perhaps you can do a modified version of the movements while sitting in a chair. *Yoga For Dummies* by Georg Feuerstein and Larry Payne (Wiley) is a great reference for beginners.

Delving into dietary, protein, enzyme, and vitamin options

Although Chapter 12 has a detailed discussion of diet and exercise, the subject of complementary therapies also involves dietary issues. Because each person plays an active, participatory role in such therapies, this section provides information about CAM diets and diet supplements.

Diet — The usual rules apply

You know the drill. With or without PD, a healthy lifestyle includes a diet rich in fruits and vegetables but low in sugar, fats, and highly processed foods (*white* foods like white bread, white flour, white rice, and such). You also want to avoid foods that have been exposed to pesticides and other toxins. (Stick with organic fruits and vegetables even though they're more expensive — you're worth it!) As we mention in Chapter 2, overexposure to pesticides and herbicides (common in nonorganic farming) may be a contributing factor in the onset of PD. For additional help, consider asking your doctor to recommend a trained nutritionist.

This professional may suggest a diet high in anti-oxidants (green leafy vegetables and the like) because ongoing studies indicate that such a diet may be beneficial for PWPs. Another diet-specific concern is whether you're getting enough calcium (osteoporosis leads to softer bones, which lead to breaks from falls). Finally, studies have shown that the intake of protein in combination with antiparkinsonian meds can be a problem for some PWP. For more on the protein factor, see the next section.

The protein factor

A common PD myth is that protein in a PWP's diet is not good. Although you certainly don't want to remove protein from your diet, your doctor or nutritionist may recommend that you limit protein intake to particular meals and take your anti-PD meds (in particular levodopa/Sinemet) on an empty stomach.

As your PD progresses, you may experience the on-off phenomenon (your meds start to wear off sooner and symptoms reappear more rapidly between doses) that's common among PWP who've taken Sinemet for several years. Some studies indicate that diets rich in protein may negatively affect the brain's ability to absorb Sinemet if meals and dosing aren't properly coordinated. In fact, levodopa is an amino acid (the building block of every protein); a high protein intake at the same time of your medication dose may compete with the absorption of your precious medications. Taking levodopa 30 to 45 minutes before meals can avoid the problem.

CoQ10 and other over-the-counter supplements

CoQ10 (coenzyme Q10) is naturally produced by the body, but it decreases with age and in people with certain chronic conditions such as PD. Available as a dietary supplement, this enzyme may slow the progression of PD for some PWP.

In 2006 the NIH announced plans to enroll recently diagnosed and early-stage PWP in a study to determine whether exceptionally high doses of this over-the-counter (OTC) enzyme may indeed affect the progression of PD. "We're looking for the aspirin of Parkinson's disease," stated Diane Murphy, head of Parkinson's research at NIH. Although some patients already take CoQ10 (with the guidance of their neurologist, we hope), the NIH dosing plan is much higher than the recommended OTC dose.

Also under study are minocycline (an anti-inflammation antibiotic available only by prescription), and creatine, an energy-boosting dietary supplement. The fact that the federal government and medical community continue to sponsor such studies is a clear indication of their willingness to consider the possibility that PD may be better managed with the use of a combination of therapies rather than a single magic bullet.

Vitamin supplements

Taking vitamins that maintain your recommended daily levels is important for PWP. For example, a good multivitamin — one that includes the key B vitamins that are so important for brain and nerve health — is a good choice. Calcium with vitamin D helps prevent osteoporosis, which is a common concern for PWP, and calcium with magnesium can play a role in relieving muscle cramps. After running some standard blood tests, your doctor may make specific recommendations. Be sure to ask your doctor about continuing the vitamins and supplements you used before your diagnosis and about adding new ones.

Several studies have looked at vitamin E as a way to prevent the onset of PD or slow its progression. The most important was the DATATOP study, a ten-year controlled trial that found no benefit in slowing or improving the disease with the use of very high doses of vitamin E. Indeed, a recent report in the American Academy of Neurology's journal stated: "Vitamin E is probably ineffective in the treatment of PD." Moreover a recent analysis of medical literature warned that high-dosage vitamin E supplementation may actually increase mortality. In other words, too much of a good thing may not be a good thing.

On the other hand, scientists have found some protective qualities in the vitamin E in foods such as green leafy veggies, whole grains, and nuts. Mahyar Etminan, a lead researcher for the Centre for Clinical Epidemiology and Evaluation at Vancouver Hospital in Canada cautions that "this is an interesting hypothesis, but it needs to be validated." Of course, eating a diet rich in natural sources of vitamin E is always a good idea for your overall health.

In general, no regimen of vitamins has shown the ability to reduce or control PD symptoms. However, because one theory about the cause of PD (see Chapter 2) involves the oxidation of free radicals, it is possible that antioxidants (like vitamins C and E) may reduce the levels of these free radicals and, therefore, provide some benefit.

Interestingly, a trial that combined vitamin C and E supplements in people with early PD showed a delayed need for drug therapy (L-dopa) by an average of two and a half years. However, more studies are needed to confirm these findings. Similarly, because PWP can be prone to bone loss, your doctor may prescribe (especially for women patients) a calcium supplement or a prescription medication for preserving bone mass. See *Osteoporosis For Dummies* by Carolyn Riester O'Connor and Sharon Perkins (Wiley) for more about this connection.

Finding the Best Practitioner

Keeping in mind that managing PD over the long haul is a team effort, be sure you talk to your neurologist about the potential benefits and pitfalls of alternative or complementary therapies you're considering. Your doctor may take a "no harm, no foul" attitude and not actually support the idea. Or she may suggest specific therapies for you to try or avoid.

Adding CAM therapy to your PD management plan requires you to carefully choose the person who'll administer that therapy. The following tips can help you in that search:

- ✔ If your neurologist endorses the idea, ask for recommendations.
- ✔ Be sure this person has received training from a respected source and passed the exams necessary to earn the appropriate degree or license.
- ✔ Acupuncturists and herbalists specializing in the use of herbs as medicine should be licensed.

Consider adapting the checklist for finding a neurologist (we provide this in Chapter 4) to guide your choice of alternative medicine practitioners.

After you've selected a practitioner, you still have a number of questions. On your first visit, ask:

- ✔ What benefits can I expect from this therapy?
- ✔ What are the risks associated with the treatment?
- ✔ Does it have any special benefits or risks related to my PD?
- ✔ What are the side effects?
- ✔ How many sessions or how long will I need to have the treatment to achieve the expected results?
- ✔ Does this treatment have any conditions that are contraindicated (to be avoided)?
- ✔ What is the cost per session?
- ✔ Will insurance pay?

You're not married to a specific practitioner. If you're uncomfortable with the treatment or the practitioner as the sessions proceed, then stop and talk the problem out. If you aren't satisfied with the response, move on.

Considering Your Approach to Life: It Too Can Help . . . or Hinder

You know the difference between the eternal pessimist (who always expects the worst) and the forever optimist (who's over the top, always anticipating the best). Somewhere in the middle is the realist (as well as a bit of an idealist, philosopher, and activist) who accepts that bad things do indeed happen to good people. This person faces adversity and then looks for ways to get life back on track.

Celebrities like Lance Armstrong, Christopher and Dana Reeve, Michael J. Fox, Muhammad Ali, and others come to mind. But chances are good that you know people within your circle of family, friends, and co-workers who also fit this positive profile. As a PWP, you're going to benefit most from this glass-half-full-and-things-could-be-a-lot-worse philosophy.

Three characteristics that most survivor-types have in common are

- ✔ A *positive* attitude.
- ✔ The ability to laugh even at the unfairness of life.
- ✔ A spiritual core that's as well-tended as their physical or mental health.

The way you approach life — and all its joys and adversities — can play an enormous role in how successfully you live that life. The very fact that you bought this book and are reading it tells us that you're a survivor and a fighter. Our message to you is that we're right here with information and ideas that can help you successfully find ways to live a full and fulfilling life in spite of having PD.

The therapeutic power of positive thinking

Life has no guarantees. But a lot of people live life more fully by rolling with the punches and taking a positive, can-do approach.

So, how do you deal with a diagnosis like PD? How do you face the progressive symptoms and side effects of the medicines? Believe it or not, the one factor that remains in your control throughout this journey is your attitude. You can expect the worst or you can fight back by choosing to live life fully and positively — as if you had never heard that diagnosis.

As a matter of fact, for some people the diagnosis creates this shift in attitude. Discovering that they have PD turns their world upside down, so now they focus more intently on the positives. The realization that life is finite after all can be a real turning point for you — if it comes with the determination to live every day to the fullest. (And if your faith tells you that God doesn't test you more than you can endure, then you can start believing that higher opinion *and* start honing those survival capabilities!)

Laughter — Still the best medicine

Face it: When you laugh, you feel better. Your outlook improves — if only momentarily. You may even feel better physically. Consider the angry, depressed man who had just gone through brain surgery. He told his wife he didn't want any visitors. But when she ran into several close friends at the elevator and told them, "Not today," the friends still insisted. "We'll only stay a moment," they promised. Within moments the woman heard the welcome sound of laughter — her husband's. As the visit went on and the friends worked their magic, that laughter couldn't be repressed.

Open up to life — Physically, mentally, and spiritually

When you face a chronic and progressive illness day after day, you understandably have times when you just want to burrow under the covers and hope it all goes away. Resist that temptation!

Because we address your physical and mental well being throughout this book, this section looks at one other dimension, your spiritual needs, and how meeting those needs can enhance your life.

Spirituality is that core inside you where your sense of well being and survival reside. For some people, organized rituals of religion can be a part of this core, but rituals can't be all of it; for other people, rituals and religion play no part at all.

Your spiritual core is also where you store your self-identity. Your body may shake and twist and your mind may play tricks with your memory and concentration, but your spirit is still there. A relative of a PWP who was in the later stages said it well: "I just believe that he's still in there somewhere, that his spirit is still aware and fighting to let us know."

Like your PD, spirituality is different for every individual. But one way to begin focusing on your spiritual well-being is by using your senses to their full effect. Consider the following suggestions:

- ✔ Listen — to a sermon, an inspirational reading, a concert, water flowing, wind in the trees, rain on the roof, your innermost hopes and dreams

- ✔ Look — at the people who surround you, love you, and care for you

- ✔ Touch — by taking a friend's hand; petting a dog or cat; hugging a loved one; stroking a leaf, a rock, a child's hair

- ✔ Smell — freshly cut grass, an autumn fire, cookies straight from the oven

- ✔ Taste — the bitter as well as the sweet

- ✔ Savor — the unique tastes, sounds, sights, scents, and feelings that form the wonders of your life

Tapping into your spiritual side takes the same focused effort as your physical and mental needs. And your willingness to push yourself on all three levels can pay off in ways you never thought possible.

Chapter 12

The Key Roles of Diet and Exercise

*Y*ou've heard it since you were a child — *eat right and exercise!* But, for people with Parkinson's (PWP) and their care partners, the importance of proper diet and a regular program of exercise can't be overemphasized. The benefits go well beyond physical fitness to bring relief from the general stresses of living with a chronic, progressive disease. In addition, a good diet and regular exercise help fight off the anxiety and depression that can accompany Parkinson's disease (PD). With or without PD, you owe it to yourself to be as fit — physically, mentally and spiritually — as possible. How else are you going to participate fully in life?

In this chapter we show you that good health isn't about training for a marathon or depriving yourself of foods you love. It's about making the choices that give you the best chance of living well and pursuing the pleasures of your life for many years — in spite of PD.

The Joy of Good Food — Diet and Nutrition

According to the National Institute of Aging, the combined effects of not making the right food choices and not being physically active make up the second largest underlying cause of death (behind smoking) in the United States. Often the element most absent from the diets of Americans is *nutrition*, foods that provide the proteins, carbohydrates, vitamins, minerals, hydration, fiber, and — yes — fats that the body needs to operate at its best. Add to that fact that PD medications and symptoms can significantly reduce the pleasures of eating, and you have a situation ripe for disaster.

This section isn't about losing that extra twenty pounds; it's about making the best food and nutrition choices to maintain optimal health as you fight the progression of PD.

Balance is the key

As a PWP, you have to perform a real balancing act when it comes to your diet. Along with the ready-made factors that impact nutrition and diet (like age, gender, and physical fitness), you have to deal with the nutritional sideshows of PD. For example, side effects of medications may include loss of appetite or even nausea. As your PD progresses, swallowing and constipation can become issues. And you may have side effects from medications for other chronic conditions, such as high blood pressure, diabetes, or arthritis.

Finding the proper balance between a healthy diet and these PD issues may require the help of a professional, so your neurologist may prescribe a consultation with a nutritionist or dietician as part of your treatment plan. If not, go ahead and ask him for a referral.

Keep in mind that timing the dosing of your medication (see Chapter 9) with meals is very important, especially for meals that include significant servings of protein. Protein — although essential for a balanced diet — can compete with the absorption of your antiparkinsonian meds. The usual recommendation is to take medication at least 30 minutes before meals unless you experience nausea or *dyskinesia* (uncontrolled twisting writhing motions) after taking your medications. If nausea is the problem, your doctor may recommend you take a low-protein snack, such as juice or saltines, with your meds. If dykinesia occurs, slowing the absorption by taking your anti-PD meds at mealtime may be exactly what you need. Be sure you and your doctor discuss the timing of meals and medications to offset this problem.

Banishing the bad and embracing the good-for-you foods

No doubt you've seen the food pyramid — which is now a bar grid — recommended by the U.S. Department of Agriculture. (See www.mypyramid.gov.) And you probably know you should hold your intake of fats and oils (not to mention desserts) to a minimum and spend most of your calories on fruits, veggies, whole grains, and dairy. (By the way, a banana split does not count in your fruit and dairy allowance!)

But this is your life, and presumably you're prepared to fight this PD that's parked like a tank in your designated space. A nutritionist or dietician can be a real help, showing you how to adapt your needs to your lifestyle. You tell her how you normally eat — on the run, in your car, at home standing at the kitchen counter, or seated with the family at the table, in fine restaurants, or fast-food joints. You reveal your food weaknesses — hate veggies, love bread, and such. Then the professional works with you to build a food plan that fits your lifestyle and your likes and dislikes.

Focus on these key issues when you start rearranging your pyramid:

- ✔ **Water, water, water!** Flavor it with a slice of lemon or a little fruit juice if you can't take it straight, but six to eight big glasses every day. (And, no, soda, coffee, and tea don't count.) Caffeine beverages may increase *diuresis* (your amount of urine output) and, as a result, cancel your efforts to hydrate your body. *Note:* Some studies have shown that caffeine may reduce the risk of PD for some people, so caffeine in moderation probably won't hurt — and may help.

- ✔ **Fiber** (whole-grain breads — not the mushy white stuff — brown rice, and whole-wheat pasta). In fact, stay away from white foods in general. Green leafy vegetables, whole grains, and nuts are rich natural sources of vitamin E that may have a protective effect against PD (see Chapter 11).

   Whole grain breads must be refrigerated, but white bread isn't. (White bread is so devoid of actual nutrients that even bacteria won't eat it. That's a pretty good clue.)

- ✔ **Bone-strengthening nutrients (calcium, magnesium, and vitamins D and K).** Think dairy products and, believe it or not, exposure to sunlight (a vitamin D source). Also, regular exercise (we discuss this later) can help you keep bones strong, maintain balance, and prevent the falls so devastating for PWP.

Although your doctor may recommend adding supplements (such as a daily multivitamin, iron, or calcium pill) to your regular diet, the key word here is *supplement*. Such products are no substitute for a nutritionally balanced diet.

But good-for-you foods can actually be more delicious and easy to prepare than you imagined. One example is the fabulous fruit smoothie: Throw berries, half a banana, a cup of fat-free yogurt, and some ice cubes in a blender. Add a teaspoon of ground flax seed for fiber, turn the blender on high, pour the milkshake-like concoction into your car mug, and you're good to go (Smoothies are also great for preventing the constipation associated with PD medications.)

Food as celebration

If, like millions of Americans, you've fallen into a rut with the when, what, and where you eat, think about spicing those meals up. The following is our list of ideas for making meals more of a celebration than an afterthought:

✔ Choose your setting to match the menu, the mood, and the season — dining room, kitchen table, inside, outside; at home or at a sidewalk café.

✔ Set the table, even if it's just for one.

✔ Think *S.H.E.* when cooking at home — simple, healthy, and engaging.

✔ Try adding special (non-salt) seasonings and flavorings to spice up your food and make it more enjoyable.

✔ Be adventurous and try new dishes you've never tasted when eating out.

Request a soup spoon when ordering items like rice or small veggies (peas, corn, and such). A large spoon makes these foods easier to manage if you have a tremor.

✔ Savor food with all your senses — the vision of healthy food presented well; the smells, tastes, and textures; even the sounds of laughter and conversation interspersed with clinking dishes and glasses.

Food is life — and as a PWP, you understand the importance of celebrating every moment.

Use It or Lose It — The Healing Power of Exercise and Activity

Plenty of research backs up the fact that regular exercise can do wonders for your health. Consider that

✔ Exercising regularly boosts the power of neurotransmittors in your brain to enhance your mood and your ability to see life in a more positive light.

✔ Exercise can relieve the muscle tension from your body's natural instinct to lock up in the face of challenges or battles.

✔ Exercise can enhance your self-image, which can lead to greater self-assurance and confidence, which can lead to a greater ability to deal with life's stresses.

Talk about a win-win!

In addition, PWP who exercise regularly seem to experience a milder and less-progressive disease process. In fact, exercise may be as good for brain function as it is for heart and weight factors. Recent laboratory experiments on animals have shown that physical exercise can potentially reduce the rate at which brain cells die. Further studies are under way to see whether regular exercise can actually slow the progression of PD.

Many exercise programs can benefit PWP. The Performance Centers of Wheaton Franciscan Healthcare in Milwaukee, Wisconsin designed the following exercises specifically to stretch and strengthen the key muscle groups for optimal flexibility and balance. Your doctor and physical therapist may fine-tune these exercises to match your specific needs, but this chapter gives you a good starting point. Begin the routine with the stretching exercises and repeat them during the cool-down period after the strengthening exercises.

The principles of a stretching/flexibility exercise program for PD are the same as those for sports-medicine rehabilitation:

- ✔ Listen to your body.
- ✔ Avoid joint pain during exercise.
- ✔ Forget the Vince Lombardi adage: No pain, no gain.
- ✔ Remember, for joint or other pain after exercise, "Ice is nice; hot is not."

Because PD frequently develops in a person's later years, other bone and joint conditions may already be present such as *osteoarthritis* (wearing of joints) and *osteoporsis* (thinning of the bones). So before you begin any exercise therapy, get the approval of your doctor and a prescription to work with a trained, experienced physical therapist.

A stretching program to enhance flexibility

The following exercises are designed to enhance your flexibility. With your doctor or physical therapist's initial guidance and ongoing monitoring, do the exercises every day, even twice a day.

If you also do strengthening exercises (such as the ones in the "A strengthening program to build muscle and stabilize joints" section later) or an aerobic activity, such as walking, bicycling, swimming, or working out on a treadmill, use these stretching exercises to warm up and cool down.

Stretching should be slow, smooth, and gentle. No bouncing allowed! And if it starts to hurt, listen to your body and ease up.

Neck stretches

Begin your routine by gently stretching the muscles in your neck, head, and shoulders.

The Chin Tuck

To perform the Chin Tuck:

1. **Looking forward, tuck your chin by pulling it in — a little like a turtle (see Figure 12-1).**

2. **Hold your chin in the tucked position for five seconds.**

3. **Untuck your chin and relax.**

Repeat this exercise five to ten times.

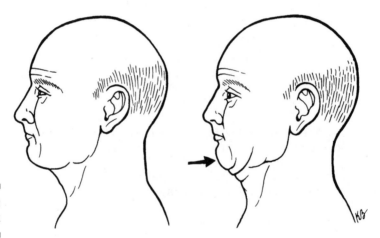

Figure 12-1:
Chin Tuck

The Head Turn

To perform the Head Turn:

1. **Looking straight ahead, slowly turn your head to the right until you're looking at the wall or view to your right (see Figure 12-2).**

   Don't force the movement; at first you may only be able to turn your head slightly to the right or left; with practice you'll become more flexible.

2. **Hold the position for five seconds and return to center.**

3. **Repeat Steps 1 and 2, this time turning to your left.**

Repeat this exercise five to ten times on each side.

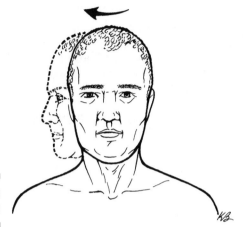

Figure 12-2:
Head Turn

The Head Tilt

To perform the Head Tilt:

1. **Looking straight ahead, bend your head to the right as if to rest your head on your right shoulder (see Figure 12-3).**

   Don't raise your shoulder — let the stretch of your neck do the work.

2. **Hold the position for five seconds, and raise your head back to straight ahead position.**

3. **Repeat Steps 1 and 2, this time bending to your left side.**

Repeat this exercise five to ten times on each side.

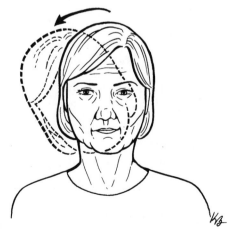

Figure 12-3:
Head Tilt

The Shoulder Roll

To perform the Shoulder Roll:

1. **Standing tall and looking straight ahead, lift and roll both shoulders back in a circular motion five times (see Figure 12-4).**

2. **Relax.**

3. **Lift and roll shoulders forward in a circular motion five times.**

4. **Relax.**

Repeat the backward and forward rolls five to ten times each.

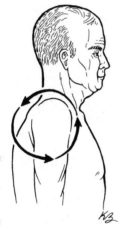

Figure 12-4:
Shoulder
Roll

The Chest and Shoulder Stretch

To perform the Chest and Shoulder Stretch:

1. **Standing tall and looking straight ahead with arms at your sides, pull your shoulder blades together (see Figure 12-5).**

2. **Hold for five seconds, and then relax.**

Repeat this exercise five to ten times.

Upper body stretches

Use the following stretches before and after your regular exercise routine to lengthen your muscles and prevent muscle pulls and tears.

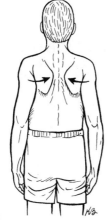

Figure 12-5:
Chest and
Shoulder
Stretch

The Posterior Shoulder Stretch

To perform the Posterior Shoulder Stretch:

1. **Reach your right arm across your chest, and place your right hand over your left shoulder (see Figure 12-6).**

2. **With your left hand, grasp your right elbow and apply light pressure to the elbow, moving your right arm closer to your chest.**

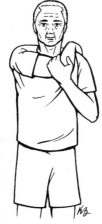

Figure 12-6:
Posterior
Shoulder
Stretch

3. **Hold for five seconds, and return your arms to your sides.**

4. **Repeat Steps 1 through 3, this time stretching your left shoulder.**

Repeat this exercise five to ten times on each side.

The Anterior Shoulder Stretch

To perform the Anterior Shoulder Stretch:

1. **Reach behind your back and clasp your hands, interlocking your fingers and keeping your arms straight, with elbows turned in (see Figure 12-7).**

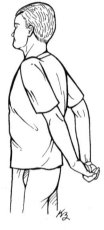

Figure 12-7:
Anterior
Shoulder
Stretch

2. **Lift up your arms until you feel a stretch (not pain) in your shoulders and across your chest.**

3. **Hold your arms in the elevated position for five seconds.**

4. **Lower your hands, and relax.**

Repeat this exercise five to ten times.

The Posterior Shoulder Side Stretch

To perform the Posterior Shoulder Side Stretch:

1. **Raise your right arm above and behind your head, reaching toward your left shoulder (see Figure 12-8).**

2. **With your left hand, reach behind your head and pull your right elbow gently in toward your head.**

3. **Hold for five seconds and relax, returning your arms to your sides.**

4. **Repeat Steps 1 through 3, this time stretching your left side.**

Repeat this exercise five to ten times on each side.

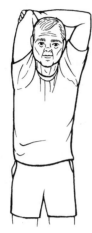

Figure 12-8:
Posterior
Shoulder
Side Stretch

The Wrist/Forearm Stretch

To perform the Wrist/Forearm Stretch:

1. **Extend your right arm straight in front of you, fingers pointing toward the floor.**

2. **With your left hand, gently pull your fingers and hand down (see Figure 12-9a).**

   Your arm should remain extended.

3. **Hold for five seconds, and then release your fingers.**

4. **Repeat Steps 2 and 3 five to ten times.**

5. **Flex your right wrist back so your fingers point to the ceiling.**

6. **With your left hand, gently press your fingers and palm back toward your forearm (see Figure 12-9b).**

7. **Hold for five seconds, and then release your fingers.**

8. **Repeat Steps 1 through 7, this time extending your left arm and stretching your left wrist and forearm.**

Repeat this exercise five to ten times on each side.

Leg stretches

These stretches work on the hips, legs, knees, and ankles. As with any stretch exercise, they're good before and after your strengthening or aerobic routine to prevent muscle-strain tears and pulls.

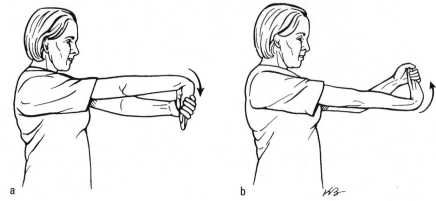

Figure 12-9:
Wrist/
Forearm
Stretch

The Hamstring Stretch

To perform the Hamstring Stretch:

1. **Sitting on the floor with your right leg straight out in front of you, bend your left leg so the bottom of your left foot rests on the inner thigh of your extended right leg (see Figure 12-10).**

2. **With your hands on your outstretched calf or ankle, slowly bend forward from the waist, keeping your back straight.**

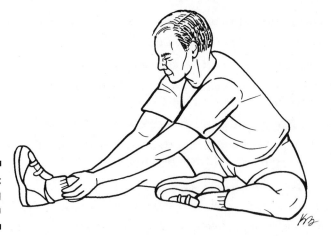

Figure 12-10:
Hamstring
Stretch

   Don't bounce. Stretch only until you feel a mild (non-painful) stretching sensation in the back of your thigh.

3. **Hold the stretch for five seconds, and then relax, releasing your calf or ankle and returning to the upright position.**

4. **Repeat Steps 1 through 3 five to ten times with your right leg.**

5. **Repeat Steps 1 through 4, this time extending your left leg and tucking your right leg.**

Do five sets of five to ten repetitions each per side.

The Quadriceps Stretch

To perform the Quadriceps Stretch:

1. **Standing beside a table, place your left hand on the table for balance.**

2. **Bending your right knee, grasp your ankle with your right hand and pull your foot backward toward your buttocks (see Figure 12-11).**

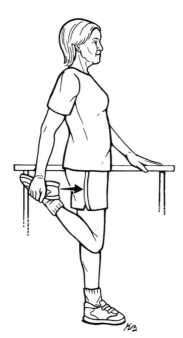

Figure 12-11:
Quadriceps
Stretch

You can also place a belt around your ankle and grasp it.

Don't lean forward. Feel the stretch in the front of your thigh.

3. **Hold the stretch for five seconds and then relax, returning your right foot to the floor.**

4. **Repeat Steps 1 through 3 five to ten times.**

5. **Turn around (or move to the opposite side of the table) and repeat Steps 1 through 3, this time bending your left knee.**

Do five sets of five to ten repetitions per side.

The Standing Gastroc Stretch

To perform the Standing Gastroc Stretch:

1. **Standing about 2 feet from the wall, lean forward so flattened palms are against the wall.**

2. **Keeping your left foot planted, bend your left knee as you step backward with your right leg; lean forward into the wall until you feel a stretch in your right calf (see Figure 12-12).**

   Your right leg should remain straight, with your heel on the floor and your toes turned slightly outward.

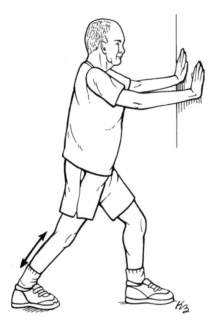

Figure 12-12:
Standing
Gastroc
Stretch

3. **Hold for five seconds and then relax, bringing your feet together.**

4. **Repeat Steps 1 through 3 five to ten times.**

5. **Repeat Steps 1 through 4, this time bending your right knee and stepping backward with your left leg.**

Repeat this exercise five to ten times on each side.

The Inner Thigh (Groin) Stretch

To perform the Inner Thigh (Groin) Stretch:

1. **Sitting on the floor, bend your knees so the soles of your feet face each other (see Figure 12-13).**

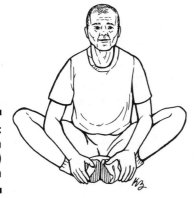

Figure 12-13:
Inner Thigh
(Groin)
Stretch

2. **Cup your hands around your toes, and gently press down on your thighs with your forearms until you feel a gentle stretch in your inner thighs.**

   Don't bounce your knees — stretch only until you feel a slight pulling sensation in your inner thigh.

3. **Hold for five seconds, and then relax.**

Repeat this exercise five to ten times.

Lower back stretches

The following stretches can protect your back from injury and help you maintain flexibility.

Knees to Chest

To perform the Knees to Chest Stretch:

1. **Lying on your back, slowly raise your right knee to your chest (see Figure 12-14).**

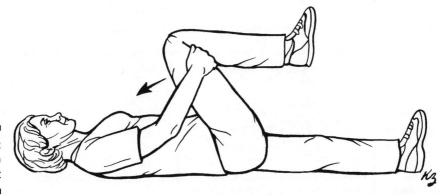

Figure 12-14:
Knees to
Chest

2. **Use your hands to hold your knee to your chest; you should feel the stretch in your lower back.**

3. **Hold this position for five seconds and then relax, returning your right leg to the floor.**

4. **Repeat Steps 1 through 3 five to ten times.**

5. **Repeat Steps 1 through 4, this time bringing your left knee to your chest.**

Repeat this exercise five to ten times on each side.

Bridging

To perform the Bridging Stretch:

1. **Lying on your back with your arms at your sides, bend your knees so your feet are flat on the floor (see Figure 12-15).**

2. **Tightening your stomach muscles, slowly raise your buttocks until even with your knees.**

3. **Hold this position for five seconds and then relax, lowering your buttocks to the floor.**

Repeat this exercise five to ten times.

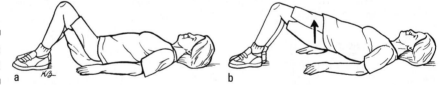

Figure 12-15: Bridging

a   b

Alternate Arm and Leg Lifts

To perform the Alternate Arm and Leg Lifts Stretch:

1. **Lying on your stomach, extend your arms over your head.**

2. **Tightening your stomach muscles, simultaneously raise your *right* arm and your *left* leg 3 to 6 inches off the floor (see Figure 12-16).**

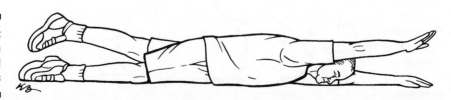

Figure 12-16: Alternate Arm and Leg Lifts

Keep both arms and both legs straight.

3. **Hold this position for five seconds and then relax, returning both limbs to the floor.**

4. **Repeat Steps 1 through 3 five to ten times.**

5. **Repeat Steps 1 through 4, this time raising your *left* arm and *right* leg.**

Repeat this exercise five to ten times on each side.

Standing Extension

To perform the Standing Extension Stretch:

1. **With both hands on your lower back, bend as far back as is comfortable (see Figure 12-17).**

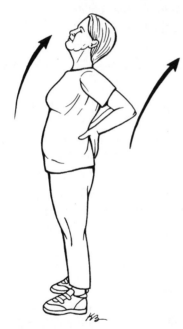

Figure 12-17:
Standing
Extension

2. **Hold this position for five seconds and then relax, straightening to the upright position.**

Repeat this exercise five to ten times.

A strengthening program to build muscle and stabilize joints

Although stretching is key to maintaining flexibility, don't ignore the benefits of strengthening your muscles — especially the muscles you need for maintaining balance and postural stability. You can perform the following shoulder and leg exercises three to five times a week to help maintain strength in these key areas.

Shoulder strengthening

The following exercises strengthen the shoulder area, especially the rotator cuff muscles (where your shoulder and arm connect). Your physical therapist can provide the stretchy exercise bands as well as help you adjust the tension and size to your needs. Or you can purchase a five-foot length of rubber tubing at a hardware store or athletic supply shop (they call it a *sports cord*). For some of the exercises, you also need a large bath towel to stabilize your arm.

Internal Rotation

To perform the Internal Rotation Exercise:

1. **Attach a band to a doorknob that's even with your elbow, and be sure the door is solidly shut.**

2. **Standing three feet from the door with your right side toward the door, grasp the band with your right hand, bending your arm at the elbow.**

3. **Place a rolled towel under your right arm, between your arm and right side of your body to stabilize your arm (see Figure 12-18a).**

4. **Pull the band slowly across your body, rotating your arm and shoulder inward (see Figure 12-18b).**

5. **Slowly return your arm to its start position.**

6. **Repeat Steps 1 through 5 five to ten times.**

7. **Turn around so your left side is toward the door (move the towel under your left arm), and repeat Steps 1 through 5, this time extending your left arm.**

Repeat this exercise five to ten times.

External Rotation

To perform the External Rotation Exercise:

1. **Wrap the ends of a sports band around each hand.**

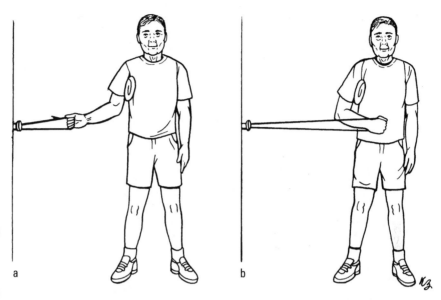

Figure 12-18:
Internal
Rotation
a   b

2. **Place a rolled towel under your right arm (between your arm and chest to stabilize your arm), and place your left hand on your left hip, keeping your right hand close by (see Figure 12-19a).**

3. **With your right hand, slowly pull the band across your body, rotating your arm and shoulder outward (see Figure 12-19b).**

4. **Slowly return your arm to its start position.**

5. **Repeat Steps 1 through 4 five to ten times.**

6. **Repeat Steps 1 through 5, this time extending your left arm. (Don't forget to place the towel under your left arm.)**

Repeat this exercise five to ten times.

Extension Pull

To perform the Extension Pull Exercise:

1. **Attach a band to a doorknob that's even with your elbow, and be sure the door is solidly shut.**

2. **Stand facing the door (about 3 feet from the door) with the band in your right hand (see Figure 12-20a).**

3. **Starting with your arm straight and forward, pull the band back by slowly lowering your straightened arm until it's at your side (see Figure 12-20b).**

4. **Slowly return your arm to its start position.**

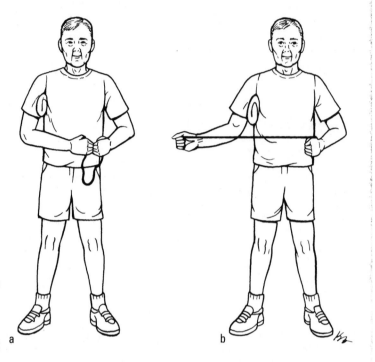

Figure 12-19:
External
Rotation

a   b

5. **Repeat Steps 1 through 4 five to ten times.**

6. **Repeat Steps 1 through 5, this time extending your left arm.**

Repeat this exercise five to ten times.

Flexion

To perform the Flexion Exercise:

1. **Place one end of an exercise band under your right foot and hold the other end in your right hand (see Figure 12-21a).**

2. **With your thumb on top of the band and your elbow straight, raise your right arm forward until it's level with your shoulder (see Figure 12-21b).**

3. **Slowly return your right arm to its start position.**

4. **Repeat Steps 1 through 3 ten times.**

5. **Repeat Steps 1 through 4, this time extending your left arm.**

Repeat this exercise five to ten times.

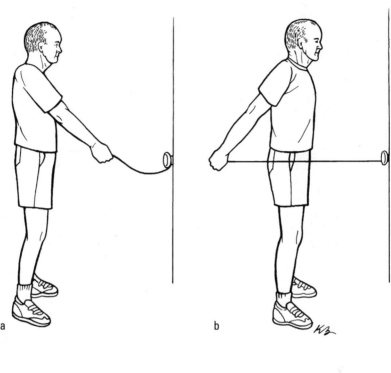

Figure 12-20:
Extension
Pull

a

b

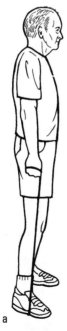
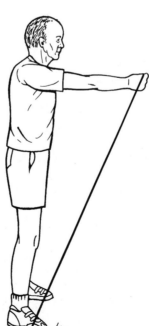

Figure 12-21:
Flexion

a

b

Horizontal Pull

To perform the Horizontal Pull Exercise:

1. **Hold the band with both hands at shoulder height (see Figure 12-22a).**

2. **With your hands close together, extend your arms out in front of you and slowly stretch the band out until your arms are wide open (see Figure 12-22b).**

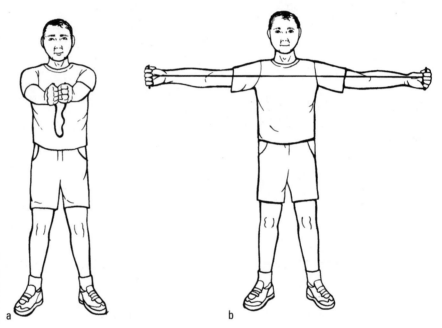

Figure 12-22:
Horizontal
Pull

a   b

3. **Slowly bring your arms back together.**

Repeat this exercise five to ten times.

Leg strengthening

Your muscles are the stabilizers for your joints. Exercises that stretch and strengthen the muscles surrounding your hips, knees, and ankles can prevent injury and possibly improve balance. Perform the following exercises at least three times a week.

Straight Leg Raise

To perform the Straight Leg Raise Exercise:

1. **Lying on your back, prop yourself up on your forearms, and slightly bend your left knee; keep your left foot flat on the floor.**

2. **Tightening your right leg's front thigh muscle, raise your right leg 8 to 10 inches from the floor (see Figure 12-23).**

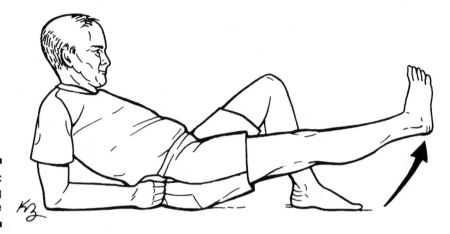

Figure 12-23:
Straight Leg
Raise

Keep the extended leg straight and knee locked as you perform the exercise.

3. **Slowly return your right leg to the start position.**

4. **Repeat Steps 1 through 3 five to ten times.**

5. **Repeat Steps 1 through 4, this time bending your right leg and raising your left leg.**

Repeat this exercise five to ten times.

Hip Abduction

To perform the Hip Abduction Exercise:

1. **Lie on your left side with both legs straight.**

2. **Slowly lift your right leg toward the ceiling to a comfortable height (at least 5 to 10 inches), keeping both legs straight (see Figure 12-24).**

3. **Slowly lower your right leg.**

4. **Repeat Steps 1 through 3 ten times.**

5. **Turn to your right side and repeat Steps 1 through 4, this time lifting your left leg.**

Repeat this exercise five to ten times.

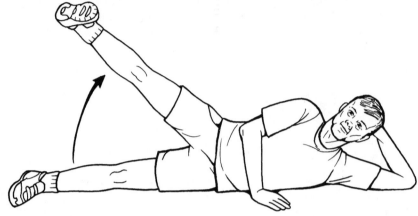

Figure 12-24:
Hip
Abduction

Hip Adduction

To perform the Hip Adduction Exercise:

1. **Lying on your right side with your right leg straight, bend your left leg at the knee so your left foot is flat on the floor in front of your right thigh or knee.**

2. **Keeping your right leg straight, raise your right leg off the ground 5 to 10 inches (see Figure 12-25).**

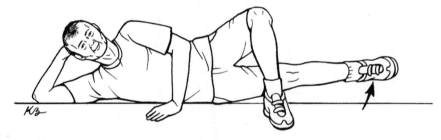

Figure 12-25:
Hip
Adduction

3. **Slowly lower your right leg to its start position.**

4. **Repeat Steps 1 through 3 five to ten times.**

5. **Turn to your left side and repeat Steps 1 through 4, this time lifting your left leg.**

Repeat this exercise five to ten times.

Hip Extension

To perform the Hip Extension Exercise:

1. **Lie on your stomach with both arms bent and under your chest.**

2. **With legs straight, and knees locked, tighten the muscle in your right thigh and lift your right leg 8 to 10 inches off the ground (see Figure 12-26).**

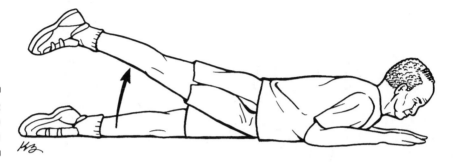

Figure 12-26:
Hip
Extension

3. **Slowly lower your leg back to the ground.**

4. **Repeat Steps 1 and 2, this time lifting your left leg.**

Repeat this exercise five to ten times.

Wall Slide

To perform the Wall Slide Exercise:

1. **Standing 12 to 16 inches from the wall and facing away from the wall with your feet shoulder-width apart, lean back against the wall.**

2. **Slowly lower your buttocks toward the floor as far as you can, but no more than your thighs being parallel to the floor (see Figure 12-27).**

3. **Hold this position for five to ten seconds.**

4. **Tighten your thigh muscles and slide back up to a standing/leaning position.**

Repeat this exercise five to ten times.

Toe Raise

To perform the Toe Raise Exercise:

1. **Stand with both feet flat on the floor.**

2. **Lift your heels and rise up on your toes (see Figure 12-28).**

3. **Hold this position for five seconds.**

4. **Lower your heels back to the floor.**

Repeat this exercise five to ten times.

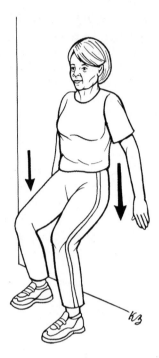

Figure 12-27:
Wall Slide

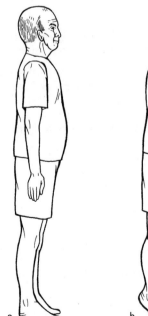

Figure 12-28:
Toe Raise

a   b

Other exercise programs that can help

After you've mastered the stretches and exercises in the preceding sections, you may be ready for a program that's more challenging and yet specifically structured for PWP. Many national PD organizations consider regular exercise so essential that they've created a variety of programs and tools to help you get started. Some of these aids are listed below. For more options in programs and equipment, be sure to check out Chapter 23.

Two programs available through the Parkinson's Disease Foundation (PDF) are:

- ✔ *Motivating Moves for People with Parkinson's*: In this program developed by movement specialist Janet Hamburg, participants sit while doing the exercises. The program is available in either VHS or DVD format.
- ✔ *The Exercise Program*: This tool by Dr. E. Richard Blonsky and a team of physical therapists specializing in rehabilitation therapy comes with audio instruction tapes and a binder with illustrated exercise cards.

Call 1-800-457-6676 for more information on either program.

The American Parkinson Disease Association (APDA) has free booklets entitled *Aquatic Exercises for Parkinson's Disease* and *Be Active: A Suggested Exercise Program for People with Parkinson's Disease*. For information, call 1-800-223-2732 or look online at www.apdaparkinson.org.

Structured exercise is important in maintaining flexibility and physical function, but equally important is maintaining an active lifestyle. Read on for ways that you can use daily physical activity to enhance your well being.

Beyond a Structured Exercise Program — PD and Physical Activity

Finding ways to redefine ourselves — especially following life-changing events such as career changes, retirement, the end of a relationship, or a diagnosis of PD — is not new to most adults. But when circumstances change the way we define our satisfaction and happiness, we either adapt or choose a less-than-satisfactory mindset, which may include depression and self-pity. Far better to work at rediscovering our identity with new resources for pleasure and purpose.

The saying "Quality trumps quantity in life" may not resonate for everyone. But if you have a PD diagnosis, then you have a choice: Bury your head in the sand or get out there and live each day to the fullest.

Enjoying recreation

Physical activity, or recreation (see how that word is really *re-creation*?), differs from exercise because recreation usually provides an element of immediate pleasure, accomplishment, or revitalization that structured exercise may not. For example, if you garden, think about the pleasure of seeing the results of your hard work. In a similar way, biking and canoeing allow us to be physically active while taking in the fresh air and scenery.

But recreation goes beyond simple physical endeavors; it includes contact with other people and opening ourselves to new experiences and information. When we were kids, we called it *playing*. But adults can still play, even when they're facing grown-up stuff like PD.

Keeping up with routine roles and activities

Chances are good that you played multiple roles before getting the diagnosis of PD. Take a moment to list them: son/daughter, spouse/lover, friend/companion, parent/grandparent, employee/employer/co-worker, community leader/volunteer. How about the roles you played at home? Cook, gardener, decorator, financial manager, handyman/woman.

Ask yourself whether you think some of these roles are no longer possible. For example, do you think you can't keep up with your current job (see Chapter 16) or do you withdraw from social functions because you don't want pity from friends and family (see Chapter 15)? Maybe you don't cook anymore because the tremors make a mess. Or maybe you're afraid of making a mistake in the checkbook, so you've handed over the finances to your significant other.

Now take a good look at Chapters 2 and 3 to see whether you find a cause or symptom of PD that says you have to start peeling away pieces of your life and abandoning vital relationships. We'll wait. . . .Did you see it? Ah hah! We knew you wouldn't!

This is a good time for you to re-evaluate those activities you may have assumed were no longer possible — employment, volunteer work, and social activities, such as card playing, sports, and the like. The harder you work to maintain your normal routine and activities, the less likely your PD will dominate your life.

True, you may need to make some adjustments in physical activities to accommodate your PD. For example, you may find that sports requiring more lateral (side-to-side) movement, such as golf and ping pong, are easier for you. Or, if you were a marathon runner, think about race-walking or just plain walking. One PWP, Parky, biked over 42,000 miles in a ten-year period by switching to a recumbent three-wheel trike. (See www.inevergiveup.org. for more about his story.) His motto: "Let's take the PARK out of Parkinson's."

The point is that you do have choices and you can take charge instead of allowing assumptions to dictate your routine. Work with your doctor and other members of your professional health team to determine the right physical activities for you.

The same advice for physical activities applies to activities that engage you mentally and spiritually. This next section suggests ways to incorporate mental and spiritual activity into your daily life.

Exercises for the Mind and Spirit

Okay, you're exercising regularly and maintaining an active and productive lifestyle. Caring for the physical body is huge for you and for those people who make this journey with you. But be sure you give attention to the mind and spirit. What's happening inside your head? For that matter, what's going on with your care partner — that person (or persons) who's been with you from the moment you were diagnosed with PD?

In fact, many PWP develop apathy, a condition defined by

- Reduced interest and participation in routine activities
- Lack of initiative
- Difficulties in starting or sustaining an activity
- Lack of concern for events and people around them

In other words, the mind and spirit seem to simply give up.

Apathy in PD is more likely a direct consequence of *physiological* changes in the brain than a *psychological* reaction to the disability. As a result, this condition is different from the other psychiatric symptoms and personality changes associated with the disease (such as depression and anxiety — see Chapter 13). In addition, PD apathy can trigger major frustration for that person's care partner especially when the care partner sees that he's working harder at keeping the PWP active and involved than the PWP is.

Basically you can approach your life's uncertainties in two ways: Devote your efforts to worrying and trying to change the situation, or devote your energy toward living the most fulfilling life you can. Although you can't control the progression of your PD, you can control your choices:

- ✔ To exercise or not
- ✔ To remain engaged in the community or not
- ✔ To set a tone for your friends and family that you may have PD but it does not have you
- ✔ To wake up every morning and make good choices all over again or not

Choices for the person with PD

Just as proper diet and exercise are the best choices for maintaining your physical health, they're also your best weapons for maintaining the health of your mind and spirit. People who walk, bike, or run often report that they do their best thinking then; they're working out mental and emotional issues as well as physical ones.

These are some exercises you can make a part of your daily (or at least weekly) routine:

- ✔ Take time out for daily spiritual renewal (see Chapter 11). Meditate, pray, read inspirational books or poetry, take a walk, attend religious services — whatever gives you a sense of renewal.
- ✔ Challenge your mind. Work a crossword or Sudoku puzzle, play along with a TV game show (preferably one that actually requires some mental effort), read a book.
- ✔ Learn something new. Take a class at the local college or community center, ask a friend to teach you a craft or new sport, attend a lecture, watch a documentary. Then share your new ideas with someone else.
- ✔ Get involved in your community by taking an active role in a cause or organization that you think is important: the local library, a museum or historical site, national projects with local chapters (such as Habitat for Humanity).

✔ Create a legacy for your children and grandchildren. Write or record your family history, research the family tree, organize photo collections into albums that truly tell the story of your family's past.

✔ Partner with your partner to find activities you both can participate in and maintain the activities you both enjoyed before your diagnosis. Go to that play, that ballgame, that festival.

✔ Join a support group — preferably one for PWP — where you can interact with other people who fully understand the problems you and your care partner are facing.

✔ Accept that life with PD has no more certainty than life before PD. Turn to the *Bill of Rights for the Person Living with Parkinson's* in the front of this book. Tear it out, read it, and put it where you'll see and read it every day.

Choices for the PD care partner

As the care partner to someone living with PD, you also live with it. It affects your daily life in ways you had never imagined or planned for. A person in your shoes may want to abandon pieces of her own life to take care of the partner. And the most likely piece to fall by the wayside is your own physical health. You eat (or maybe don't eat!) as a reaction to your worries rather than as a source of nourishment. And when you add the responsibilities of caring for someone with PD to your full calendar, something's gotta give; the most likely candidate is your own regular exercise. *Stop!*

Before you go any further, take a moment to consider the following:

✔ Someone you love has PD and will *eventually* need help.

✔ You partner is managing fine with the present treatment plan. You understand that this plan can last for years by monitoring the disease and using medications.

✔ You have a choice:

- Project the worst as you try and control the future by making life-changing decisions right now.

- Make reasonable plans and preparations by educating yourself about options and then living the life that's still reasonably normal.

If you elect the second option, congratulations! Plan to familiarize yourself with the information in other sections of this book, especially Parts 4 and 5.

Now, about *your* body, mind, and spirit. Start by following the same guidelines we suggest in the "Exercises for the Mind and Spirit" section. Then read the Bill of Rights for the PD care partner in Chapter 19.

You don't have PD. You have a life beyond caring for this person — just as the PWP has a life beyond living with it. Mental and spiritual well being for each of you depends on maintaining normalcy as long as possible. The greatest danger is surrendering your potentially good and happy years to anxiety and depression, which can be a major factor with PD. Check out Chapter 13, where we address that concern in depth.

Chapter 13

Combating Anxiety and Depression

. . . .

In This Chapter

▶ Getting on top of the downside: Anxiety, depression, and apathy

▶ Looking for help in all the right places

▶ Thinking positively for you and your care partner

. . . .

You've gotten some bad news: It's Parkinson's disease (PD). At the moment, you don't know a lot — about the disease, about its impact on you and those you love, about so many questions. You're trying to come to terms with a diagnosis that means your life has changed and will keep changing as the years roll by. Of course, you have anxious moments — maybe some full-blown panic attacks. And news like this doesn't exactly put a smile on your face or a lot of sunshine in your outlook. When reactions like these last for a short time and then pass, that's normal human behavior.

On the other hand, feelings of anxiety, panic, and depression that persist for days, weeks, or even months are not normal. And for people living with Parkinson's (PWP), the anxiety and depression can be complicated by their PD — a combination of living with a chronic, progressive illness *and* the neurochemical changes occurring in the brain.

This chapter looks at the ways PD plays a part in the onset of anxiety and depression, and we provide a host of proven solutions — some of them admittedly a little unorthodox — that can bring you relief.

Recognizing the Mental Downside to PD

Anxiety and depression are serious — but treatable — medical conditions that can affect your quality of life and ability to function as you adapt to living with PD. And a number of circumstances (like stress, side effects of meds, and lifestyle changes due to PD) can trigger an episode that sends you reeling.

Don't take the symptoms of anxiety and depression lightly, and — just as important — don't postpone getting to the appropriate professional for treatment! (See the section "Finding and Accepting Help" later in this chapter for specifics about professional help.)

Anxiety is normal — to a point

Some situations naturally warrant anxiety and worry (the meeting with the boss, for example, or giving a major presentation or party). However, when the panic, terror, and outright impending doom aren't relieved by time, accomplishment, or common sense, something's wrong. Are you normally easygoing, self-confident, and optimistic? If you suddenly (and regularly!) find yourself dealing with dread or disproportionate fear, these feelings need attention.

Research studies confirm the following facts about anxiety for PWP:

- ✔ It affects up to 40 percent of PWP.
- ✔ It can be one of the first symptoms that make the PWP seek a doctor's care.
- ✔ It often goes hand in hand with depression.

Identifying the source of that anxiety

Anxiety can be brought on by any number of circumstances and generally takes one of several forms:

- ✔ **Generalized anxiety disorder (GAD):** A condition in which the person lives day in and day out with an underlying sense of worry that something will go wrong, but the worry has no real basis.
- ✔ **Social phobias:** When that persistent worry focuses on a specific situation or circumstance related to the social environment (such as a fear of failure or of interacting with other people).
- ✔ **Panic attack:** When anxiety strikes unexpectedly, suddenly, and hard. Usually a panic attack comes complete with major physical symptoms (such as a racing heartbeat, shortness of breath, and even chest pain). In fact you may think you're having a heart attack.

Circumstances leading to anxiety may include a particularly unsettling and stressful event (such as a diagnosis of PD); personality traits (such as low self-esteem and poor coping skills); or the presence of an additional mental condition (such as depression).

One way to identify the circumstances that cause anxiety is to be mindful of your own *fight-or-flight* mechanism. (*Fight-or-flight* is the most common reaction when people face situations that bring on stress, anxiety, or outright panic. In other words, they either stand and fight or take off.) Think of the times when you faced that choice. For example, if your boss confronted you about a missed deadline and you simply accepted his blame, that's flight. But if you listened and then explained exactly why the delay was unavoidable, that's fight.

So as a PWP, what sets off your fight-or-flight alarm? How persistent is it? Is your first instinct usually to take action, find answers, seek knowledge? (That's fight.) Or do you wait for others to direct you? (That, of course, is flight.) It's perfectly understandable that you'll have times when you just want to crawl under the covers and let somebody else live with PD for a while. But the more you adopt the fight mentality, the more likely you are to maintain independence and control over your life.

Measuring your level of anxiety

Although doctors use professional tools to diagnose anxiety, a short self-evaluation of your symptoms can help determine whether you should seek professional help. Which feelings in the following list do you experience on most days and for much of the day?

- ✔ Anxious or nervous
- ✔ Afraid (for self or others)
- ✔ Out of control
- ✔ Panicky or jumpy
- ✔ Short of breath or pounding heart
- ✔ Dizzy or faint
- ✔ Flushed or sweaty
- ✔ Unable to concentrate or take action
- ✔ Unable to remember
- ✔ Sensing impending doom

If you answered "Yes" to five or more of these symptoms, talk to your doctor. You may be suffering needlessly from anxiety.

Anxiety disorder includes additional categories such as post-traumatic stress disorder and obsessive-compulsive behavior disorder, but these are less common among PWP.

Depression — More than just sad and blue

According to the National Institute of Mental Health, depression can strike anyone, but PWP may be at greater risk. This section can help you consider your symptoms and determine whether it's time to take action.

Keep in mind that some PD symptoms (such as the masked facial expression, slow movement, and lack of energy) can actually be symptoms of depression — and vice versa. But when these symptoms accompany anxiety, apathy, or loss of interest or pleasure in activities and relationships, consider the possibility that you have a *treatable* mental health condition.

Recognizing the symptoms

The National Institute of Mental Health lists the following as symptoms of depression:

- Persistent sad, anxious, or empty feelings
- Feelings of hopelessness and pessimism
- Feelings of guilt, worthlessness, or helplessness
- Loss of interest and pleasure in hobbies and activities
- Fatigue, feeling slowed down, or decreased energy
- Difficulty concentrating, making decisions, or remembering
- Insomnia or oversleeping
- Appetite or weight gain or loss
- Restlessness and irritability
- Thoughts of death or suicide; suicide attempts
- Crying, especially over little, seemingly incidental issues

Ask yourself these questions

Although we definitely don't recommend self-diagnosis or treatment, ask yourself these ten questions if your feelings (mental and emotional) concern you on a daily basis:

- Are you discouraged or sad?
- Are you moody or irritable?
- Are you feeling isolated or lonely?
- Have you lost interest in activities you can still do?
- Have you pulled away from interactions with friends and family?
- Is your outlook affecting your ability to work, make decisions, or make choices?

> ✔ Has your mood affected your sleep (for example, sleeping more in the day or not sleeping at night) or energy level?
>
> ✔ Have you experienced changes in appetite and weight?
>
> ✔ Have you lost interest in sex or intimacy with your partner?
>
> ✔ Have the people you trust suggested that you seem depressed?

If you've answered "Yes" to five or more of these questions, you need to raise the possibility with your doctor that you may need treatment for depression.

Dealing with apathy and lack of motivation

Many PWP develop *apathy*, a condition defined by

> ✔ Reduced interest and participation in routine activities
>
> ✔ Lack of initiative; having difficulty starting or sustaining an activity to completion
>
> ✔ Indifference or a lack of concern
>
> ✔ A flattening of affect (the mind and the spirit seem to give up on all emotions: good, bad, pleasant, or painful)

In addition to these symptoms, the PWP's apathy can trigger frustration in family, friends, and the care partner. When those around an apathetic person begin to realize that they're working harder at fighting your PD than you are, the tendency is to think that the person suffering from apathy doesn't appreciate their efforts or help. The end result can be that family and friends gradually go back to their own lives, leaving the person with apathy (and the care partner) more isolated and in need of help than before.

Apathy can be associated with several neuropsychiatric illnesses (such as Alzheimer's dementia, PD, and stroke). In PD, however, apathy is more likely a direct consequence of physiological changes in the brain and lack of dopamine than a psychological reaction to disability. Although professionals can distinguish apathy from psychiatric symptoms and personality features (particularly depression and anxiety), it's not an easy task. Consider these subtle but distinguishing characteristics:

> ✔ Like people with depression, apathetic patients may be sluggish, quiet, and disengaged. They may talk slowly or not at all.
>
> ✔ Unlike depressed patients, apathetic PWP deny being sad, feeling guilty, or having suicidal thoughts.

Recognizing apathy and differentiating it from depression in PWP is important because the medical treatment for the two conditions may be different. Patients with apathy are not lazy and may respond to a series of strategies that include gentle encouragement to initiate activities as well as schedules and routines to keep them busy.

For example, consider a PWP who's always loved going to the ballpark. When his best friend invites him to a major league game for his birthday, he says he wants to stay home in front of the television. But when the friend insists, they go to the park, and the PWP has a good time all day. However, he immediately turns the television back on when he returns home.

Ask your primary care doctor or neurologist about the differences between apathy and depression and what symptoms you (and your care partner) should watch for in either case.

Finding and Accepting Help

You may have experienced depression or anxiety before the onset of PD, or your first episode may come after the diagnosis. But the chicken-or-the-egg question doesn't really matter. What does matter is that the symptoms (see the previous sections) are unnecessary hardships when you're dealing with PD.

Ask your doctor to recommend a consultation with a mental health professional who'll work closely with your doctor to assess your depression in the context of your PD.

Taking medication may help

In most cases, PWP tolerate antidepressant medications well. But medications can take weeks to have a real effect, and the right medication can take trial and effort. As a result, many doctors recommend a combination treatment plan that may include or take the place of antidepressants. Combo possibilities include

- Talk therapy (the services of a professional counselor)
- Changes in diet, exercise routines, and sleep habits

Before you take any medication (prescription or over-the-counter) to treat symptoms of depression or anxiety, be sure your prescribing doctor is fully aware of all your other medications. Some over-the-counter (OTC) supplements can interact in a negative or even harmful way with your other medications.

Seeking a professional counselor

Your doctor may recommend a professional counselor who helps you talk through the feelings and fears that are at the foundation of your depression or anxiety. In looking for the right counselor, keep in mind the different categories:

- **Psychiatrists:** Medical doctors with training (at least four years) beyond their medical degree. These doctors are board-certified by the American Board of Psychiatry and Neurology and licensed in the state where they practice. They can prescribe medications and coordinate a total care plan for any mental or emotional health issue.

- **Psychologists:** Counselors with a master's degree (MA or MS) or a doctoral degree (PhD or PsyD) in psychology and/or counseling. Psychologists are board-certified by the American Board of Professional Psychology and licensed by the state where they practice.

  Psychologists are less focused on biological causes of depression and anxiety and more focused on treating your symptoms.

- **Clinical social workers:** Counselors who are licensed or certified by the state and usually hold a masters degree in social work and/or counseling. Some social workers have advanced training in psychotherapy and may have the title of Licensed Clinical Social Worker or LCSW.

- **Other counselors** include

  - **Psychiatric nurses or clinical nurse specialists** (CNS) who are registered nurses (RN), with additional training in psychiatry

  - **Family therapists** who hold a title or degree but focus primarily on counseling within the context of a family group

  - **Pastoral counselors** who, in addition to religious training, have training in counseling

Finding a counselor

Therapy to treat depression, anxiety, or a mental or emotional condition should be a collaborative process. More than with any other healthcare professional, you need to feel a real sense of trust and rapport with this person.

Keep in mind that your therapist will push you to examine and confront sometimes unpleasant and even painful issues. She's not trying to be mean, but she is trying to get you past roadblocks that may hamper your ability to accept PD in order to live a fuller, more satisfying life.

Any mental health professional has the ethical (in some cases, legal) responsibility to keep your therapy discussions confidential *unless* you threaten to cause harm to other persons or property.

Choosing the right counselor for you

In addition to checking his credentials and experience, take time to really consider the connection you'll have with this therapist or counselor. The following are key steps to follow:

✔ Be sure your primary care physician (PCP) has already ruled out medical causes for your depression or anxiety symptoms.

✔ Consider specifics (such as the therapist's age, gender, ethnic or religious background) that may be important to you and make those known when you ask for referrals.

✔ Get at least two (and preferably three) referrals from your primary care doctor, neurologist, or support group facilitator.

✔ Be sure to consider location. You're going to see this person on a regular (perhaps weekly) basis over several months. The last thing you need is an inconvenient journey to and from the appointment.

✔ At your first appointment

- Ask the same questions you ask your other specialists. (See Chapter 6 for these questions.)

- Be prepared to describe the symptoms that led you to seek help.

- Listen to the therapist's possible plan for treatment (medications, talk therapy, or both).

    Listen for language like "in cases like yours . . ." that suggests a generalized rather than a customized approach to therapy. If this one-size-fits-all seems to be the therapist's approach, keep looking.

✔ After the first appointment, keep in mind that a genuine trust and connection with this person is key to successfully conquering your symptoms. Give yourself time to think about the first meeting — what went well and what disturbed you — before keeping a second appointment.

Check with your insurance provider (or Medicare/Medicaid if appropriate) to find out what services are covered. If your insurance provider doesn't cover mental health services (or only covers a portion), ask the therapist whether he has a sliding fee scale based on income.

Sharing the emotional journey with a support group

A support group can be a real lifesaver for many people with a chronic, progressive condition (and their care partners). Through these gatherings, you can hear about valuable coping skills and keep up with the latest myths and bona fide medical advances. Generally, each group has a facilitator with professional experience in working with PWP and their care partners. This objective, outside facilitator has the following responsibilities:

- Keeps the discussion moving
- Doesn't allow a few outspoken participants to highjack the meeting so quieter personalities fade into the background (and eventually leave the group)
- Covers the logistics: Meeting place and time, special speakers or programs, and notices of meetings

The most successful groups determine their own personality and style. The following are examples of group formats:

- Participants talk about PD news and personal updates. They support one another emotionally and offer ideas for coping.
- A speaker presents a specific topic for discussion.
- The group has a political focus, such as getting Congress to allocate research dollars that will put PD on the front burner for finding a cure. (See information on the Parkinson's Action Network in Appendix B.)
- Some groups include all of these formats, alternating support with specific programs and advocacy projects.

 PWP and their care partners are indeed fortunate to have a number of national organizations that offer support groups through their regional or state chapters. To see whether such a group is available in your area, check www.parkinson.org or www.caregiver.org.

Two other possible resources are the community education and outreach department of your local hospital or the local PD exercise class we describe in Chapter 12.

If your area has zero groups specifically for PWP or their care partners, consider starting one. See the sidebar "Building a support group: From *me* to *we* in five easy steps" to get started.

Whether you join an established group or start one yourself, support groups can enrich your life beyond anything you can imagine because you

- Connect with people who truly understand the challenges of living with PD.
- Have the opportunity to laugh and cry together.
- Can advocate for better treatments and a cure.
- Can make an enormous difference for yourself and for those who love and care for you.

Building a support group: From *me* to *we* in five easy steps

The steps for starting a PD support group are relatively simple:

1. **Ask your doctor or neurologist to tell other PD patients and their care partners that you're interested in organizing a group**.

   Provide cards with your contact information for the doctor to give to interested PWP. These people can then contact you (not the other way around).

2. **Gather the following information:**

   ✔ Ask your local hospital or home care agency whether they have anyone qualified and willing to facilitate the group.

   ✔ Find out whether your local library, bookstore, coffeehouse, or medical clinic has a room available for 10 to 12 people for two hours once a month at no charge.

3. **Consider initially combining PWP and care partners in the same group.**

   As the group grows, you may hold separate meetings for the PWP and care partners.

4. **When at least four people have expressed interest, call an organizational meeting and ask these people to invite other PWP or care partners.**

5. **At the first meeting:**

   ✔ Have nametags and perhaps light refreshments.

   ✔ Ask attendees to briefly introduce themselves and state what they're looking for in a support group.

   ✔ Establish the working details for the group: when and where to meet; how often; for how long; dues, if any, to cover cost of refreshments or mailings; and programs or format style of the group.

   ✔ If possible, ask an experienced support-group facilitator to lead this meeting.

   ✔ If you don't have a trained facilitator, consider professionals speakers to lead the first several meetings. Then alternate the leader role and assign responsibilities (meeting room, program, and participant notifications) for the next three months.

   ✔ End the meeting by checking everyone's contact information and allowing time for people to socialize and get to know each other better.

Making lifestyle changes to improve your point of view

Two words: exercise and diet. (But you can check out Chapter 12 for a few more words.) It's no secret that research shows how regular exercise and a properly balanced diet can work wonders for your health. But just in case you need a refresher on some of those wonders, did you know that exercise can

✔ Boost the power of neurotransmitters in your brain to enhance your mood and your ability to look at life more positively?

> ✔ Relieve muscle tension when your body's natural instinct is to tense up in response to a challenge?
>
> ✔ Enhance your self-image, which leads to greater self-assurance and confidence, which increase your ability to deal with negative stress?

Not a bad return on an investment of only 30 to 60 minutes a day!

As for diet, start with a simple choice like lessening stimulants (such as caffeine and chocolate) that can contribute to your anxiety. Ready to kick it up a notch? Educate yourself about the mind-enhancing powers of certain food groups. (For more information on diet and nutrition, see Chapter 12.) When you combine these power foods with regular exercise, you have the right formula to make an enormous difference in your emotional state of mind and self-image.

Alternative therapies (such as relaxation and meditation) and mind-exercise programs (such as T'ai Chi and yoga) can also be enormously effective in relieving the symptoms of anxiety and depression. See Chapter 11 for more info on each of these techniques.

Don't worry — Be happy

No doubt you'd like to remind us that PD isn't exactly humorous. But at least one of us (the author with PD) knows all too well that finding humor in the mishaps and misadventures with PD is no different from finding humor in other life challenges (like the impossible in-law or the service people who don't show up and then don't give much service when they do get there).

The following sections provide a few tips for ways you (and your partner) can fight anxiety, depression, and apathy.

Just say the word

One PWP came up with the acronym *S.O.F.A.* (as in "Get off the sofa") to remind himself that anxiety, apathy, and depression were dangerous areas for anyone with PD. *Sadness* can lead to *Obstructions* (of physical and mental abilities) that lead to a *Fall* (the danger for any PWP), so the only cure is *Ambition* (to get moving — physically, mentally, and spiritually). This acronym may not work for you, but try one of your own — a password that empowers you and your care partner when anxiety and depression start to rear their ugly heads.

The crème' de la comedy

Renowned essayist and editor Norman Cousins pioneered the idea of laughter as medical therapy. In his book, *Anatomy of an Illness*, Cousins describes how he watched hours of classics like the Marx brothers and *I Love Lucy*. As a result of his and other researchers' work, laughter is now a respected therapy that supplements mainstream medicine.

It's not all about you: Ways to look beyond your PD

One sure way to get past the poor-pitiful-me piece is to focus less on yourself and ramp up your attention to other people. This simple change can also remind other people to stop viewing you as someone with an incurable condition and start seeing you as the vital, loving, and giving person you've always been.

Fresh out of ideas? Not surprising. But, hey, that's why we're here. Pick any one of the following and see what happens:

- ✔ If a clerk or service person gives especially good service, tell him and then tell his boss.

- ✔ Offer to trade seats on a bus, train, or plane to let a family or couple sit together — even if you end up with the dreaded middle seat.

- ✔ Find old pictures of family members, frame them, and send them to the person with a note that recalls what the photos mean to you.

- ✔ Look beneath the surface. When a friend's in a crummy mood, know that it probably goes well beyond the surface. Acknowledge that she seems to be having a bad day and ask if there's anything you can do to help.

- ✔ Pass along a good book you've just finished or make special scrapbooks or family recipe books for the children in your family.

- ✔ If you're a gardener and need to divide your perennials, offer the new neighbor some plants from your garden. (They can do the digging!)

- ✔ Put an extra coin in an expired meter.

- ✔ Call the clerks and other service people that you regularly see by name.

- ✔ Take a treat to your co-workers, even if you have to buy rather than bake it.

- ✔ Use the magic words, "Please" and "Thank you," and make a big deal out of someone going the extra mile for you.

Focusing on other people — caring for and about them — is possibly the simplest way to move beyond your self-pity and angst about PD. Of course, it's not a cure for clinical depression or anxiety, but caring for others is a major first-step in changing your destructive, negative self-talk to something far more positive and life-affirming. Bottom line? It is indeed better to give (care and concern) than to receive (pity and avoidance).

Did you hear the one about . . .

At your next support group meeting, suggest the group indulge in some laugh therapy for 15 to 20 minutes by sharing funny incidents. After all, who else can understand the ridiculousness of trying to shave (if you're a man) or pulling on a pair of pantyhose (if you're a woman)? Who else but PWP can laugh out loud and not seem cruel when you describe yourself hurrying to catch an elevator?

The humor you find in PD is, of course, bittersweet, but don't permit the bitter to overpower the sweet. Choosing to laugh at yourself — and the frustrations and mishaps with PD — offers a healthy dose of the absurd that'll work better than any pill. The ability to laugh can work miracles.

Tapping into the power of positive thinking

The ability to enjoy life — to be content — is often bound up in the need to be in control. But how much can anyone really control? The next hour, day, or year? Nope. The only control you really have lies in how you choose to react to life's circumstances and challenges. And when you choose to react with a sense of humor and a positive life outlook, research suggests three possible benefits:

- You'll greatly reduce your physical and emotional stress and greatly enhance your relationships with other people.

- Your outlook will be contagious. By setting the tone (as we suggest in Chapter 5), you can help your care partners (professional and personal) accept the diagnosis and move forward with you.

- You'll have an aura of self-confidence that also inspires people around you (who may be tempted to nurture or baby you) to step back and let you take the lead. They'll be more inclined to make decisions *with* you than *for* you.

Your attitude can very well be the difference between taking control of this disease and allowing PD to control you. How much better to hear people marvel at your incredibly upbeat and positive attitude toward PD than to hear them talk in tones of pity and sympathy!

So how can you change a glass that's half-empty into a glass that's half-full? More to the point, is it even possible to change it, given your PD diagnosis?

Optimists tend to believe that good things do happen and bad things are just temporary challenges. Fortunately, enhancing your optimistic side is within reach. Check out these tips for becoming more optimistic:

- Find the joy — in work, in relationships, in everyday stuff like preparing a meal, cleaning, repairing something, getting dressed, and meeting the day head-on.

- Surround yourself with people who are positive, upbeat, and optimistic.

- Commit random acts of kindness (not original to us, but we like the sound of it!) by looking beyond yourself to the needs of others (see the sidebar, "It's not all about you: Ways to look beyond your PD."

- Accept and work through situations you can control; let go of those you can't. (Does the word *serenity* come to mind?)

- Be aware of your reactions. Banish negative self-talk ("I can't," or "I never . . ."), and look for underlying traits you admire (or even love) in the family members and friends who irritate you.

- At the end of every day, write or tell yourself three good things (okay, they can be really little) that happened that day.

As Garrison Keillor, author and host of the popular radio program, *Prairie Home Companion,* once said, "They say such nice things about people at their funerals that it makes me sad that I'm going to miss mine by just a few days."

A Word for the PD Care Partner

Given the nature of depression, anxiety, and apathy, it's most likely that you — not the PWP — will need to be vigilant about recognizing symptoms and getting help to break the cycle. These are a few actions you can take:

- ✓ **Pay attention.** Look at the PWP's body language. Listen to what she says (or doesn't say). Sure, that mask (lack of facial expression) or stooped posture may be a result of PD, but is something else at work here? If the person you love seems persistently uninvolved and disinterested in the normal routine you two once enjoyed, those clues need your attention.

- ✓ **Don't be afraid to ask questions.** Your PWP may have a logical but curable reason for appearing to be depressed, apathetic, or anxious. Through gentle questioning, maybe you can get him to admit his concern so the two of you can talk about it (and address it with his doctor). On the other hand, if his answer to all your questions is something like "There's nothing wrong," he may have more troubling him than he can manage. In that case, you can:

  - Offer information from PD Web sites (see Appendix B) and books like this one that clearly demonstrates how such feelings are common for PWP and can be treated.

  - Suggest that he talk to his neurologist about his emotions and ask whether these unusual feelings are treatable.

- ✓ **Talk to the experts.** If the PWP refuses to address your concern that he may be depressed or suffering from anxiety or apathy, contact the neurologist yourself and ask for help. Or ask the care partners in your support group whether they've dealt with these issues. If they have, ask for some suggestions on how you can follow through.

Don't forget to take care of you

Being the primary care partner for a PWP will — over time — become a natural piece of your life. Before you realize it, the role is more than a daily routine; it's part of your identity. "That's Joan Sutton. Her husband has Parkinson's," someone may say, implying that your husband's condition somehow identifies you as well.

The processes of partnering in care and caregiving requires constant adjustment. Understandably you'll have days (and weeks) of exhaustion, frustration, and depression. But, interspersed will be moments of such high drama, joy, and sharing that you find the will and energy to fight on. You make an enormous difference for the PWP. The support and care you provide is vital, important work.

The danger comes when you try to do it all (or at least more than you should), and you burn out. The signs of burnout aren't that different from depression (see the earlier section, "Depression — More than just sad and blue"). Decide now to watch out for these signs and give yourself permission to take a break, hand off some of the responsibility to others, and most of all, have a life of your own.

Positive steps you can take

We recommend the following ways to help you hang in there:

- **Identify and nurture your personal support system.** You need people to be there just for you — to listen to and comfort *you*. You're dealing with a host of feelings including grief and bereavement. If you feel so isolated that you can't think of anyone to talk to, you need to consider seeking some counseling. Ask your primary care doctor to recommend a counselor, or perhaps your clergyperson is able to help.

- **Join a support group!** We can't stress this enough. The underlying cause of depression in care partners is a sense of isolation. The people you meet in a support group don't replace your best friends, but they do give you a place to vent and share PD war stories.

- **Give yourself a break** — an actual physical break — every day if possible. Use your support network to come in and take over for an hour. Take this time for yourself. Go for a walk, watch a movie, grab some coffee. Don't use your personal time for tasks like paying the bills or calling the insurance company.

- **Keep your priorities straight.** Your health is vital to the PWP, so exercise, eat a balanced diet, and maintain your own social interactions and activities.

Chapter 14

Clinical Trials and Your Role in the Search for a Cure

....

....

*I*t's one thing to say that a new drug or treatment works in a monkey or mouse, but it's quite another to take that next leap and declare the product safe and effective for people. Research scientists make that leap by conducting *clinical trials* (experiments) that use human volunteers.

Okay, interesting, you say, but not exactly a priority for you at the moment. But maybe it should be. Why? Because you can make a difference — for yourself and for those who follow you down this path of Parkinson's disease (PD) — by getting involved. Want to know how? Read on.

What Is a Clinical Trial and Why Should You Care?

Clinical trials (also called *clinical research studies*) answer certain questions related to a specific health condition. They're also an important hurdle before new therapies for the treatment, management, and cure of a disease can be approved and marketed. Without such trials, therapeutic advancement is impossible. But eventually these studies require human participation. That's where you and other people living with Parkinson's disease (PWP) come in.

Recently major PD organizations have formed an alliance to build awareness of clinical trials among PWP. In addition to making more persons with PD (and their physicians) aware of clinical trials for treatments — and even a cure — these organizations offer some good reasons for participation:

✔ If more people living with PD volunteer to participate in a trial, the testing and marketing periods (on average 12 to 15 years) can be cut in half, a whopping 6 to 7 years shorter.

✔ If the testing and marketing periods can be cut, then new therapies can be available sooner and at a lower cost. (For you curious souls, the average cost to bring a single new medicine to market is approximately $800 million.)

The statistics tell their own story. According to a presentation at the 2006 World Parkinson's Congress, only 1 percent of PD patients participate in a study compared to 5 percent of the total cancer community. Although both stats seem small, the National Cancer Institute estimates that, if they can double the number of participants in clinical trials for cancer, many studies can be completed in one year (rather than the current three to five years). Simply doubling the numbers can have an enormous effect on the researchers' and the industry's ability to understand PD (its causes and course), find advanced treatments, and make those treatments available sooner.

But, before you volunteer, you need to understand how clinical trials work as well as their benefits and risks. The following sections explain this process.

Taking a Close Look at the Process

This section explains in a nutshell how the clinical trial usually unfolds. Like most topics in the world of medicine and science, the subject of clinical trials comes with its own unique vocabulary, so we clearly define each term when we introduce it.

First, to get a clinical trial underway, a team of research scientists must determine the general category of their clinical trial. Their options include

✔ **Interventional trials:** Scientists test experimental treatments and drugs or new ways of using existing therapies with groups of patients under controlled conditions.

✔ **Observational trials:** Researchers study a specific health issue (such as aging or stress) with a large group of people in their natural home, work, or community setting.

Note: In this chapter we discuss only an interventional trial, but you may participate in either type of trial for PD.

Next, the team applies for approval from an Institutional Review Board (IRB) to conduct the clinical trial. The IRB is a group of physicians, statisticians, researchers, community advocates, and others that meets independently of the research group and ensures that the trial protocol is ethical and that the rights of study participants are protected.

After the IRB approves the trial, the team follows the study's *protocol* (roadmap), which outlines the process, establishes timelines for completion of each step, and describes the profile of participants. The research team evaluates the safety and effectiveness of the trial drug, but the protocol specifies safeguards for monitoring the overall health of participants throughout the trial.

Researchers conduct studies in phases.

✔ Phase 1 usually tests the therapy on a small group (20 to 80) of healthy volunteers to assess potential side effects and risks.

✔ Phase 2 tests the therapy on a larger group of people (100 or more) who have PD and evaluates the effectiveness and side effects of the therapy.

✔ Phase 3 tests the therapy on at least 500 volunteers with PD and compares the new therapy with therapies currently available.

Although trials may go through several stages and take years to complete, they're still the fastest, safest way to discover and test any new treatment, medicine, and medical device before these products are available to the general public.

In every trial the research team establishes certain qualifiers for selecting participants. These are the *exclusion/inclusion guidelines* for the study. For example, the study may include people over the age of 60 but exclude anyone under that age. Or, if liver problems are known side effects of the drug, then individuals who already deal with liver problems are excluded. Criteria can cover gender, age, even weight or geographical location. Such guidelines are included in the trial's description.

After participants are selected (that's you!), they sign a document of informed consent (which we discuss in more detail later in the chapter in "Considering the Benefits and Risks Before Signing on") and are assigned to a *treatment group* (where everyone receives the same form of treatment). The study may include one group for the experimental drug, one for an existing drug that's the current preferred treatment, and one for a *placebo*.

A placebo is a medicine with no active ingredients — no way of medically effecting change either for better or worse — so your symptoms remain unchanged. (You may have heard people talk about the *placebo effect,* meaning the observed effects arise from the patient's expectations rather than from the treatment itself.) In clinical trials, researchers want to remove that placebo factor from the equation. However, as many as 30 percent of patients who receive a placebo in a trial report improvement. This result seems to be especially true in PD because the just the possibility of getting a better medicine can create the expectation of a reward and liberate *dopamine* (the chemical in your brain that controls movement). This placebo effect is one reason that research for PD is so difficult and takes so long.

In other words, trial participants usually go into one of two treatment groups: participants who receive the real treatment or drug and participants who receive a treatment that only *looks like* the real deal but doesn't have any of the active ingredients.

Double-blind studies are the preferred design for testing new therapies today because they assure objectivity throughout the study. In double-blind studies, participants don't know which treatment group they're in, and the researcher doesn't know which group is getting the test therapy. In *single-blind* studies, only the participant or the researcher (but not both) knows which group is receiving the placebo and which is taking the actual drug. In *open label* studies, both the doctor and the study subject know what drug is administered.

Clinical trial researchers must adhere to the strict standards of the Food and Drug Administration (FDA), the government bureau that monitors trials and approves research to move on to the next stage. After the trial progresses through its stages and is successful, the FDA signs off, and the new treatment (or medicine or medical device) becomes available to the general public. (There's a lot more red tape involved, but you get the gist.)

Considering the Benefits and Risks Before Signing on

By taking part in a clinical trial, you're

- ✔ Taking that proactive role that we've encouraged throughout this book.
- ✔ Gaining access to new therapies before they become available to the general public.
- ✔ Contributing to the cure for a disease that you wouldn't wish on your worst enemy.
- ✔ Getting the expert attention of scientists and healthcare professionals.

These benefits are fairly impressive but, of course, they come with risks, and those can be major. Although major risks are rare, you still need to know what you may be up against before you sign up. These are some possibilities:

✔ The treatment may have unforeseen side effects.

✔ The experimental treatment may not work for you.

✔ The trial may have costs associated with participating — travel to and from the trial site, for example.

Before you decide to participate in a trial (assuming you meet the needs of the study and have been invited to participate), you'll be asked to sign a document of informed consent. This document is your agreement that you've received the key information about the clinical trial (its purpose, how long it will last, what's expected of you, and the names and contact information for the research team). Your signature on this document also indicates that you're aware of the risks, potential side effects, and potential benefits of the treatment. Take your time. Talk the document over with your family, your doctor, and even your attorney to get a full picture of what you're agreeing to. *Note:* If the document has way too much *fine print,* ask for a *large print* version — literally and figuratively.

The informed consent is *not* a contract or legally binding document for you or the company/institution conducting the trial. You have the right to withdraw from the trial at any time you choose. But keep in mind that participation of people like you brings us closer to a cure — faster.

Although the informed consent is intended to protect the patient, you're still responsible for understanding all you can about the trial before agreeing to participate. You must ask the important questions such as what happens (to your body and brain) during the trial and, more importantly, what the risks are and how the team handles any adverse reaction. Answers to these questions are especially important if you're participating in a study for surgical treatment of PD.

Taking the First Steps into Volunteering

To volunteer, you first have to know where to look. Clinical trials start all the time all over the country. The key is to find a trial that's convenient for you, that's actively enrolling participants, and that you and your doctor believe may help your individual situation. Ready to get started? Read on.

Finding clinical trials for PD

The most efficient way to shop for clinical trials is the Internet. Two excellent Web sites are www.PDtrials.org and www.clinicaltrials.gov. Both sites give you important base information about locations of trials, exclusion/inclusion criteria, and other facts that can help you rule out certain studies right away. If you don't have access to a computer, ask a friend who has one to help you, or go to your local library and ask the librarian to assist you in browsing these sites.

Also you can call PD Trials at 800-801-9484 and request to be on the mailing list for periodic information and updates related to PD trials and studies.

Volunteering to participate

Volunteering to participate in a trial is not as simple as volunteering at your local library or school. Each study or trial works under a strict set of guidelines and standards, and participants must meet certain specific criteria. These restrictions assure that new therapies are tested under the most appropriate conditions to prove or disprove the study team's theories.

Don't get discouraged or take it personally if your application is denied. Keep trying to participate because the future of new treatments (and perhaps one day a cure) needs you!

These are the steps you need to take to be part of a clinical trial:

1. **Find a trial through the resources we list earlier in this section.**

2. **Read the description and record the number that begins with NCT (the official assigned trial number) and all contact details.**

3. **Call or e-mail the contact; include any initial questions you have and request more detailed information about the study or trial.**

4. **Discuss your interest in volunteering for this trial with your neurologist and your family; if possible, talk with people who've participated in past clinical trials.**

5. **If you don't qualify for a certain trial (or the trial has the full quota of participants), ask the coordinator to stay in touch.**

   The trial may need more participants as it moves forward, or the contact person may become aware of other trials that better match your profile.

6. **Keep a record of your calls, e-mails, and conversations, noting dates and responses. Make follow-up calls if you haven't heard back from the coordinator in a timely manner — within two to three weeks.**

Trial coordinators are juggling many calls and details, so be patient about a reasonable response time. On the other hand, be persistent and ask when you can expect a response.

Why prescription drugs cost so much

Unless you've been living on another planet for the last decade or so, you already know that prescription medications don't come cheap. Of course, we can assume that pharmaceutical companies are not in business for the good of mankind — at least not entirely. These companies are businesses and, by definition, they want to make a profit. ("But do they need to make such a *large* profit?" you ask. The answer depends on who you ask. All we're going to say is that, in America, capitalism remains king.)

Seriously though, the journey to discover and develop new therapies for treating disease is long, costly, and fraught with uncertainties. Nearly half of all new medicines and therapies come from laboratories and clinical studies in the United States. The system may be cumbersome, but it works.

European countries often get bogged down by each country having its own approval protocol;

a drug readily available in one country may be years away from approval for distribution in a neighboring country. That situation would be like taking the approval process away from the FDA in the United States and handing it over to the individual states. In that case, the drug you need may be approved for distribution in California, but you live in Maine, where it's still three years away from final approval.

Think of it this way: Every purchase has a value beyond its dollars and cents cost. Ask yourself what the value of a new therapy for PD means to you and your family. Ask yourself the value of finding a cure. Like those ads for the credit-card company: a prescription that relieves symptoms — $xx; a new medical device that enhances movement — $xxx; a cure for PD — priceless. Keep in mind that your health and safety through the course of that journey is also priceless.

Never volunteer for a trial just because you think you may get *free* medicines because you may end up in the placebo group. And always question any trial that offers you significant monetary reward if you join. Payments for expenses and medical care are one thing; pay-outs to get you in the door are something else entirely and should raise a huge red flag. Similarly, if your doctor seems overly anxious to *sell* you the idea of participating, you need to question the doctor whether he's receiving an incentive from the trial sponsor to recruit patients.

Asking Important Questions Before Committing

An invitation to participate or an approval of your eligibility for a study doesn't obligate you to sign up. Before you make that decision, gather as much information as possible. Address your questions directly to the research team even though many of the answers are in the informed consent document (check the "Considering the Benefits and Risks Before Signing on" section earlier in this chapter for more on this document). We suggest you ask the questions in person, not over the phone or via e-mail, so you can judge for yourself exactly how on board they are with the information in the informed consent. Most people can't imagine buying a car or home without meeting the dealer or realtor face-to-face. Participating in a clinical trial can be far more important than a car or a home.

For that meeting with the team, come prepared with your questions in writing. Bring someone along to act as scribe so you can focus on listening and assessing the unspoken responses of the team. Better yet, bring along a tape recorder and record the meeting so you can play it back later as you make your decision.

In a face-to-face meeting, you want to ask:

✔ **What's the purpose of the study?** According to the National Institutes of Health, studies may be conducted for one or a combination of reasons:

- Testing experimental drugs or approaches to therapy

- Testing to determine ways to prevent disease

- Testing to discover new ways of diagnosing a disease

- Testing ways of detecting a specific disease

- Testing ways that patient comfort and quality of life may be improved in chronic illness

✔ **Who's sponsoring the study?** Sponsorship for a clinical trial can come from a variety of sources including pharmaceutical companies, private foundations, universities and medical centers, biotech companies, or even the government. When you know the sponsor (read that as *funding source*), you can better determine whether it's a reputable and reliable source with the funds necessary to see the research through in spite of any glitches along the way.

✔ **Who's conducting the study?** The members of the research team should be well qualified to manage the study and safeguard the health and well being of participants during the study. Because the study team has been approved by the IRB (see the earlier section "Taking a Close Look at the Process"), you may want to ask this question simply to better identify the role of each member.

✔ **Why does the research team believe the therapy or research question will be helpful or effective in the treatment or management of PD?** The answer should cover information about previous studies. Perhaps they've already tested animals; maybe researchers in another country have tested (or even used) the therapy.

✔ **In what ways does this therapy differ from the current treatment regimen for PD?** The answer can help you gauge whether the difference between your current therapies and the new drug or treatment is substantial enough to warrant your participation in the test.

✔ **What tests and treatments will be performed in the course of the study?** With this answer you start to get specific information about their expectations of you.

✔ **Where will those tests and treatments be administered?** The convenience of the study site is important because you need to be there during the course of the trial. An important follow-up question is, "How often will I need to come to the site?"

✔ **During the study, who will be in charge of my PD care and my general healthcare?** The answer should make it crystal clear that someone is going to take charge of your general care during the trial.

✔ **Will hospitalization be necessary at any time during the trial?** If the answer is *yes*, be sure to ask about the length of stay, where you'll be hospitalized, and who'll pay the bill.

✔ **What are the risks — potential side effects — of the treatment or study?** One of the primary reasons for the trial is to determine the risks and side effects. Still, the team has some idea of what they anticipate, and you should know these facts before you agree to participate.

✔ **How will your current treatment be affected during the trial?** You need to know whether your current medication regimen for managing your PD symptoms will be interrupted, changed, or stopped altogether during the study.

✔ **How long will the trial last?** Trials can last for a matter of weeks, months, or even years (usually the longer trials focus on quality-of-life issues). The research team needs to be clear about the time this study will take, but only you can decide whether the time is reasonable for you.

✔ **What will it cost and who will pay?** You can reasonably expect expenses directly related to the study to be covered during the course of the study. In addition, you may receive a stipend for some indirect costs, such as mileage to and from the study site. You should not expect the study to cover the costs of managing your general health. In other words, a study for a new PD therapy probably won't include payment for that dental crown you've needed.

✔ **Under what circumstances would the trial or study be stopped?** Trials may be stopped for any one of several reasons. In the most serious circumstances, the government can stop a trial because side effects and risks become too common and serious. In another case, a company may halt a trial because a competing drug has been approved and is coming to market. Follow-up questions here are: "How will participants be notified if a trial is stopped?" and "What follow-up can participants expect?"

For example, will there be regular (as in quarterly or annual) check-ups to see how you're doing and will you have a contact person in the event of a change in your reaction to the medication or therapy down the road?

✔ **After the trial's complete, will you still have access to the trial therapy if it's worked for you?** Especially if you're participating in an early phase of the trial and the new therapy seems to make a difference for you, you want to know that you'll be able to continue taking the medicine or receiving the treatment.

✔ **What if you agree to participate but you change your mind after a few weeks?** You always have the right to leave a study. Ask this question to understand how your decision to leave in the middle of a study may affect the overall results.

As you collect the information and ask any follow-up questions, pay attention to details such as how they refer to you and other participants; you want to be the *patient, subject,* or *participant* and never the (heaven forbid!) *number.*

Following this interview, check with these people before you make your final decision about volunteering:

✔ Your doctor(s) to discuss the potential benefits and risks of participation.

✔ Your family to discuss any reservations they may have.

✔ Your attorney to review the document of informed consent.

As you weigh your decision, remember that you're a key stakeholder in this process. Don't be a passive participant; instead, take your place at this table as an equal player. The research team may have the degrees and fancy titles, but you're the key to that treasure — finding new and more effective therapies for PD and, one day, its cure.

Part IV
Living Well with PD

The 5th Wave

By Rich Tennant

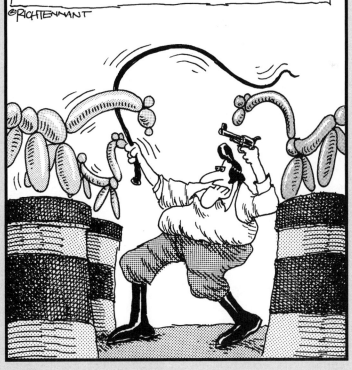

Attempting to reduce the stress in his life to help his Parkinson's disease, Waldo 'Whip' Gunschott goes from being a wild animal trainer to a wild balloon animal trainer.

In this part . . .

Having Parkinson's disease may well change your lifestyle, but it doesn't have to be a life sentence. In this section we explore ways that you can maintain the relationships and activities that give your life meaning and purpose. We also pass along ideas on the best ways to manage your PD on the job. Last but not least, we take a look at adapting and adjusting to the changes that a progressive condition can bring.

Chapter 15

Maintaining Healthy Relationships

- -

In This Chapter

▶ Renewing your relationship with your significant other

▶ Keeping kids — young and old, near and far — in the loop

▶ Maintaining close ties with the grandchildren

▶ Accepting help from your first family

▶ Letting friends be friends

▶ Keeping your sense of self

- -

*Y*our relationships with family and friends (as well as those you'll create with healthcare professionals, support group members, and others along this journey) can hold the key to successfully managing your Parkinson's disease (PD) symptoms over the long haul. In sharp contrast, shutting yourself off from people or permitting those who have loved and supported you to drift away can only make matters worse — for you and for them.

But your relationships will change. The shifts you see in balance and roles will be healthy for and vital to maintaining a full, productive life. In this chapter, we take a more in-depth look at these key relationships. After seeing how your PD can affect each of these relationships, we offer suggestions for bringing those relationships back in line so that you (and the other people) understand that your bond hasn't changed just because you have PD.

Normal is a relative term in life. With any luck, it includes the people and activities that bring satisfaction and contentment to your days. But having PD doesn't mean you need to start from scratch on a new definition of *normal* — the fundamentals are still there. Although you do need to get creative as you adapt your routines to PD, you don't need to abandon those people and activities that brought you happiness before your diagnosis.

Life, PD, and Your Significant Other

Your relationship with your significant other is likely your most important and cherished relationship. This person is the one you can trust with your deepest (and sometimes most unpleasant) feelings and thoughts; who'll be there in spite of your anger, fear, and bouts of self-pity; who'll laugh with you when your performance of some task borders on the ridiculous. This person is the one who'll act as your advocate when speaking for yourself is difficult, who'll remind you that you both have lives outside of PD, and who'll affirm that you're the same person you always were. This person is your primary care partner and, perhaps one day, your caregiver.

Sharing the journey

When one partner in a relationship gets a diagnosis of PD, that diagnosis may seem to be for both of you. Both lives will be affected every day. But how the two of you face that fact and prepare for the inevitable changes can be the difference between strengthening your relationship and straining it to the breaking point. The good news is that for most couples, facing a challenge like PD as partners actually strengthens the relationship.

If this relationship is new and relatively untested by life's normal challenges, be sure each of you knows what living with PD will likely mean. And if the relationship is longstanding but was beginning to show signs of wear and tear before the diagnosis, both of you need to face that at the outset.

Sharing the PD journey is bound to put an extra strain on the relationship — at least part of the time. In either case (that is, new but untested or established but shaky), seek the counsel of a trusted and objective third party before leaping into full-blown care-partner mode. If it's not a good fit with your significant other, you need to discuss what role your partner can manage and then decide who else in the family or close circle (perhaps an adult child, sibling, or extremely good friend) can step up.

When you get the confirmed diagnosis (see Chapter 5), each of you needs time to digest the news and react. And the first reaction for one or both of you may be denial. Or maybe your partner will become overprotective and treat you as if you're gravely ill. Underneath your partner may first feel cheated out of the life you had planned and then angry at such a selfish thought when you're the one facing a debilitating illness. Financial concerns may pop up; your partner may wonder about the costs and sacrifices involved.

Neither you nor your partner may admit any of these feelings initially. Big mistake. (Again, check out Chapter 5 for more specific information about the pitfalls of the early days after diagnosis.)

Warning! Trouble ahead!

After you've both had time to let the diagnosis sink in, you need to prepare to face some common pitfalls that can result when one partner has PD and the other remains healthy. Here are three of the most common:

✔ **Changes in the dynamics of your partnership:** With PD in the equation, roles can shift. For example, now that you have PD, your wife's job is more important than ever because your health insurance is through her employer. Understand that this puts added stress on your partnership. Not only is she facing a new role as your care partner, but she's also facing the stress of performing her best at work so her job (and that vital insurance) is secure.

At the same time, your traditional role as the head of the house and breadwinner (if you bring home the larger paycheck) is also stressed. You both need that paycheck, but how will your PD affect your ability to perform at work and for how long? (See Chapter 16 for a full discussion of PD in the workplace.) Your best bet is to prepare for such role changes by talking them through — with a counselor if necessary.

✔ **Co-dependency (not a good thing):** Co-dependency occurs when your care partner is more invested in managing your PD than you are. The danger here lies in your partner abandoning major pieces of his own life in order to take control of the situation, to fulfill what he perceives to be your needs and wishes. When his perception and your needs don't jive, resentment quickly follows.

He resents doing his best but not being appreciated (plus he's surrendering pieces of his own life to offer you this unappreciated gift!). You resent fighting as hard as you can to maintain independence and autonomy, and you feel guilty for adding to your partner's anxiety and frustration by refusing — however gently — to accept his solutions.

✔ **"But everyone else manages so well" syndrome:** Remember Jackie Kennedy after the assassination of JFK? In the face of this unspeakable personal tragedy, she held a nation's hand through the sheer force of her grace, courage, attention to detail, and devotion to her children.

Spousal care partners may remind you of Jackie Kennedy and her remarkable achievements. These men and women seem to do it all — and do it with style. She works full-time, cooks, cleans, does the yard work, manages the finances, provides the most complex level of personal care for her partner, deals with the professionals, and maintains an active family and social life. And the most annoying part is that she does it all with an aura of serenity and calm that's intimidating to say the least.

Beneath the most serene surface lie whirlpools of unspeakable pain, anxiety, and even anger and resentment at the havoc PD is wreaking. Even Jackie Kennedy's calm façade cracked behind closed doors. Just like super-partner, you and your partner do your best and that's more than enough in most cases to sustain the partnership during this difficult time.

The next section offers a couple of concrete suggestions for avoiding the pitfalls and getting on with living life.

Avoiding the pitfalls

In any life-partner relationship, certain passages come with the territory: transitions, such as children growing up and going on to lives (and families) of their own; lifestyle changes, like a bigger house, a better job, retirement, and downsizing; and tough times, great times, chaotic times, and calm times. Through it all, you and your partner have formed your own unique ways of managing each passage. Now you face life with PD. It's one more challenge — but a big one, and one that'll affect the rest of your lives.

Here are two keys to avoiding the pitfalls in your partnership while managing the stresses and strains of living with PD:

- ✔ **Communication and caring = coping:** You'll both have times when you struggle to adapt to the changes caused by PD. Your partner may feel stressed by all the extra responsibility. As the PWP, you may be depressed and anxious for good reason. Take time to talk it out, to state your needs, to listen to your partner's concerns — even if you can't immediately solve the problem. If you're seeing a counselor to manage depression and anxiety (see Chapter 13), ask that person for tips for improving communications during especially stressful times.

- ✔ **Mutual respect — the foundation of successful relationships:** Think about all the reasons the two of you teamed up in the first place. You loved her bubbly outgoing personality — so different from your shy, quiet demeanor. She loved your take-charge-in-a-crisis style. The activities that gave you individual identities also strengthened you as a couple. You aren't clones; you complement (complete) each other. Now one of you has PD and the other has been cast in this new role of care partner. Just as you adapted in the past (when the kids came along or one of you changed jobs), you can do that again.

Few relationships remain stagnant (at least those that survive and thrive don't). So chances are good that the dynamics of your partnership would have changed and shifted whether or not you had PD. So, don't permit yourself (or your partner) to stress out about the possible changes you'll face as the years pass. And for heaven's sake, don't allow PD to keep you from enjoying the intimacy that comes with living in a loving partnership.

Keeping the magic alive — Sex and intimacy in spite of PD

For some couples, one of the most challenging shifts can come in the area of intimacy. You and your partner can either surrender to a loss in this area or you can get creative and find new ways to share your love.

Humans take a certain amount of pride in their physical, mental, and even emotional attractiveness. The diagnosis of a lifelong, debilitating condition can play havoc with a person's sense of self, and it can be especially devastating for his or her sense of sexuality. The relationship you may have enjoyed with your significant other for years — even decades — suddenly comes under question. Can I adequately satisfy the needs of this person I love? Is this person humoring me by pretending that nothing's changed? Why don't I feel like being intimate even though I love this person? Doesn't this person deserve a *whole* lover?

Okay, just stop it. Take a moment to get the facts before you leap to unfounded (and, in some cases, unnecessary) conclusions. These are the facts:

- ✔ When sexual needs and desires change, the root cause usually responds to medication or other therapy. Check first with your primary care physician to see whether the cause is treatable.

- ✔ If the change comes on the heels of the diagnosis — well, duh! You just got some tough and depressing news. Talk about a mood crasher!

- ✔ As a matter of fact, depression and anxiety may well be symptoms of your PD (see Chapter 13), so your sexual concerns may result from the disease itself. And what about those prescription meds for depression? Read the label. Most likely they list sexual dysfunction as a side effect.

- ✔ Certainly people with PD may experience performance anxiety, given the facts that PD is a movement disorder, and good sex often involves coordination and flexibility.

- ✔ Women's fluctuating hormone balance in the perimenopausal years can affect desire. Women with PD should be sure their gynecologist and neurologist work together to regulate hormone replacement and antiparkinsonian medications.

- ✔ Unfortunately the effects of PD can play havoc with self-image. The *mask* (inability to show facial expression) is one example. Struggling to manage basic grooming (shaving your legs, styling your hair, putting on make-up) can also make a woman feel less than desirable.

- ✔ If you're male, you may experience episodes of erectile dysfunction — another sideshow of PD — because the brain needs to work with the body for you to maintain an erection.

So what to do? Well, you don't want to ignore any problem that may have a solution. And sexual dysfunction is one of them. Let your doctor know because treatments are available. For example, if depression is behind your change in sexual interest, counseling may be the answer.

And for both your sakes, talk to your partner. Your partner may be having problems as well. For example, when faced with a loved one's diagnosis, some partners leap light years ahead to the day (that may never come) when the loved one can't function at all. As a result, your partner goes into serious protection mode and tries to avoid any activity that he or she thinks may cause you more stress (and that includes sexual relations).

Yes, you and your partner may need to explore new ways of being intimate. Gee — experiment with new ways to kiss, to hold each other, to touch, to. . . . Sounds like a good thing!

Retaining personal space for each of you

Receiving a diagnosis of PD may draw the two of you even closer together, but don't make the mistake of abandoning your individual activities and contacts. As much as you love and cherish each other, you still need some personal space from time to time. The richness of relationships is often rooted in the fact that each has interests (and friends) that are unique. You may share news about these activities and people with each other, but you both accept that this is *my* activity or *my* friend and that's okay.

In these early weeks, you have a lot to take in (tests, doctor's appointments, therapy sessions, and such). But if your partner has enjoyed a weekly card game or volunteer activity for years and hasn't been able to get back to it for months now, this is a problem. And *you* need to lead by example. Take stock of those individual activities and contacts you've let slide and get them back on your calendar. Then insist that your partner do the same.

A second time that you and your partner are in danger of surrendering your personal space occurs when your PD symptoms become more troublesome. As your need for assistance and care escalates, your partner may become so entrenched in caring for you that her own physical, mental, and emotional well-being is jeopardized. Make it your job to prevent that problem from happening. Prepare in advance for ways each of you can protect your life beyond PD. This strategy isn't an act of selfishness; in the long run, this separateness can bring the two of you closer and enrich the life you share. (Check out Chapter 23 for more ways to care for your care partner.)

PD and Kids — Adult or Younger

For people with Parkinson's (PWP) who have children, the change in your relationships will depend in part on the age of your children. A person with young onset PD (see Chapter 8) may have very young children. But if your PD was diagnosed later in life, your children may have children of their own (your grandchildren) who will also need your attention. Regardless of their age, children can become confused or alarmed when they hear that a parent has PD. Some of that initial response comes from a knowledge base (or lack of one) about PD and its progression. And some of the response can be normal self-concern about life changes now that a parent is ill. In either case, you need to reassure your children and include them as you and your care partner make decisions that may affect their lives.

Addressing their fears about the future

"What if they need to use my college savings fund for Mom's medical bills?"

"I thought we'd have more time before I needed to be there for my parents."

You and your significant other need to discuss early on how to deliver the news of your diagnosis to your children (see Chapter 7). After you tell them, look for obvious and not-so-obvious reactions, such as withdrawal or slipping grades when she was an honor student before the diagnosis. If you see mood changes (such as increased irritability) or personality changes (your little extrovert suddenly becomes quite the introvert), talk it out. You may consider taking your preteen and teenage children with you to the next neurologist's appointment so they can raise their own questions. Or consider going with your child for some talk therapy with a counselor.

Regardless of your children's ages, your positive outlook and sense of humor will go a long way toward reassuring them that life won't change much just because you have PD. As time goes by (years — not weeks) and the PD becomes more difficult to control, your children will adapt with you.

In the following sections, we give you some tips on discussing your PD with your children, both young and adult.

When your children are young

If your children are very young (under age 10), keep your information simple. But if young children ask questions or change their normal behavior toward you, then those concerns need your attention. Just be careful not to blow problems out of proportion. For example, your child's very simple concern, "Can I catch Parkinson's like a cold?" may have an easy answer, "No."

Middle-schoolers (ages 10 to 13) need a more direct approach. Kids today can get a lot of information through the Internet. The problem is when they check sites that scare or worry them. Consider giving these children an assignment; put them in charge of staying on top of and reporting the PD e-news from the trusted sites listed in Appendix B. A specific assignment like this can help a child feel a part of the solution. It's vital that you avoid allowing children of any age feel as if they're being kept in the dark.

Teenagers (ages 14 to 19) are fully capable of participating in a family discussion (see Chapter 7) and plan of action for managing household changes. When included from the beginning, teens are more likely to take ownership and responsibility for additional chores or tasks. Whenever you and your partner reassess the plan and discuss necessary changes, include your teen.

A great way to empower children who are struggling with a parent's illness is to encourage them to raise funds for a national organization that's searching for a cure. Maybe your child can participate in a run or bike ride and ask for donations. How about a lemonade stand? Kids like action. Help them take an active (and proactive) role to raise awareness or money for research.

When your children are adults

Adult children may live at home, nearby, or miles away. They may be single, married, have children of their own, have promising and demanding careers, be in college or graduate school, or have a combination of these. The point is that they've moved on (even if they're still in your house) into lives of their own. You're a part of that life but not in the way when they were younger.

After your diagnosis, chances are good that your adult children feel (even if you don't) the roles have shifted; they may now consider taking care of you instead of the other way round. Such ideas can make for some interesting relational conflicts. Your best tactic is to clearly demonstrate through words, actions, and — most of all — attitude that you do need their support and concern but you're still fully capable of deciding how you'll live with PD.

If you don't ask, they won't help

Maybe your natural instinct as a parent is to protect your kids from worrying about you. If you constantly respond to your children's concern with, "We're doing fine," then don't be upset when your kids take that at face value and get on with their lives. But here's a news flash — they're probably worrying anyway *and* frustrated that you won't let them help. Give them a chance to help by stating your needs! (Check out Chapter 7 for more on this step.) The worst result is that you'll be disappointed by the reaction. The best result is that your child steps up to the plate and delivers a solid hit by taking on some chore, visiting more often, or bringing the grandkids to see you more often.

When they live nearby

Adult children who live nearby can be a blessing for you and your care partner — especially when your PD progresses and you can use a little more help. Establish some new family traditions, like potluck or ordered-in dinners once a week for you, the kids, and grandkids. This ritual can

- ✔ Help your children and grandchildren adapt to the impact of your symptoms on your normal life

- ✔ Open the door to the more intense regular contact down the road

Because PD tends to progress slowly, you'll probably read the signs that your symptoms are getting worse. (For example, your meds may not work as well and routine tasks become a struggle.) When you recognize these new limits on your abilities, consider a family meeting (see Chapter 10).

The following suggestions can help you in that meeting:

- ✔ Offer specific ways your adult children (and older grandchildren) can pitch in.

- ✔ Clearly demonstrate that you appreciate their busy schedules.

- ✔ Start small. For example, can your grandson cut the lawn? Can your daughter cook up a casserole once a month for the freezer?

Ask yourself whether you would have been willing to commit to this responsibility when you were your kids' ages. Would you have cheerfully taken on additional weekly tasks? Would you have put this ahead of everything else on your schedule? If the answer to these questions is "No," then perhaps your ideas about what and how much responsibility your children can handle is overly optimistic. Far better to start out with smaller, less time-consuming tasks such as loading the dishwasher or taking out the garbage and then add more responsibility as time (and your PD) progress.

The goal: Involve your adult children almost from the beginning so that, as your needs escalate, they are already a part of the routine. Be sure you include them in the decisions and planning. Ask for their opinion and input. The decision is ultimately yours, but including your children in the discussion permits them to feel a vital and valued part of the whole process.

If some adult children live nearby and some live farther away, don't take the assistance of nearby children for granted. In many families, visits from far-away kids and grandkids are a cause for celebration, but in-town children who provide regular hands-on help (at some personal sacrifice) also need to feel appreciated. Call your in-town daughter specifically for the purpose of thanking her after she's rearranged her schedule to do something for you. Comment on how much you appreciate something specific that each of your children (in-town and out-of-town) does for you when you're all together.

When they're far away

Adult children who live far away may suffer some guilt from not being available. When they visit, you may want to plan some major project (changing the storms and screens, cleaning the basement, or painting the kitchen) so they become a part of that hands-on care routine. You want them to realize that they're not your guests — they're your children. Even though they can only offer sporadic hands-on help, you still need them to come through for you and your care partner.

Be sure to include these adult children in family meetings and conferences (even if only by e-mail or phone). Ask for their input and include them as you come to a decision. In short, distance can shut down lines of communication even with today's cell phones, computers, and such. Make a personal commitment to keep all your adult children in the loop. They need to hear your news, including major decisions or changes, from you (or your care partner) — not from a sibling.

PD and Grandchildren

Your first step with your grandchildren is to consult with their parents before you talk with them about your PD. How do the parents want you to handle their children's questions? What have the parents told your grandchildren already, and how did they tell them? After you know those answers, show your grandchildren through your interactions that nothing has really changed. You are still Grandma or Grandpa. Keep your routine with them as normal as possible.

If you've played games or gone apple-picking with them in the past, keep that up. If those tasks aren't possible for you now, find new activities. Perhaps make a game of doing your exercises with your grandchild. Or go to the apple farm and buy the apples, bring them home, and make applesauce with your grandchildren. Most of all, reassure them with simple but honest answers to their questions, and let their parents know whether you see signs that your grandchildren are holding questions or concerns inside.

Children are wise beyond their years and extraordinarily tuned in to the moods and vibes of the adults in their world. They may not fully understand what's going on, but they know when you're upset, sad, depressed, or angry. And more often than not, they mistakenly think they're to blame or that your mood has something to do with them.

We're not suggesting you fake a happy-go-lucky attitude around the young ones. But don't sell them short. You're the adult here. You know when your frustration causes you to lash out or withdraw. Pay attention to your reactions and to the reactions of the child you're with and speak up. "Sorry I snapped at you. Sometimes I just get so frustrated when I can't do the things I used to do. Do you ever feel sad like that?" Now you've opened the door to a dialogue with the child and perhaps to a conversation that can reveal some of their own angst about your PD.

Children and grandchildren of all ages can be good medicine. Their curiosity and sense of adventure can be contagious in a good way. Their belief that they're indestructible and immortal can be inspiring. The way that kids pack 40 hours of activity and energy into a single day can serve as an important reminder: This is the day we get — live it or lose it!

PD and Parents and Siblings

If you have children of your own, you realize that nothing's as terrible as discovering that your child has an incurable and progressive condition. Regardless of your age, you will always be your parent's child.

If the parent-child relationship is such that you can confide in your parent, allow your parent to play the role of mentor and counselor as you face this new challenge. Seek advice for balancing the demands of PD with your other life responsibilities. A good way to start this discussion is to remind your parents of difficult challenges they've faced over the course of their lives.

However, if your parents are more emotionally fragile and thrown by the news of your illness, your role may become one of reassuring them rather than relying on them. But, because you really don't need more emotional responsibility at this time, consider asking a sibling to reassure Mom and Dad. This arrangement can be especially helpful if your brothers or sisters are looking for ways they can offer you support and tangible help.

Considering parents and siblings, remember that you have a longstanding history with these people. If you never could please your mother or if your brother always had to live up to your example, those facts have colored the way your family interacts. Don't make the mistake of expecting the foundations of your relationships to magically change simply because you have PD.

Over the course of your life each of you has found ways to adapt to those unique interactions. Perhaps you handle your Mom's apparent disappointment in you by simply enduring her comments and moving on. Good choice. Likewise your brother's sense of insecurity (and inferiority) is his issue — not yours. Be sympathetic but understand that he's no more likely to step up now than he has before.

If your sister or brother becomes your primary care partner, the two of you need ground rules about the relationship just as if your care partner were your spouse or significant other. For example:

✔ You both need to acknowledge and then set aside the familial roles you may have assumed throughout childhood. For example, if she always played the big sister role and you followed her lead, that relationship needs to change. The way you choose to handle life with PD is your decision, and she needs to be willing to follow your lead.

✔ You both need to face the fact that you're adults, which means you've probably gone in different directions philosophically and may have different approaches to a variety of issues.

Having said that, you need to focus on the reasons having your sister as your care partner makes sense: She brings strengths to the table that you counted on when the two of you were growing up. You've chosen her for those strengths. She's agreed because your history tells her that she can work with you the same way the two of you faced challenges together as children.

For people diagnosed with young onset PD (see Chapter 8), the chances are very good that your parents are still living. If your parents' health is compromised and you're providing some care for them, you and your care partner need to consider how best to incorporate your dual role as adult child with PD and caregiver for aging parents into an already busy life.

PD and Close Friends

No matter what your friendships are like, there's nothing like a chronic, progressive, and eventually debilitating condition for sorting out friends who'll be there from those who'll eventually drift away. And discovering who's who in this process is usually surprising. The guy you thought would be there no matter what may not handle the idea that you can't enjoy the vigorous sports activities the two of you have always shared. Even though you assure him that it may be years before that happens, he doesn't hear you. Meanwhile a co-worker you've always seen as a casual acquaintance (nice to have a beer with after work and such) steps up, intuitively understanding how to be helpful but not intrusive for you or your care partner.

The following suggestions help you make this transition with your friends as smooth as possible:

✔ **Tell it like it is:** Friends may want to help but don't know how. And, like everyone else, they'll take their lead from you. If you repeatedly assure them that everything's fine and reject their efforts to understand PD and figure out how to help, then shame on you. And if you shut them out with self-pity, depression, and a nobody-can-help attitude, don't be surprised when they drift away.

It's all in how you look at it

At the foundation of your ability to maintain healthy relationships is your ability to maintain a healthy sense of self. With respect to PD, you certainly have an impressive roster of celebrities to emulate (Muhammad Ali and Michael J. Fox to name the most obvious). But, to understand the importance of this sense-of-self on a personal level, go to a PD support group meeting and look around.

Joan sits over there in a corner. Diagnosed two years ago, her symptoms are well controlled with medication. Yet Joan is always looking for the downside; her conversations project a dire future. She likes to report disastrous cases, like the person who fell, hit his head, and became demented almost overnight. (Take this opportunity to move on as quickly as possible!)

You notice Charlie in another part of the room. He's had PD for over a decade. His hand shakes uncontrollably at times, he has trouble swallowing, and you have to lean in close to hear him. But you discover that he still runs his own business, attends social functions with his wife, and is an active volunteer in the fight to find a cure for PD. He's telling a story about his latest doctor's visit:

"Doc asked whether I had vivid dreams . . . and whether I was in my dreams," he says. "I told him I was in my dreams, and I didn't have PD — just me moving freely with no tremor."

You ask Charlie what the doctor said about that and Charlie replies, "He said I must have one whopper of a positive outlook!"

You can be Joan, you can be Charlie, or you can be someone in between. The choice is yours. No doubt Charlie has his bad days. But how he's chosen to get through those days is worth finding out.

✔ **Treat me the same:** Okay, you don't want to lose your friends, but you also don't want them treating you any different. Tell them that. Be open to their questions. Give them the facts. Seriously consider their suggestions for treatments, doctors, and such before you reject them out of hand. Let your friends know you'll have good days and bad. And then decide together how they can best support you.

✔ **Lend me an ear:** Friends are terrific at playing the role of confidante for you and your care partner. And, by the way, we hope you and your care partner have one really good friend (not the same one!) that you can trust to hear you vent, whine, and feel sorry for yourself now and again.

✔ **Know their strong suits:** Recognize that some people are good listeners and counselors and others need to offer hands-on help. Surely you know these folks well enough to know the difference. So when the inevitable question of "What can I do to help?" arises, be prepared with concrete and specific ideas — just as you try to with your children and other family members.

✔ **Keep a balance:** Beware of accepting too much help. Some people (friends and family) may start strong, practically smothering you with their help. But the odds are good that these people will over-promise and under-deliver, eventually burning out. By the same token, the more you permit other people to do for you — especially early on — the less you push yourself to remain active and independent for as long as possible.

And Then There's YOU

Having Parkinson's is a life-changing situation — one that will continue to affect you for the rest of your days. But are you a PD patient, or are you still the same active, involved, in-charge person you were before you had PD? You can choose to allow a diagnosis of PD to dominate your daily routine even in the early stages or you can take the proactive approach — doing what it takes to adapt PD to your lifestyle.

Consider these two questions: How many hours do you average each work-week? Between what times do those hours occur? For most people, the answer to the first question is between 40 and 60 hours, and the second answer is between 8 a.m. and 6 p.m. So, one way to look at adapting PD is to focus on those daytime hours and how to use them in meaningful ways.

Although you certainly can't schedule your PD symptoms, the basic idea of adapting PD to fit your lifestyle has some merit. You're still the same person you were before you got diagnosed. Your life's activities may need to change over time — just as they do for everyone with or without PD. But for now, your normal routine is probably still viable.

As a matter of fact, you may be able to get back to some activities you had dropped when your PD symptoms went untreated. Perhaps your stiffness and slowness can be partially relieved through physical therapy and a regular exercise routine (see Chapter 12). Maybe those feelings of anxiety, persistent sadness, and depression that you thought were job-related are treatable with therapy and counseling (see Chapter 13). And maybe your hand tremor can be managed with medication (see Chapter 9).

The point is that you and those around you had a life before you were diagnosed, and you still have that life. You may have to accept changes, but your ability to participate in those activities that gave your life purpose and meaning are still possible.

Chapter 16

PD in the Workplace

In This Chapter

▶ Get ready, get set: Understanding your work potential

▶ Timing is everything

▶ Approaching your boss with the news

▶ Checking in with Human Resources

▶ Getting the right word out to co-workers

▶ Tapping into private and government programs that can help

*A*dapting to life with Parkinson's disease (PD) works best when you can partner with other people. We hope you're already partnering with your healthcare team (see Chapter 6) and your primary care partner (along with your family and friends — see Chapter 15). The third angle of this partnering triangle is your partnership with your employer and co-workers, a relationship that permits you to stay on the job and takes into account your employer's need to run the business effectively. In this chapter, we offer some ideas for delivering the news and building the workplace version of that team-oriented partnership.

Don't assume that our suggestions are exactly right for your situation. Every employer-employee relationship is unique, just as your PD is different from other people's PD. You know the specific climate that surrounds your workplace, and only you can decide the best approach for telling your employer that you have PD.

Doing Your Homework

If there's one message we pound home in this book, it's this: Your best course of action in all facets of managing your PD is to prepare, prepare, and then prepare some more. That advice is never more true than when you're about to tell your employer that you have a chronic and progressive condition. And those words are exactly (and probably only) what your boss is likely to hear. Therefore your job is to prepare to fight that misperception with every resource you can muster.

Before you tell your employer, you have homework — and yes, we do mean you! In broad strokes (with details to follow), here are your assignments:

- Put together an honest assessment of your position requirements and whether or not you can continue to fulfill them.

- Discuss your job responsibilities with your neurologist and get a medical evaluation of your ability to perform those duties.

- Research what the company can offer to accommodate your changing needs and has offered other employees in the past (such as a different workstation configuration or a flexible schedule so you can work when your symptoms are well managed or work from home).

- Familiarize yourself with options that may be available through the Americans with Disabilities Act (ADA) or other government programs.

Honestly assess your ability to continue in the job

Before you start spreading the news that you have PD to your boss and co-workers, decide how and if you'll be able to continue working. To do this, you first need a clear understanding of your job requirements and performance demands. You and your neurologist both need this information so you can honestly assess your ability to continue in the job as your PD progresses. For example, if your job requires fine hand-work and you already have a significant tremor in one hand, you can't ignore this problem.

Keep in mind that PD progresses at different rates for different people and neither you nor your doctor can really predict its course. However, two ways to acquire the information you and your doctor need in order to make the best possible assessment are:

- Reviewing the written job description from when you were hired

- Taking advantage of recent or upcoming performance review sessions where your employer restates the expectations and requirements of the position

If you didn't receive a printed job description or your next performance review isn't in the near future, then consider asking for an informal conversation with your supervisor — especially if she's not the same person who hired you. Her expectations for your performance may not be the same as your former supervisor's were. Keep the meeting informal and conversational. If you say something like, "I wonder whether you'd give me a written, detailed description of my position," you're going to raise all sorts of red flags (especially if you've been working there for some time already).

If you have no job description and can't have a chat with your immediate supervisor, take time to think through the tasks required of you — physical, mental, and emotional (stress-related). Be as specific as possible.

This is the time — *before* you sit down with your supervisor to deliver the news that you have PD — to be brutally honest. For now, no one else is asking these questions or listening to your answers. But if you try and fudge the answers when you know your PD's already making some tasks difficult, you're only harming yourself.

Ask yourself the following questions:

- ✔ Do you have a desk job, a manufacturing job, or something more physical?
- ✔ How many hours a week are you scheduled?
- ✔ How much overtime or work at home do you typically have in a week?
- ✔ What are the physical demands of the job (Standing most of the time? Sitting at a computer? Moving around — perhaps teaching small children — much of the workday? Traveling? Needing fine motor control?)
- ✔ What are the mental demands of the job? (Quick decisions? Complex problem-solving? Coordinating the efforts of several other people?)
- ✔ What are the stressors of the job? (Bottom line expectations of employer? Deadlines? Balancing several projects at the same time?)
- ✔ What are the emotional challenges of the job? (Supervisor is in over his head, making your job harder? Working in healthcare with patients who are ill or infirm? Balancing the demands of your job with your role as a spouse or parent and your PD symptoms?)
- ✔ And finally, do you see your schedule getting less intense? More intense?

At your next appointment with your neurologist, discuss your job requirements and how to adapt your PD symptoms — those you're experiencing now and those that are most likely to occur over the next year or so — to the demands of the job (and vice versa). Take notes. If you think your employer may have safety concerns but your doctor indicates that you can continue the job, ask your doctor for a letter stating that you're capable of performing the tasks in question.

Consider options that may be available

Depending on the size of your company, you may have an entire list of options to help you stay on the job and perform effectively — or you may have no options at all. If you work for a larger company, your employer may be able to offer flexible hours, job-sharing, working from home one or two days a week, or a reduced workload (which, of course, may have a reduction in pay).

But even the small business owner may still have some options. For example, if you work in a restaurant that's busiest at breakfast and lunch, your employer has little leeway for adapting your hours. But is it possible for you to work a later shift when the restaurant has fewer customers to serve?

Think outside the box. Your employer's not the only one responsible for devising options for you. The employee who needs to be on the job by seven but struggles with getting up, dressed and out the door in time to meet that start time may need to get up an hour earlier and talk to his doctor about adjusting the timing on his medication routine to accommodate his early morning start time.

If you work for a larger company, you probably received an employee handbook as a part of your new hire information. As part of preparing to tell your boss about your diagnosis, dig this employee handbook out and read it. Better yet, go to the company's internal Web site and get the latest version. If your company (or the company your care partner works for) provides group insurance for employees, read those policies. Make notes so that in the meeting with your boss (and eventually the person from Human Resources, HR) you have a firm understanding of the company's policies regarding special accommodations or coverage for short- or long-term disability.

Deciding When to Disclose Your Diagnosis

Although PD is progressive, it isn't one of those you've-got-six-months-to-live situations. You have some time to tell your employer about your PD. On the other hand, you also want to choose the best time for your specific situation. We help you make that all-important decision in this section.

From your perspective

Only you can decide the appropriate time to tell your employer. The goal is to minimize the fallout from sharing this kind of news.

Consider the effects of these two scenarios:

- ✔ You rush in to your boss's office within days of the diagnosis and announce that you have PD.
- ✔ You withhold the news until your symptoms become more difficult to control and begin to affect your performance.

In the first case, the danger lies in your employer (and co-workers) viewing you *and* your performance differently. In other words, well before your PD symptoms have any effect on your ability, other people may perceive a problem and attribute it to your PD. Inadvertently you may be labeled and pigeon-holed (possibly passed over for a better position) because of other people's misperceptions.

In the second scenario, you may think you're controlling your symptoms, but your news comes as no surprise to your employer or co-workers. If your boss has been aware of a change in your performance for some time, she may wonder why you took so long to come forward. Worse, if facial *mask* (lack of facial expression) is one of your symptoms, she may have interpreted that symptom as disinterest or apathy and then attributed the decline in your performance to that misinterpretation.

If your supervisor has expressed concern about your recent job performance (via questions like "Is everything all right?" or "How's everything going at home?" or even at a more formal review of your performance), that's a good hint that he's concerned about you and the work he needs from you.

Depending on your job, it may be years before your PD has any real impact. In the meantime, make use of the initial days and weeks following your diagnosis to accept that you have PD and that it's going to be a factor in every facet of your life, including your work. (See Chapter 5 for more specific ideas on getting through those first weeks after diagnosis.)

If you know that safety will eventually become an issue, stay ahead of the curve by considering other positions within the company that you can handle as your PD progresses. If training for such positions is available, take it to maximize your options. Prepare and plan ahead.

From your employer's perspective

Keep in mind that bosses can't look at a situation in isolation. Employers must consider how your situation affects other people and, yes, ultimately, the bottom line. This fact of life may seem harsh, but the point of opening a business is to make enough money to reinvest in the company's future and keep the business going. Most employers want very much to maintain good employees. If you're a person who delivers on the job and adds value to the company, your employer will probably be eager to help you stay on the job for as long as possible.

If safety is relevant to your position, your employer can't put the company, you, or your co-workers at risk. And in this case, the bottom line isn't about making a profit; it's about security for you, your co-workers, and your families.

The first person to tell at work is your immediate supervisor (and then the folks in your HR department). In rare circumstances, employers can be short-sighted when it comes to supporting employees in tough personal situations. Maybe you and your supervisor already have an adversarial relationship, so you're concerned your PD will tip the situation over the edge.

In such cases you may be tempted to go around your superior and seek out someone in the company that seems more supportive. But this plan only makes the problem worse and can actually backfire on you. Your supervisor may resent being passed over and make it more difficult for you to convince other people that you're still a valuable asset to the company.

Telling Your Boss

Okay, the moment's at hand. It's time to deliver the news of your PD to your employer. Here are some steps to consider:

1. **Request a meeting.**

   This can be informal if you and your supervisor have a relationship that permits you to say, "Do you have 20 to 30 minutes today or tomorrow? I need to talk to you about something." If the request needs to be more formal, follow the company process for requesting and scheduling a meeting with your supervisor or manager. Allow at least 30 minutes for the meeting.

2. **Prepare and practice your talking points — those key points you want your boss to hear after you've said, "I have Parkinson's."**

   Keep the points short and simple. This is no time to try to educate your boss about the intricacies of PD. Ideally, you'll take a positive and proactive approach. For example, you may say, "I've been diagnosed with Parkinson's disease." (Allow time for a short response — hopefully a sympathetic one.) You continue, "The good news is that progression is slow and my doctor agrees that it may be some time — even years — before symptoms really have an impact."

3. **Demonstrate that you've done your homework.**

   Your boss may hear very little after you say, "I have Parkinson's." And inevitably he'll start thinking of its short- and long-term impact on the business. This may be a good time to offer him a simple fact sheet about what PD is (and is not).

   This is also a good time to produce a copy of any letter your neurologist has provided that states your ability to continue in the job.

   Follow up with a few simple comments that demonstrate the effort you've already given the situation: You've reviewed the job description and performance expectations set out for your position; you've met with your doctor and gone over the demands of the job; and your doctor has given you the letter. This is where all your homework and advance preparation pay off, but keep it short and simple. You don't want to inadvertently raise red flags by saying something like, "And as for the travel piece of my job, well, I'm pretty sure that won't be a problem as long as the travel doesn't increase."

Note: You don't want to come off as threatening or adversarial at a time like this; you don't want the message to be, "I have PD, and I know my rights." Instead, say something like, "I know this raises all sorts of questions, but I'm confident that together we can find answers and solutions that will allow me to continue to contribute effectively."

4. **Maintain a positive and can-do attitude throughout the meeting regardless of the response you get from your manager.**

   Understand that your manager is going to need some time to take this all in, so don't agree to any firm offer or accommodation your supervisor may offer off the top of his head at this initial meeting. Acknowledge any such offer as a possibility but one that you should both discuss after he's had time to digest the news — the same way you needed some time to digest your diagnosis.

   You know that having PD is a challenge but not a deal-breaker when it comes to your ability to contribute. Your job in this meeting is to demonstrate through your can-do attitude that this is just one more challenge you can conquer.

5. **Address the subject of co-workers at some point in the meeting.**

   One suggestion is to meet with the members of your immediate department and give them the news. Show your manager a brief fact sheet that answers frequently asked questions about PD. (One excellent handout is available online at www.ninds.nih.gov/disorders/parkinsons_disease.) Tell your employer that, with permission, you want to tell these co-workers about your diagnosis, give them the fact sheet, and ask them to help squelch rumors or misinformation as the news spreads.

6. **Let your manager know that you'll be contacting the HR department to gather information about your benefits and options.**

7. **Thank your manager for his support and concern and ask whether the two of you should set a time to meet again or you should wait to hear from HR. Then get back to work.**

Getting the Facts from HR

Your HR department can provide answers to most questions related to your insurance options and work options if you're no longer able to do your job. But just as you prepared for your meeting with your manager, prepare a list of questions for this meeting, and be ready to write down the answers (or get printed materials that provide the information).

The Americans with Disabilities Act — your golden parachute — maybe

According to the Equal Employment Opportunity Commission (EEOC), the Americans with Disabilities Act (ADA) gives civil rights protections (similar to those for race, color, sex, national origin, age, and religion) to individuals with disabilities. The ADA prohibits discrimination in all employment practices: job application procedures, hiring and firing regulations, promotion opportunities, benefits, and compensation.

The broad protection given by the ADA sounds very promising. But keep in mind the fine points as well — points that can affect your rights under the law. Examples are:

✔ If your workplace employs fewer than 15 people, you may not be covered under this legislation.

✔ As a person with PD, your disability must "substantially limit major life activities such as seeing, hearing, speaking, walking, breathing, performing manual tasks, learning, caring for oneself, and working."

✔ You must be qualified to fill the requirements of the job, and your employer maintains the right to establish performance and production standards that all employees must meet, disabled or not.

The ADA further requires your employer to consider whether you can continue to do your job with certain "reasonable accommodation." Examples of this requirement include special products (such as voice-activated computers), changes that make your existing workspace more accessible, or restructuring the job itself.

Because every disability and its effect on an employee's ability to do a specific job is slightly different, keep the following suggestions in mind:

✔ Your employer will rely on you to speak up and suggest possible solutions. If you don't have a suggestion, do some research and work with your employer to find one.

✔ Understand that the company is expected to pay for any equipment or necessary accommodation, but your employer isn't required to provide an accommodation that causes an *undue hardship* on other employees or the business. If cost is a factor (and you can afford it), you may consider offering to pay part of the cost.

✔ The ADA doesn't give you a free ride. Your employer can hold you to the same standards of performance and production as people without disabilities. You have a responsibility to be honest with yourself and your employer about your ability to meet those standards.

We strongly urge you to

✔ Become familiar with the pros and cons of the ADA for your situation.

✔ Not assume an adversarial or threatening attitude with your employer when it comes to applying ADA regulations to your situation.

Managing your PD is a team effort between you and your health team, you and your care-partnering family and friends, and you and your employer.

For more information about ADA, call 800-514-0301 (voice within USA), 800-514-0383 (TTY), 202-514-0301 (outside USA) or check out www.ada.gov.

When you meet with your HR representative, you're actually on a fact-finding mission. You're not necessarily going to act on any of the following factors right away, but you need to clearly understand your employer's policy related to:

✔ Disability

✔ Early retirement

✔ Availability of any pension/401K funds

✔ Government programs, such as COBRA

✔ Health savings accounts (HSAS)

✔ Social Security disability benefits

✔ Medicare and Medicaid

✔ Any available state health insurance pools

The Americans with Disabilities Act (ADA) can be a real resource of options as your PD progresses. But be aware that the ADA doesn't apply to all employers, and it does have limitations. (See the sidebar, "The Americans with Disabilities Act — your golden parachute — maybe.")

Positioning the News for Co-Workers

The type of job you have and the people you work closely with will influence what and how much you tell your co-workers. Here are two possible scenarios:

✔ You are in a management or supervisory position and have several people who report directly to you. After you've told your boss (and gotten his agreement that you need to break the news to your team), call a meeting of your group. Keep it informal. (In some business settings, this meeting is called a *huddle,* like a football team huddling to get the play before going into action. The huddle's a great analogy for the kind of atmosphere you want to create for delivering this news.) Consider taking these steps:

    • Deliver the news. Do it with humor, if possible, but keep it direct and simple.

    • Hand out the simple fact sheet about PD (see the earlier section, "Telling Your Boss").

    • Lay out the ground rules for what aspects may change, but emphasize that it will be business as usual — you're still a team.

- Offer some guidelines for how you expect your team to handle any gossip or rumors they may hear about you or PD. (Remind them that they can squelch any such nonsense using the simple facts you've provided.)

- Let your co-workers know that they can come directly to you with any concerns or questions, assure them that you are most definitely still you, and send them back to work.

✔ You're part of a close-knit group whose ability to succeed relies on everyone pulling her weight. Your teammates react to the news with one of two attitudes: "Poor Mary. How will she manage? What can I do to help her?" or "Poor me" (as in "This is going to end up meaning more work for me."). Be prepared for either reaction by:

- Maintaining that same upbeat, can-do attitude you demonstrated when you told your boss

- Offering the fact sheet and stating outright that, according to your doctor, you're going to be around for years to come

- Assuring everyone that you're not expecting special considerations from them and you'll continue to pull your weight on the team

The manner in which you deliver the news of your PD to your manager and co-workers forms their attitude as they carry that news forward. If you're positive and upbeat, they're more likely to assure others that you have a real handle on it. And that image is exactly the one you want to project to everyone.

Taking Steps to Protect Your Income

Working people have a variety of ways to protect themselves and their dependents if they can no longer work. The following list describes the more common methods.

Although this list provides general definitions of a variety of options, we aren't recommending any one of these programs. If you need to leave your job and rely on other sources for your income, consult with a qualified financial planner or counselor (see Chapter 21).

✔ **Income-generating plans:**

- **Employer Disability Plans**: Such plans can be short- or long-term, and eligibility requirements differ from one employer to another. In general these plans allow employees to purchase short- and long-term disability insurance as a part of their overall company-sponsored benefit package. If you need to leave work because of a disability, the plan pays you a percentage of your salary while you're disabled. Some plans pay that full percentage even if you're also eligible for and receiving benefits from Social Security (see the next bullet); other plans may prorate their payments based on what you receive from the government. (For specific information of disability benefits, talk to your HR department.)

- **Social Security Disability Plans**: This segment of Social Security is different from the more common retirement benefit payout. Two programs are available: Social Security Disability Insurance (SSDI) and Supplemental Security Income (SSI). Both programs have stringent eligibility requirements.

  SSDI is for people with an established work history; the amount received is determined by that history and specific earnings.

  SSI is based on financial need and serves people with little work history and very limited financial assets. (For more information on becoming eligible for either program, call 800-772-1213 or go to www.ssa.gov.)

✔ **Insurance coverage options:**

- **The Consolidated Omnibus Budget Reconciliation Act (COBRA)**: This option permits employees who lose their employer-sponsored benefits to pay out-of-pocket for the same health insurance coverage they received while working. The normal period you can pay for coverage is 18 months after you leave unless you're determined to be disabled, in which case you can extend coverage to a total of 36 months. (For more information, talk to your HR department.)

- **Long-Term Care (LTC) insurance:** LTC insurance plans provide coverage for care necessary to help a person with the basic activities of daily living, such as bathing and dressing. Benefits are usually available for a range of settings — the home, an assisted-living facility, or a nursing home.

  A growing trend among employers is to offer an LTC insurance option as a part of the employee benefit package. If your company provides this option and you haven't taken advantage of it, check into it again. If you aren't eligible, your care partner may be. (For more information on LTC insurance, talk to your HR department or call your state Office on Insurance.)

- **Medicare:** People under the age of 65 can qualify for Medicare (the federal health insurance and drug coverage plan). For current information on qualifying if you aren't yet 65, call 800-633-4227 or go to www.cms.hhs.gov. (For a more complete explanation of the Medicare program, see Chapter 21.)

- **SHIP Programs and Medicaid:** Every state has some form of a State Health Insurance Counseling and Assistance Program (SHIP) to help its citizens find the best insurance options regardless of the person's financial or health situation. In addition, every state offers Medicaid, the federally funded and state-managed program that provides health services based on financial need. (For more information on Medicaid in your state, go to `www.hcfa.hhs.gov/medicaid`.)

Chapter 17

Adjusting Your Routine as Your PD Progresses

....

In This Chapter

▶ Easing into new routines and daily rhythms

▶ Keeping the family up to date and in focus

▶ Befriending your friends

▶ Going public *and* enjoying it

▶ Making room for R&R

▶ Going forward with your care partner

....

*I*n the early months after the onset of your Parkinson's disease (PD) symptoms, you may be surprised how little accommodation your symptoms require. In fact, if your doctor's recommended regular exercise and a balanced diet and you've followed her advice, you may be feeling better than you have in some time. Your symptoms may actually be more of an annoyance than any real concern. Now that you think about it, you may have avoided going to see the doctor for that reason — the symptoms weren't really interfering with your routine.

As time goes by, however, your symptoms will become troublesome enough to affect your life and routine — perhaps significantly. But this doesn't mean you can't live a full and active life. In this chapter, we offer tips for managing your symptoms — even as they worsen — *without* letting PD be the driving force in your life.

You're the same person you were before the diagnosis. You hold the same importance to your family and friends and retain many of the talents and skills you developed through your life. You may need to adapt — doing activities a different way, at a slower pace, or even with the help of others — but nothing about your essential identity has changed.

Exploring Ways to Make Daily Activities Easier

You can take a number of positive and proactive steps to keep your daily routine from overwhelming you. In this section, we look at some key ways that you can stay in control — as long as you're willing to adapt and not dig in your heels with a my-way-or-the-highway attitude!

Do not allow other people's expectations or your own internal demands to direct your activity. The added stress of trying to compete or live up to last year's successes (big and little) can have an adverse effect on your overall health. Stress and performance anxiety can actually inflame your symptoms and incapacitate you even more — at least momentarily.

Timing your activities

The main difference in your life now is timing — it can be everything. Your ability to understand when you can and can't do something may be the key to continuing many (or most) activities you've always enjoyed. We're not talking about timing your meds (which you and your doctor need to work out together) or your activities for your *on* times (see Chapter 9). We're talking about accepting and understanding that *everything* is a matter of time. You take longer to get ready to go places and longer to get from here to there. You take longer to do a task (like dressing or brushing your teeth) that you used to knock off in a matter of minutes.

Even if you take four or five times longer, you're still independent. It's important that you continue to perform these basic activities with little (if any) help for as long as possible.

Those around you — family, friends, employer, co-workers — also need to understand this need for extra time. Working out an appropriate time schedule for tasks you perform personally or on the job is important. Be realistic. If you used to take 15 minutes to do something, you may now need an hour.

Reserving your energy

Accept that your energy is limited and must be conserved and used wisely. This attitude can help protect your right to live independently and fully for as long as possible. Some days you'll just be downright pooped, unable to complete the list of activities you'd planned. So what? Are you saying you never fell short of completing an ambitious list *before* the onset of your PD symptoms?

Yeah, right. Everyone overestimates the potential for accomplishment from time to time. You're just wise enough to say, "Okay, I'll tackle that tomorrow — or the next day."

Approach each day with an I-don't-have-to-do-everything-but will-do-as-much-as-I (and my PD)-can attitude. These are a few more tips to help you manage your energy bank:

- ✔ Take the time to think through the demands on your schedule each day; prioritize the list by what you need to tackle and what you can put aside for later.

- ✔ Schedule important tasks for when you're at peak-performance.

- ✔ Discuss with your doctor the advantages of regular exercise and diet changes for improving your levels of energy; implement his suggestions.

Taking tips from other PWP

Your ability to manage basic tasks may vary greatly from hour to hour and depend on where you are in your medication dosing cycle. But the ingenuity of 1.2 million people with PD (PWP) in the United States and a history of nearly two hundred years can provide you with more than a few tricks to make your life with PD easier. The following sections share ways other people with Parkinson's (PWP) maintain independence in spite of their symptoms.

Your occupational therapist (OT) can offer ideas and explain proven techniques for adapting your routine to accommodate your symptoms. Appendix B also recommends a number of resources and devices available to make life easier.

Strategizing

Your determination to be as independent as possible — no matter how long a basic task takes — begins with curiosity and imagination. Take advantage of these general tips to make each day run a little more smoothly:

- ✔ Try to approach each situation as a separate challenge and break each task into individual steps. Focus on one step at a time. Try to start with the simplest one; after you've conquered that, move on.

- ✔ Keep in mind that timing is everything — coordinate the timing of these tasks with your medication routine to avoid *off* symptoms (see Chapter 9) that can make each step even more frustrating.

- ✔ Let your partner know that the difficulties you face are as frustrating for you as they are for her, but it's important that you continue to try. Discuss ways she can help without taking away your opportunity to do as much as you can. For example, your partner can put toothpaste on your toothbrush and leave it out for you. Or while you shower or bathe, your care partner can remain nearby in case you need help; she can also lay out your clothing for the day.

Grooming

Personal grooming is probably so much a part of your day that you barely think about all the individual tasks. Brushing your teeth, washing your face, shaving (if you're a man), applying makeup (if you're a woman), and combing your hair are routines you've performed for decades.

But now your symptoms are making these simple tasks next to impossible and even exhausting. Are you at the point where you need to ask for help? Not necessarily. Give these proven techniques a try:

- ✔ Sit down instead of standing — you'll not only conserve energy but also lower the risk of losing your balance and falling.

- ✔ Prop your elbows on the counter to steady your hand and support your shoulders as you shave or apply makeup.

- ✔ Use electronic appliances — razor, toothbrush, and so forth — that do a lot of the work for you.

- ✔ Try a hairstyle that's easier to manage and dries quickly without a hair dryer. In a pinch, try one of the dry-shampoo products available at drugstores or beauty supply shops.

- ✔ Treat yourself to a weekly (or bi-weekly) shampoo and styling at a discount hair salon or local beauty school. (This tip is also great therapy for relieving stress!)

- ✔ Suggest a certificate for a professional manicure or pedicure when people ask for birthday or holiday gift ideas. Or check with a local beauty school for a less-expensive session with a student.

Other people respond more positively to the person who takes an interest in the way she looks. And looking your best empowers and keeps you in control of your own destiny. So make the effort — put your best face and foot forward every day.

Dressing

Before your PD symptoms started getting in the way, you probably never thought about the many balance and flex movements that are necessary just to put clothes on.

Before you begin breaking down this task into manageable steps, take the time to go through your closet and assess your wardrobe. Are the clothes easy to put on and take off? Consider these suggestions:

✔ Look for pieces with closures that are easy to manage. Try an elastic waist in place of a button and zipper, for example.

✔ Consider replacing the buttons on a favorite shirt or blouse with magnetic snaps or Velcro closures.

✔ Consider having the buttons sewn closed when clothes are loose or stretchy enough to pull on over your head.

✔ Use elastic shoelaces (or shoes with Velcro closings) to avoid tying your shoes.

Avoid clothing items that only make life more difficult for you, no matter how much you love them. For example,

✔ Stay away from fabrics that tend to cling or stick to other fabrics (flannel, velour, corduroy, and such).

✔ Avoid sweatpants that have elastic at the ankles.

✔ Get rid of bedroom slippers (use non-skid socks like hospitals have), and avoid heavy-weight shoes (wingtips, for example).

✔ Women: Abandon pantyhose in favor of knee-highs or socks, and forget the high heels.

Think through the steps of dressing — from choosing what to wear to putting on each item — and allow plenty of time. These tips make the tasks easier:

✔ Prepare the night before: Choose your clothing and lay out all the pieces (from underwear to accessories).

✔ Sit on a sturdy armchair (not a rocker or the edge of the bed) and use the arms for support as you dress.

✔ Have a small footstool close at hand to provide support when you put on socks and shoes.

✔ Lie down on the bed if that makes it easier for you to put on certain items such as pants or socks.

Try to look your best — it can make a difference. When you look good, you feel good — or at least better. Some days you may think, "What's the point of getting dressed? I'm not going anywhere and no one's going to see me." Yes, you are going places — even if it's just around the house. And your family (and any friends who happen to stop by) are hardly *nobodies*.

Bathing and showering

Bathtubs and showers can be falls waiting to happen, so your first step is to make them as safe as possible. Your OT can help assess the need for safety bars, tub mats, shower chairs or stools, non-skid rugs, and such. (Read more about OTs in Chapter 6.)

The next step is to determine whether your normal bathing routine still applies. For example, when you consider the extra effort a shower or bath takes with PD, is your former daily routine realistic or even necessary? *Note:* One symptom in the mid-to-later stages of PD is excessive perspiration. If this is the case, at least a daily sponge bath is indeed necessary.

Because of the danger of falling, never attempt a shower or bath when you're home alone. Although you may want the privacy of managing this routine on your own, your care partner or someone in the family should be close enough that you can call for assistance if you need it. (Besides, what's so bad about having someone else wash your back?)

Whatever schedule you and your care partner decide is best, these additional tips can make bath time less stressful:

- ✔ Cut down on trips that can drain precious energy by gathering everything you need (soap, towels, shampoo, robe, and such) in one place — perhaps a plastic container in the bathroom can keep it all together.

- ✔ Check that the bathroom is free of drafts and that the water temperature is comfortable. Your bath time should be a pleasant, relaxing time, not a time when water that's too hot or too cold surprises you and can lead to a dangerous loss of balance or a fall.

- ✔ Undress and, using the techniques you practiced with your OT, get into the tub or shower. If your neurologist hasn't prescribed occupational therapy and you're beginning to struggle with such movements as getting in and out of the tub, ask for an OT referral. The OT can come to your home to work with you. In the meantime, be safe. Let your partner assist you in and out of the tub or shower, or plan to take sponge baths.

- ✔ Take your time — the sensation of washing yourself should be a pleasurable one. If holding onto a bar of soap is difficult, consider using a bath mitt, which is a glove-like washcloth that's available at most drugstores. And speaking of soap, go easy on the bath oils. They can make the shower or tub floor slippery (even with a rubber safety mat). Better to rub on bath oil as part of the drying process after your bath.

- ✔ Dry yourself thoroughly when you've finished. Again, take your time. Apply any lotion or cream to dry or chafed skin, and put on your robe. In fact, a thick terrycloth robe is a super way to dry yourself when the flexibility needed to towel dry becomes more difficult.

Don't attempt to get even partially dressed in the bathroom; the danger for falling as you attempt to dress in such close quarters is huge. Put on your robe and go back to your bedroom to dress, following the guidelines in "Dressing," earlier in this section.

Thinking outside the box

You may have heard the old joke about the patient who says to the doctor, "Doctor, if I follow your treatment, will I be able to play the piano?" When the doctor says, "I don't see why not," the patient replies, "Great. I always wanted to be able to do that."

Dr. Gary Guten — yes, the guy whose name is on the front cover — had battled PD over a decade when it occurred to him that playing the piano may be a way to maintain flexibility and coordination in his fingers and hands. Over the years, Gary — an orthopedic surgeon, marathon runner, and expert in the field of sports medicine — has found several innovative ways to meet the various challenges of his PD. Taking up the piano is just one more *therapy* he's devised to deal with the advancement of symptoms.

In the process, Gary and his teacher developed various techniques — like placing 2-pound weights on Gary's wrists to help steady his hands and creating a system for remembering notes and reading music. After several weeks of lessons and practice, Gary joined 20 other students (average age of 13) to present his first recital. As Gary said, "At my age and at this stage of my PD, what else could I do to earn the applause of 75 people?"

Early in his PD, Gary discovered that ski-pole-like hiking sticks (available at www.exerstrider.com) help him maintain an even stride and balance, allowing him to walk with rhythm and relative confidence. He also discovered that lateral twisting movements (from side to side) are easier than straight-on movements. As a result, he plays golf and ping-pong (which use a lot of lateral movement) to remain active — and athletic.

You may not be an athlete or a musician, but Gary's advice is to remember the words of the famous writer Gilbert Keith Chesterton: "If a thing is worth doing, it is worth doing badly." Like Gary, you and your healthcare team can get creative about what works for you in the fight to maintain your balance, mental alertness, and independence. By keeping a there-must-be-a-way attitude while you hold onto your optimism and good humor, you may have won half the battle against advancing PD.

Personal hygiene

One symptom PWP can develop as their PD progresses is urinary incontinence (see Chapter 18 for a discussion on the impact incontinence may have on your PD). This problem is not only a health concern but also a real hygiene issue due to the potential for odor. Of course, your first step is to discuss these problems with your doctor. Also consider these tips:

- ✔ Try using one of the disposable products (such as sanitary pads available in varying degrees of thickness) on the market today. Many of these are far more discreet than wearing an adult diaper product.

- ✔ Make certain that the pathway to and from the bathroom is well-lighted and free of obstacles. Or ask your doctor to prescribe a portable commode that you can place near your bed to avoid trips to the bathroom at night.

✔ Keep moist towelettes, disposable pads, and other products within easy reach in your bathroom so you can clean yourself as needed.

✔ Keep a few pre-moistened disposable wipes and an extra set of clean underwear and clothing in a plastic bag in your car, in a bag, or in a backpack for whenever you go out, just in case.

Maintaining the Family Dynamic

Collaborative management is a relatively new term in managing the symptoms of a chronic condition such as PD. In medical circles it applies primarily to the healthcare team (see Chapter 6) that helps you plan for and manage your PD symptoms. But it's also a useful term for families that need to include a chronic and progressive condition into their daily routines. The elements of collaborative management within a family unit may include:

✔ **Defining** the issues to be managed (medical, mental, and physical health) as well as the emotional impact of PD on the PWP and the family. For example, if the PWP's been the family's chief financial manager, this is a good time to train another family member in the details of managing the finances, paying the bills, investing and saving, and so on.

✔ **Targeting** each issue by establishing realistic goals, achievable objectives, and a satisfactory plan of action for the PWP and the family. Goals can be simple and short-term such as planning a family trip. If the PWP has always handled the planning, preparations, and details, then other members of the family need to step up and define ways they can take on some of those tasks.

✔ **Supporting and encouraging** the PWP's autonomy and independence through medical interventions, lifestyle changes, and emotional support systems so the PWP and her family can maintain as normal a routine as possible. Often a family member will respond to the PD diagnosis by jumping in and trying to do everything for the PWP. Because that person wants to deal with this challenge through action, find ways she can contribute. For example, maybe she can prepare a salad or side dish for dinner while the PWP — an accomplished cook — makes the rest of the meal just as she did before PD.

✔ **Monitoring** (through ongoing and open communication) the status of the PWP's role within the family unit and the family's ability to adapt to the presence of PD. Regular weekly or bi-weekly family meetings (see discussion of initial family meeting in Chapter 7) can accomplish this goal and provide a safe haven for members to voice concerns. The agenda starts with an update from the PWP. Then other family members engage in a round of *concerns and joys* in which each person can talk about possible needs or red flags and then mention something that is working well or has brought special delight since the last meeting.

As much as the challenge of living with PD may appear to be all about you, in fact it affects every family member. Whenever you have these family gatherings, make sure that *you* listen to your family's honest concerns (and sometimes outright frustrations). Acknowledge the concern, focus on the specific issue rather than the emotional overtones, and, opening the discussion to everyone, seek the best solution together.

Socializing with Friends

Every circle of friends has the person or persons who drive the social calendars of getting together, going places, calling, e-mailing, and the like. Each circle also has people who wait to be called, e-mailed, and the rest. Before your diagnosis, which role did you play? Were you the extrovert or the introvert? The social butterfly or the hermit?

If you're an introvert by nature, maybe the friends you counted on to call and set up get-togethers seem to have turned into a bunch of loners. If you were the social cheerleader of the group, maybe you've dropped that ball now that you have PD — not wanting to impose yourself and your symptoms on your friends.

Get over it! If your friends are real, they're waiting for you to show them the way. If the usual extroverts seem to be hanging back, call them and clear the air. Chances are they've been hanging back while trying to figure out what you want. If you were the social leader, get back in the game. Call the old gang together and have an open discussion about your PD, how you're handling it, and most of all, how you hope *they'll* handle it. Then get back to doing whatever you did together before your diagnosis.

Whatever activity you decide on, do *not* make your PD the focus of (or reason for) getting together. The purpose here is to bring the relationships back to some semblance of normalcy. After your friends see you in action and enjoying the activities you've always enjoyed (maybe with a bit more effort and a little less speed), they'll relax and the friendship can move forward.

Going Out and About in the Community

You may as well get used to it. You'll have times when total strangers stare at you with pity (or worse, disgust), children point and snicker, and people even cross to the other side of the street to avoid passing you on the sidewalk. Some people will misread your balance symptoms as intoxication. Others may read your facial mask and lack of expression as a sign of mental illness or not being very bright. (This is fairly obvious because the person speaks ver-r-ry slowly and loudly as if instructing a small child or a non-English speaker.)

You can choose to take this ignorance and lack of good manners personally, or you can choose to understand that this stranger is the one with the problem — and then get on with your day. In either case, what do you care about the opinions of strangers? Are you going to permit people like that to stop you from living normally? Aha! We didn't think so. The following sections provide some tips for maintaining your activity in the larger community.

Attending public events

Try to schedule your medication timing and dosing to your greatest advantage during the planned outing. (Talk to your doctor about your plans and let him suggest any modifications to your normal dosing routine). If you're going to a play, movie, concert, ballgame, or restaurant, some simple steps may help:

- ✔ Call ahead to get answers about accessibility (ramps not stairs, seat on the aisle if preferred, room for a wheelchair if necessary, and so on).
- ✔ Get plenty of rest before the event.
- ✔ Allow plenty of time to get ready.
- ✔ Arrive early so you can be seated and settled without rushing.

Social outings should be as enjoyable for your care partner as they are for you. This is not the time for you to try and prove your independence. For example, if helping you get ready (such as putting on your shoes for you) allows more time for your care partner to get ready, accept the help — *appreciate* the help. If using a wheelchair makes life easier and the occasion less stressful for your care partner, use a wheelchair. Think of this acceptance not as a surrender of your autonomy but as a gracious way of caring for your care partner.

Traveling

Taking a trip requires careful planning to make the trip a pleasurable experience rather than a hassle. As with everything else, when you consider taking a trip, break it down into more manageable steps:

- ✔ Choose where you'll go. At this point in your PD journey, what's realistic (a theater tour of NYC?) and what's not (scaling Mt. Everest?)? Talk to a travel agent about special tours available for folks traveling with a disability.

  The Web site www.travelconsumer.com/disability.htm provides links to special topics (such as recreational vehicles [RVs], tour groups for people with special needs, and cruises) and a link to _Travelin' Talk_, a network of people with disabilities around the world who are in regular contact and gather firsthand information about accessibility in a particular area.

✔ Figure out the transportation. Plane, bus, car, train? Or maybe all of the above? If you go by car, you and your travel companions are probably well aware of your limitations and needs. If you're taking a plane, train, or bus, contact the company well in advance to discuss provisions they offer special-needs travelers.

✔ Be very specific about your needs. For example, you may need your seat to be close to the bathroom. On the other hand, navigating the entire length of a jumbo jet as you board just so you can be close to the economy-class facility may be more trouble than it's worth. Ask whether you can have a seat closer to the front and permission to use the closer facility in business or first class. **Note:** If you'll be using a wheelchair — not a bad idea to conserve energy as you get from place to place within airports and train stations — the carrier needs advance notice.

✔ Select your overnight accommodations carefully. You may love an old, historic bed and breakfast, but is that realistic if you have to navigate stairs (which in old buildings can be steep, winding, and narrow!)? If you're fine with a traditional hotel and it publicizes _accessibility_ for people with special needs, do _not_ take them at their word. Call and ask specific questions. For example, does the bathroom have grab bars and a walk-in shower (not a shower in a tub)? Are the doorways wide enough to accommodate a wheelchair or walker?

✔ Plan to get out and about. Most tourist attractions in major cities around the world are well-prepared to accommodate visitors with special needs. But often the trick is to locate those entrances, facilities, and other special services. Call ahead and gather complete information about available services. Then on the day of your visit, call again and let the staff on duty know that you're on your way. (You may want to call the day before to give advance notice.)

If you or your traveling companion holds a membership in the museum or site, call the member-services department and let them know you're planning a visit. They may be able to offer you and your party more than the standard accommodations for special-needs visitors.

✔ Be prepared — just in case. Emergencies happen even on vacation, so take the following suggestions seriously:

• Always hand-carry your medications, don't put them in your baggage.

• Always take along an extra supply (two to three days' worth) of your medications _and_ their prescriptions in case you have to replace medications.

- Always carry a list of your medications (including over-the-counter products) and the emergency information listed in Chapter 9.

- Ask your neurologist to recommend a colleague in the place you're visiting (or check online at www.aan.com for a complete listing of certified neurologists worldwide).

Volunteering — The double blessing

Giving back to your community and making a real difference in the lives of other people pays double dividends. Not only are you contributing to the betterment of society — locally, nationally, or globally — but you're permitting yourself to turn your attention away from your own problems.

Whether you were an active volunteer before your PD or never had the time because of work and family responsibilities, now is the time. When you give of your time and energy in spite of your own challenges, you inspire other folks and give them hope. If you can manage your PD *and* mentor a troubled teen or manage the volunteer program for the blood drive or coordinate a fundraiser for your church, then you move other people to action. And that's something. As one song says, "You can hang a life on that."

And speaking of getting involved, don't overlook this golden opportunity to really make a difference for yourself and other PWP. See Chapter 24 for ways you can build awareness of and increase knowledge about PD locally or even nationally. The national PD community is active, organized, and inspiring — not to mention a great deal of fun.

Taking a Breather — Respite for the Weary

Living with a chronic, progressive condition (and living with someone who has such a condition) can become stressful and even overwhelming as the months and years go by. The warning signs are right there:

- Communication problems, like increased frustration, irritability, short tempers

- Physical symptoms, like stomach upset, shortness of breath, headache

- Unhealthy lifestyle behaviors, such as overeating or not eating enough, increased smoking or alcohol use, sleeping too much or too little

- Emotional symptoms, such as depression, anxiety, feelings of deep anger or sadness

The trick is not to lose control of these symptoms before you take action. But the real trick is to plan regular respite for yourself and your care partner — separately and together — as part of your daily routine. (Even the lowest-paid laborer gets fifteen-minute breaks a couple of times a shift!) In addition, you and your care partner need to consider the following:

✔ Your diagnosis doesn't require the two of you to be joined at the hip. You had separate activities before (and probably enjoyed telling your partner about the experience). That arrangement shouldn't change simply because one of you has PD.

✔ You both need to identify (in some cases, *remember*) the ways you individually relaxed and found respite before PD. Perhaps your partner spent an afternoon with the grandchildren. Maybe you had a regular card game. Maybe each of you gave time to a favorite charity.

✔ Try to plan vacation-type respites together. You'd be surprised how the travel industry has begun to accommodate the special needs of travelers like you. Check out the Web sites we list in the "Traveling" section earlier in this chapter.

If long-distance traveling becomes more stressful than fun, then perhaps going on *vacation* in your own community is a possibility. Ever notice how much you enjoy the special sites and events of your community when you have out-of-town company? Treat yourself — move to a hotel or accessible Bed and Breakfast for a few days; eat meals out at restaurants you've been meaning to try; visit a tourist attraction such as a concert, play, or sporting event, and buy souvenirs for the grandkids. Just remember to pace yourself and get the rest you need to enjoy the *trip*.

✔ As your PD progresses, you may find that you don't have the freedom to physically *get away*. Respite for you may come in the form of alternative and complementary therapies such as meditation or yoga, which we discuss in Chapter 11. And you may be surprised to discover how regular exercise can also be a respite therapy (see Chapter 12).

A Word for the PD Care Partner

Watching your loved one struggle to perform simple tasks can be frustrating and even emotionally painful for you. You may instinctively want to do whatever you can to make the task easier. That compassion certainly isn't bad, but you really need to fight the follow-through.

Managing the symptoms of PD means the PWP must fight to maintain as much movement, flexibility, and independence as possible for as long as possible. If you permit yourself or your loved one to give up on an activity that she can still do, you're actually (in a small but significant way) accelerating the process for real hands-on care.

Instead, discuss ways you can help without taking away her ability to manage on her own. For example, show your complete confidence in her ability by assuming she will be the one behind the wheel (as usual) when the two of you go out. At the local coffeehouse, if the PWP's tremor makes you shudder every time she tries to transport a cup of coffee from the counter to the table, *ask* if you can carry it for her. If she refuses, accept that.

Respite is vital for you and the PWP as you face the progression of current symptoms and the onset of new ones (see Chapter 18). Take advantage of available support so you can care for yourself without guilt. You have every right to do this. Those supports may include:

- ✔ Family and friends who assume the role of primary care partner for brief periods while you take a break

- ✔ In-home or respite care or adult day care programs (see Chapter 20) when care partnering becomes caregiving

Part V
Coping with Advanced PD

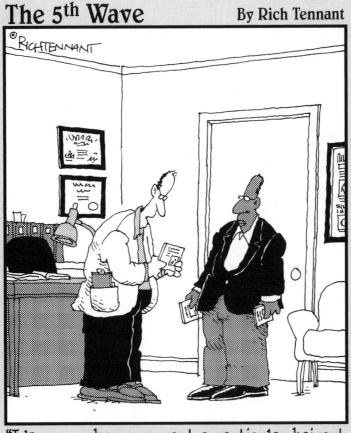

The 5th Wave   By Rich Tennant

"I know – when you want a particular haircut, you bring the barber a picture. But this is vocal surgery – bringing me CDs of Pavoratti isn't going to work the same way."

In this part . . .

Over the years you and your care partner will continue to adapt your lifestyle to the demands of PD. So it's wise to prepare and plan for circumstances that may come in the later stages. The chapters in this part help you do just that. In this part we look at the financial and legal matters that everyone (even people who don't have PD) needs to work through. We give you information that helps you remain in your home for as long as possible, and we set out options for the time when staying at home may no longer be a good idea. Perhaps of most importance, this part includes a chapter about a care partner's role shift to caregiver.

Chapter 18

Facing the Progression of PD Symptoms

....

....

*S*ooner or later the time will come for you to accept that a progressive disease like Parkinson's disease (PD) is reluctant to remain in the background of your life. In this chapter, we tackle the symptoms that may be brand new for you — perhaps even unexpected. Or maybe you've been dealing with some of them already. Our suggestion? The best defense is a good offense: Decide to fight back by:

✔ Discussing any changes in your condition with your neurologist

✔ Exploring options for additions to your current treatment or therapy

✔ Preparing for lifestyle changes that may become necessary (such as relying on a cane or walker or changing your living space arrangements)

On the follow pages, we look at PD symptoms that usually occur later and we also suggest some realistic ways to combat these symptoms.

Noticing Changes Caused by Your Meds

You may face a couple of challenges after you've been on meds that control your PD symptoms for a while.

The first medication-related challenge is *wearing-off*, which occurs when your medication can't control symptoms over several hours. In this case,

✔ Symptoms simply return earlier than usual, initially on a predictable basis (for example, you notice the symptoms return half an hour or an hour sooner than they used to).

✔ An unfortunate evolution (the *on-off syndrome* discussed in Chapter 9) occurs where you can't predict the length of symptom control from one dose to the next. Some people with PD (PWP) get to know the pattern and may elect to simply live with the *off* times rather than increase medication.

Another challenge brought on by the meds is *dyskinesia,* that twisting, writhing movement (see Chapter 9). Dyskinesia is the result of a complex interaction in the brain between the disease progression and the chronic administration of dopamine medication. As a result, dyskinesia

✔ Usually appears after you've been on the meds for some time (somewhere between two and ten years)

✔ Affects PWP in varying degrees that range from mild to severe, depending on the progression of their disease and their dose of levodopa

Your neurologist may be able to lessen or control your dyskinesias through a change in your medication routine. If the situation becomes intolerable, your doctor may suggest DBS surgery. (See Chapter 10.)

The best way to help your doctor control your symptoms is to keep a diary of the symptoms, including the time of medication intake and the time you feel the symptoms begin to return.

Doctors treat on-off problems in a variety (or combination) of ways:

✔ Prescribe medication doses closer together

✔ Add a second medication

✔ Increase the dose to reduce wearing-off or reduce to control dyskinesia

Whenever you notice a different reaction to your antiparkinsonian medications, talk to your neurologist before making any changes in your dosing routine on your own.

When Communication Becomes Difficult

For PWP, *dysarthria* (problems with speaking clearly, understanding, reading, writing, telling time, or using numbers) can be especially disheartening. These problems in communicating can become downright depressing and frustrating. The following sections break down two major problems: vocal and written communication.

The challenge to vocal expression

You can recognize changes in your normal communication by paying attention to the dynamics of a conversation. Consider the following scenarios:

- People (not just your significant other) seem to be leaning in or straining to hear and understand what you're saying. They do a lot of nodding and smiling but don't appear to comprehend your ideas.

- People often ask you to repeat what you just said or to speak up.

- People seem to be talking over you or finishing statements for you.

- You're frustrated from a normal conversation because you're asked to repeat yourself, or worse, you're ignored.

Do these situations seem all too familiar? Try to minimize these frustrations by asking your family and friends to do the following:

- Be patient and look directly at you when the two of you are talking.

- Try to conduct conversations away from background noises such as televisions, car radios, or other competing conversations.

- Keep in mind that your *mask* (lack of facial expression) doesn't reflect your level of interest in the conversation. (See Chapter 3 for an earlier discussion of this symptom.)

You can help yourself, too, by taking care of your voice:

- Take a deep breath and project, without straining or shouting.

- Allow time to rest your voice.

- Slow down if your words come out too fast.

- In any case, use it (talking, reading aloud, and singing). Use it or lose it!

As symptoms progress, you may want to seek help outside of yourself and your care partner. We help you explore your options in the following sections.

Speech pathologists

Speech pathologists (specially trained speech therapists) have the training and tools to improve symptoms or delay their worsening by using therapy in conjunction with your medication regimen. Your therapist can assess your needs, design a program of exercises to help strengthen your voice, and offer tips for making communication a more productive and pleasant experience.

If you have no speech professional in your area, consider ordering one or more of the following tools:

✔ *Parkinson's Disease: Speech and Swallowing:* A free booklet from the National Parkinson Foundation that includes exercises to help you strengthen vocal and facial muscles. (Available online at www.parkinson.org or call 800-327-4545.)

✔ *LSVT (Lee Silverman Voice Treatment) Alive!:* An interactive vocal exercise video. (Available at www.lsvt.org or call 888-606-LSVT [5788].)

Special devices

Several devices (such as message boards or more complex voice-activated software for your computer) can also help by amplifying your voice or making communicating easier. *Note:* These devices can be expensive and awkward to carry around and use. Your speech professional can advise you on these tools or you can contact the American Speech-Language and Hearing Association (ASHA) at www.asha.org or 800-638-8255.

Amplifiers that you wear to facilitate communication are also available. Also, to improve communication via telephone, phone companies offer special equipment at very low prices and at no cost for customers who qualify. For more information, contact your phone provider.

Handwriting — Telling the story of your on-off cycles

Micrographia is characterized by writing that starts out normal-size but becomes increasingly smaller and more cramped. This symptom may appear early in the progression of your PD, later, or not at all. When medications are managing symptoms well, handwriting may appear normal. But as medications wear off and the PWP gets closer to the next dose, the fine motor skills may be compromised. When this happens, your writing may start strong and normal but quickly trail off into small, cramped letters and words.

Consider these tips to help you compensate for the writing challenges:

✔ Ask your neurologist to have you write a sentence and then repeat that exercise at each check-up to see how much (or whether) your micrographia is progressing.

✔ Talk to your occupational therapist (OT) about tips to help you manage this symptom.

✔ Use an electric typewriter or computer for your written communications.

✔ Use lined paper that's sold with school supplies (several sizes are available) to help your pen stay in line.

Swallowing: You Can't Take It for Granted

In some PWP, *dysphagia* — swallowing difficulties — becomes a problem as PD progresses. You may try to write the symptoms off to an unrelated condition, but these need to be evaluated by a doctor, speech therapist, or speech pathologist. Don't ignore the onset of swallowing difficulties. Watch for these symptoms:

- Difficulty in eating and the need for a beverage to wash food down
- Episodes of food going down the wrong way or food seeming to get stuck in the throat
- Coughing or throat-clearing during or immediately after consuming food
- Unexplained weight loss
- Refusal of food or drink because swallowing is too difficult and eating has become an unpleasant experience
- Fever due to aspiration in the lung
- An increase in saliva or thickened mucous-like saliva
- Drooling — a little or a lot

Problems you may have with both saliva and drooling are likely due to your lack of regular swallowing. Two tips to prevent drooling and control saliva include the following:

- Keep your head up and your mouth closed when you're not talking or eating.
- Take frequent sips of water throughout the day. Doing this not only reminds you to swallow and keeps you hydrated but also waters down that thicker saliva.

Your doctor or speech professional may perform an X-ray procedure using barium to assess the swallowing muscles in action. You may be asked to eat a sample of various foods and beverages so that the doctor can evaluate how different foods and drinks affect your ability to swallow. And you may be tested at various times in your dosing cycle to determine how your medications may be affecting your swallowing.

After the evaluation, your doctor can recommend ways to ease your swallowing difficulties and make eating and drinking easier. Possible suggestions include:

✔ Timing your meals during the on cycle of your PD medications

✔ Cutting food into small bites, chewing thoroughly, and taking a sip of water before the next bite (yup, the old dieter's trick)

✔ Blending fruits and veggies to create a drink — the popular *smoothie* that may be easier to swallow.

These may sound like simple solutions, but don't attempt to self-diagnose a swallowing problem. It could be a condition completely unrelated to your PD.

Your Vision: A Bump in the Road

Another significant problem that can crop up as your PD progresses is the potential for changes in your vision — blurred vision, difficulty focusing (and reading), dry eyes, and such.

Some of these conditions are frequently a part of the aging process and have easy solutions. For example, your doctor may prescribe a special eye drop or suggest an over-the-counter (OTC) product for dry eyes. Blurred vision may also be nothing more than the need for a change in your lens prescription.

On the other hand, your dry eyes may result from the decreased number of times you blink due to your PD. Fortunately the irritation and discomfort respond to the same artificial tears product your doctor recommends for similar problems related to aging.

Other vision problems that can affect PWP are spasm of the eyelid or excessive blinking (blepharospasm) and double vision. Interestingly, the popular cosmetic injection, *Botox,* can treat the problem of excessive blinking. Double vision may be the result of the slowed and uncoordinated movements of your eyes, and it can be controlled by special lenses (prisms). Wearing a patch over one eye can help while you wait to see the eye doctor.

As with any health issue, do *not* attempt to self-diagnose or treat. See your eye doctor, describe your symptoms, and let the expert prescribe a solution.

To Drive or Not to Drive

Changes from the progression of your PD have the potential to seriously impair your ability to safely operate motorized vehicles, and that can be huge for a PWP. Added to vision problems is the potential for

✔ Wearing off of your meds at inopportune times

✔ The possible worsening of your rigidity that impairs the coordination necessary to operate a motor vehicle

✔ Slowed reaction timing — hazardous for any driver

What to do? How to continue to drive in spite of your PD? How to know when it's no longer an option? Follow these suggestions to assure your safety (not to mention the safety of other people) before you get behind the wheel:

✔ **Be smart about when you drive.** Consider limiting (or eliminating) driving after dark. This isn't solely a PD issue; lots of people struggle with night driving as they age.

✔ **Don't drive if another driver's available to take the wheel.** This includes public transportation when it's available.

✔ **Don't drive after consuming even the smallest amount of alcohol.** You really can't predict the effects of combining a drink with your meds.

✔ **If you (or your partner) question your ability to drive,** play it safe by asking your occupational therapist (OT) to refer you to a Driver Rehabilitation Specialist (also an OT but with expertise in this area). Let that person assess your ability and, if possible, recommend changes (such as not driving at night or for long distances) that permit you to keep driving.

✔ **For legal reasons, if your PD isn't a factor in your driving ability,** have your doctor note in your chart that you're capable of driving — day or night. This written verification can protect you if an accident occurs and you're not at fault.

Especially for men, driving is a mark of independence — that macho thing. Get over it. If the end of your driving days isolates and depresses you because you refuse to consider alternatives, that's on you. You have choices, including asking a friend or family member (who just happens to be looking for a concrete way to help) for a lift.

Freezing and Rigidity: When Your Head Says "Go," but Your Body Says "No"

Advanced PD often affects your ability to walk safely. What used to be unconscious, easy maneuvers that you took for granted are now major hurdles, just waiting to trip you up. This section discusses three of the most common problems: freezing, festination, and rigidity. Also, it includes suggestions to minimize the greatest concern — your risk of falling.

Freezing and festination: It's all in the legs

You're walking along fine and then — Bam! — like the cartoon character who steps in glue, you're stuck! *Freezing* is the sudden inability to step forward, and it typically happens in three situations:

- ✓ **As you step out:** *Start* hesitation classically occurs when you attempt to take the first step forward. The feet are glued to the floor and you may feel like you're walking in place. While the feet are stuck, the rest of the body may lurch forward, placing you at great risk for falling.

- ✓ **In mid-stride:** Even after you get started, freezing often happens in doorways or when you need to take a step as you perform another action, like turning the doorknob.

- ✓ **When stopping or turning:** Freezing and hesitation can really complicate the act of turning around or changing direction — another circumstance that's ripe for a fall.

A growing number of products are designed specifically to address the problem of freezing, such as some of the walking aids listed in Appendix B. In addition, exercise videos and booklets offer programs specifically for PWP. Check out Appendix B as well as Chapter 12.

Another typical walking problem in advanced PD is *festination* (from the Latin word *festinato* or *haste*) where you take several short, almost running steps in an effort to regain your balance. This usually occurs as you break out of an episode of freezing.

You can use several tricks to maintain the rhythm of your walking:

- ✓ March in place or hum a marching tune.

- ✓ Take a step to the side before attempting to move forward. (This change in direction seems to interrupt the freezing sensation and allows you to continue your forward movement.)

- ✓ Step over an imaginary line on the ground.

- ✓ Visualize your foot moving through space three feet forward.

Rigidity: When your whole body locks up

Rigidity (stiffness in the muscles and limbs) as we discuss in Chapter 2 may first become evident in a reduced arm swing when walking or as the mask, loss of animated facial expression (see "When Communication Becomes

Difficult" earlier in this chapter). As PD progresses or if medication becomes less effective, the severity of rigidity can escalate. Rigidity can also result in muscular pain. In normal movement, activating one muscle (the *agonist)* is offset by relaxing the muscle that performs the opposing action (the *antago-nist*). In rigidity, the opposing muscle fails to relax.

Your doctor can determine the degree of rigidity by gently moving the arm, leg, torso, or shoulder while you're standing or sitting in a relaxed position. One classic type of rigidity is known as *cogwheel,* where the arm, for example, can move only in short, jerky, or ratchet-like movements. Cogwheel rigidity is usually associated with resting tremor (tremor is present only in times of inactivity). Another common type of rigidity is *lead pipe*, when the muscles feel heavy and weak and using them causes fatigue.

A program of regular exercise and stretching (see Chapter 12) can be the most effective weapon to fight increasing stiffness and rigidity. Many communities offer special exercise programs through the local YMCA or hospital for people with conditions that cause muscle stiffness, weakness, and rigidity. Talk to your physical therapist (PT) or support group about the availability of such a program in your area (or about getting a program started).

PD and Falling — A Tricky Balancing Act

The greatest risk as PD advances is the danger of falling. By some estimates, two-thirds of all PWP experience falls in the mid-to-later stages. This percentage is significant because falls are the number one cause of hospitalization for the PWP due to fractures or head injuries, and because they're the precipitant factor in worsening of symptoms or even death due to onset of pneumonia.

Your PD symptoms contribute enormously to your possibility of falling. Think about the following scenarios:

✔ Your shuffling gait practically begs for the opportunity to trip over a rug or uneven pavement.

✔ Your general stiffness and slowness affect reaction time, so you can't stop yourself from falling by grabbing onto something.

✔ Your tendency to overcompensate for impaired balance by swaying backward when you turn or stand compromises your balance.

As a PWP, you're at risk to fall from four sources. The following sections cover those sources and the steps you can take to reduce your risk of falling.

Mind those meds

Most medications to manage PD symptoms have side effects, including "may cause dizziness." Medications for other health conditions (such as high blood pressure) can add to the problem. If you experience any change in maintaining your balance (stumbling, dizziness, lightheadedness, overcompensating to stay upright, and so forth), report these changes to your doctor immediately. And if you're experiencing new symptoms of dizziness or imbalance and you've had a recent change in meds, the change may be contributing to the problem. Don't try to guess — call the doctor.

Anything you can do to prevent a fall is worth the effort. The following suggestions may help:

✔ Ask your doctor to order an assessment of your current status by a PT and OT. (See Chapter 6 for info on these specialists.) Ideally the therapist(s) can compare this assessment to one you had shortly after your diagnosis to evaluate the amount of change.

✔ The therapist can evaluate your movements and risks for falling and then suggest changes in your home environment to prevent falls. (See Chapter 21 for tips on making this home survey yourself.)

✔ Ask your doctor whether your meds come in a dissolving tablet (you take them without water) so you can take a dose before you get up. At some point, you may want to ask your doctor to prescribe a hospital bed that you can raise and lower for greater assistance.

Steady as she goes

Training and adaptive devices (including the proper cane or walker) can help you move safely and independently. Please don't just assume that Uncle Dan's old cane is right for you. Ask your therapist to properly fit a device to you.

Falls (and possible injuries that require hospitalization) can lead some people to pull back on activity. If your fear of falling limits your activity, you may be doing more harm than you think because staying active — physically and mentally — goes hand in hand with staving off PD symptoms (and thus preventing more falls). Talk to your doctor about the possibility of a PT or OT assessment and therapy that helps you adapt and get active again.

Make adjustments along the way

Impaired balance can be part of your PD's progression (due to your increasing muscle stiffness, rigidity, a stooped posture, and more frequent episodes of freezing). See the earlier section "Freezing and Rigidity: When Your Head

Says 'Go,' but Your Body Says 'No.'" Never is your team of professional care partners more important than now. Your doctor, PT, and OT can assess your needs and make recommendations to help you maintain your balance. In the meantime, this short list of suggestions can help you prevent a fall:

✔ Use that cane or walker that your doctor or PT ordered and customized for your needs.

✔ Avoid footwear with rubber soles that may stick to the floor. Ask your PT to suggest the best footwear for you.

✔ Use a recommended trick for maintaining a rhythm as you walk (see "Freezing and festination: It's all in the legs" earlier in this chapter).

✔ Focus on walking rather than distractions. For example, don't try to talk on a portable phone and walk around at the same time.

✔ Take time to turn (TTT). Walking a few extra steps to make a wide turn is far better than pivoting suddenly and losing your balance.

Overcoming Sleep Disturbances

Anything that causes a disruption of normal sleep on an ongoing basis and prevents you from getting the rest you need is considered a sleep disturbance. Disturbances may have a number of causes: genetic or environmental factors (such as shift work), age, medications, and diet.

PWP are particularly prone to develop sleep disturbances for a wide variety of symptom-related reasons:

✔ Difficulty turning in bed or medication-induced dyskinesias may disturb the level of muscle relaxation necessary to sleep.

✔ Urinary urgency and frequency may force you to visit the bathroom several times during the night.

✔ Medication to treat your PD symptoms, if taken too close to bedtime, may cause vivid dreams or agitation that awakens you.

✔ Anxiety and depression, which frequently affect PWP (see Chapter 13), can make falling asleep difficult (anxiety) and can cause you to wake early or sleep too much (depression).

In addition, PWP may experience a number of specific sleep disturbances. The most important one is *rapid eye movement (REM) sleep behavior disorder,* a condition that makes you act out your dreams, unknowingly talk out loud, move your limbs, and sometimes even hit your bed partner! All of these actions can create a state of chronic sleep deprivation that leads to fatigue, excessive daytime sleepiness, and visual hallucinations.

However, keep in mind that many sleep disturbances can be improved simply by developing better sleep habits. The American Academy of Neurology offers the following tips:

✔ Sleep only when drowsy and only in the bedroom.

✔ Keep lights and noise low when trying to sleep, but keep a night light on to prevent falls if you need to get up in the night.

✔ Limit your intake of tobacco products, caffeine (chocolate, coffee, non-herbal tea, and such), and alcohol.

✔ Don't eat a heavy meal or participate in strenuous exercise for four to six hours before bedtime.

✔ Make use of relaxation and stress relief techniques (see Chapter 11).

Of course, like any new or troublesome symptom, discuss a sleep distur-bance with your neurologist. The problem may be a side effect of your med-ications or a signal of a more serious condition such as sleep apnea syndrome, which requires specialized management.

Those Embarrassing Constipation and Urinary Issues

The good news: Although a nuisance for PWP, urinary and bowel issues are often treatable and manageable even with the progression of PD.

As we note in Chapter 17, never automatically dismiss urinary or bowel prob-lems as unrelated to your PD. If incontinence or constipation becomes a problem as your PD progresses (or you've had issues in the past but they seem to be worsening), tell your doctor. While both conditions are common side effects of many medications (even common OTC meds), simply stopping or changing meds may not relieve symptoms.

In some cases PWP may suffer from an overactive bladder and feel an urgency to get to the bathroom as soon as possible, especially at night. Other PWP may experience an inability to fully empty the bladder, so they need to go again within a short time. Malfunction of the bladder isn't uncommon in PD. If you're experiencing such symptoms, you need to tell your doctor. In males, the problem can be an enlarged prostate gland; in women it may be an infec-tion (called a *urinary tract infection* or *UTI*). In either case, your doctor may recommend that you see a urologist to rule out other causes.

The slowed movement that is a core part of PD can make constipation a rela-tively common problem for PWP. Because of other issues that can crop up with the progression of PD (swallowing difficulties that lead to a poorer diet, not drinking enough liquids, and infrequent exercise due to increased impairment to movement and balance control), constipation can become a recurrent problem for many PWP.

Let your doctor know of any changes in your normal bowel or urinary habits. In the meantime, you know the routine (your mother probably drummed it into you when you were a kid):

- ✔ **Drink plenty of water:** Yes, even if you need to *go* all the time.

- ✔ **Eat your roughage:** Also known as fiber (fruits, veggies, and whole grains). See www.mypyramid.gov.

- ✔ **Get daily exercise:** No, reaching for the remote doesn't count!

Dealing with the Big "D" — Dementia

Dementia may be one of the most frightening and unsettling words in the English language. Just to be very clear, the term means

- ✔ A person's intellectual function is impaired to the degree that it affects normal and routine activities (such as decision making, balancing a checkbook, and such) and relationships with other people.

- ✔ Possible changes occur in behavior and personality. A person with dementia may experience delusions or hallucinations.

- ✔ At least two normal functions of the brain (including memory, reasoning, perception, judgment, and such) are affected. Memory loss by itself is not dementia.

Dementia — senile or otherwise — isn't a normal part of aging.

Probably the question uppermost in your mind is: Is dementia part of PD's progression? The answer is: It may be, but it may not necessarily be true for you. In general, dementia seems to more frequently affect patients over the age of 70 and those in the late stages of the disease.

Everyone experiences the progression of PD in a unique way. So learn what you can about dementia and consider how you and your care partner may handle its possible onset. Then get back to living your life.

PD is not Alzheimer's disease

Today Alzheimer's disease (AD) is one of the most commonly recognized conditions associated with dementia. A person with AD faces a progressive loss of intellectual and mental function. Dementia in AD is a *primary* dementia. This means it doesn't result from any other disease or condition.

In contrast, for people with conditions that affect movement or other functions (such as PD), dementia is a *secondary* dementia. That is, it appears to arise from a separate source. For example, a person with PD may also have high blood pressure or other cardiovascular conditions and may develop symptoms of dementia related to those conditions. This form is then termed *vascular dementia*.

PWP may develop AD in their later years, or they may develop *Lewy body dementia,* a disturbance of their cognition characterized mainly by fluctuations in attention and alertness, executive dysfunction, and recurrent visual hallucinations. (When dementia occurs very early in PD, the term *Lewy body disease* indicates a separate disease in its own right.) But whether the onset of the secondary dementia is *linked* to PD or simply *co-exists* (like PD plus diabetes) is currently unknown. Recent studies of brains at different stages of PD suggest that dementia may be the very last pathological stage of the disease.

The point is this: The onset of dementia in a PWP isn't a foregone conclusion, and it isn't the same as AD. You need to report any sign of cognitive malfunction to your doctor, because your sudden hallucinations or excessive sleepiness and dull mind may have a perfectly logical (and treatable) explanation.

Reviewing those cognitive symptoms

Although Chapter 3 has a full discussion of cognitive symptoms, a quick review is helpful in this chapter's context of PD progression.

Having some cognitive symptoms doesn't necessarily mean you're headed for full-blown dementia. Don't panic, but do talk to your doctor if you're experiencing any of the following:

- ✔ **Anxiety or depression** are part and parcel of PD. Focus on the fact that they're treatable. If you ignore or refuse to acknowledge these symptoms, shame on you. (If you haven't read Chapter 13, do it soon.)

- ✔ **Executive dysfunction** can include troubles with balancing your checkbook, following directions, making routine decisions, and such. Fortunately, you can strengthen and exercise your mind and possibly keep this problem at bay. (See the following section "When Medical Treatments Are Limited.")

- ✔ **Hallucinations** (seeing objects that really aren't there — perhaps a child or animal passing quickly by your door or simply feeling the presence of a person without actually seeing that person) can be a side effect of your medications. But as your PD advances, these visual (and usually harmless) hallucinations maybe associated with a cognitive disorder. As with everything that seems out of the norm, you (or your care partner) need to let your doctor know. Simple medication changes or adding others medications to block hallucinations may help.

When Medical Treatments Are Limited

Identifying the various symptoms that may worsen or appear as your PD advances is only one piece of the puzzle. Another piece is addressing those changes. What options do you have when medical treatments can't provide the answer?

You have a number of resources — all within your grasp — for fighting back if you have to face the onset of new symptoms or the progression of your present symptoms. The following guidelines can help you stay the course:

- ✔ Continue to eat a healthy diet rich in antioxidants (see Chapter 12).

- ✔ Continue your daily exercise program (also discussed in Chapter 12).

- ✔ Continue to exercise that mind! Mental activities (no, TV doesn't count) can help to keep your mind agile.

- ✔ If possible, consider taking a class or starting a new hobby.

- ✔ At the very least, remain socially active and engaged in the world and the community around you.

Yes, you may be approaching the point where you rely on other people more. But this doesn't mean you have to surrender all decisions and control. Your lifestyle and life choices can play an enormous role in your ability to postpone your PD's progression. Keep fighting! Keep moving! Keep living!

A Word for the PD Care Partner

As your partner's PD progresses, you may face some tough challenges like having to persuade him to give up driving or acknowledge that he's showing more and more signs of cognitive impairment that can impact his safety. Such challenges can seem even more difficult because you've both been living with PD for a number of years. Obvious symptoms that the PD is getting worse can add strain to the relationship. The following tips may help you hold it together as you and your PWP enter this new phase of living with PD:

- Acknowledge changes as they come and seek the advice of the neurologist especially if you notice any unusual progression of symptoms (like sleep disturbances or onset of visual hallucinations) or recurring behavior (excessive eye-blinking or increased urinary urgency).

- Continue to prepare for potential lifestyle changes that may become necessary (such as a change in living accommodations) and check out availability of options in your community.

- Let someone else be the villain when it comes to taking away driving privileges. If you're concerned, let the PWP's doctor know. The doctor can order a driving evaluation and make recommendations based on that.

- If the doctor doesn't respond to your concerns about your partner's driving, contact a representative in your state motor vehicle department and ask her to require a road test as a step in renewing the license.

- If *you* begin to feel overwhelmed with more and more of the responsibilities (financial, physical, emotional), talk to your support group contacts or facilitator, your clergyperson, or the counselor you found when you and your PWP set up the healthcare team (see Chapter 6); ask for some concrete tips for coping.

- Realize that you're in danger of burning out. Attending to your needs for regular short-term breaks and an occasional long-term respite are keys to keep on keeping on. Plan for these breaks and consider them as vital to living with PD as your partner's timely medications.

If you and your partner have prepared for this day, you've already discussed some difficult decisions. Your partner now needs to accept and appreciate that you're simply carrying out those decisions you made months or years ago. If your partner is incapable of understanding (or appreciating) that fact, remind yourself that he's still in control. But you need to remember: Having made the choices together, you're now simply carrying out his wishes. (For more advice on coping with progressing care, read Chapter 19.)

Chapter 19

When Care Partners Become Caregivers

*Y*ou're likely to live for many years in spite of your Parkinson's disease (PD). The prognosis is hopeful and every day brings us all closer to a cure. But as your PD progresses, the day may come — most likely following a fall and maybe a fracture that requires hospitalization — when you'll need more hands-on, direct care.

We hope you've had a care *partner* as you've made your PD journey to this point. But that can be good and bad news. The good news is that this person is the most likely candidate to become your primary caregiver, and he or she is probably very familiar with you and the path your PD has taken. The bad news is that you've gotten pretty used to being in charge. Handing off that control will take some adjustment.

As your need for care increases, you'll almost certainly be surrounded by different tiers of care. Your primary caregiver is the person who takes the lead, manages your care day-to-day, and acts as your spokesperson if you can't speak for yourself. But you'll also need secondary caregivers. These people (usually other family members and friends) take on a specific role, like handling your finances or doing the grocery shopping.

In this chapter, we consider that transition from partnering to receiving the care of another person because of your symptoms' progression (see Chapter 18 for more on these). This chapter covers specific changes in your caregiver's new role and how your relationship with that person may adjust. We also offer alternative arrangements that may be necessary over time, give you a heads-up on the biggest challenges of this transition, and suggest ways to develop your secondary caregivers. Finally, we offer straight talk and important suggestions for your care partner.

Understanding Your Primary Caregiver's Role

By definition, caregivers provide some type of hands-on assistance to other people. That assistance may be in the area of handling finances, managing legal affairs, providing emotional support, attending to routine chores, administering personal care, or any combination of these categories. According to the Family Caregiver Alliance, as many as 52 million family caregivers in the United States provide care for an adult (age 20 and over) family member or friend. Most caregivers (75 percent) are women, and about half of all caregivers are employed elsewhere full-time.

Your caregiver is the person who takes primary responsibility in providing more intensive home and personal care assistance. This person is who you trust to abide by your wishes — the ones you made clear in better times — and to speak for you if you're unable to speak for yourself.

Your caregiver isn't the person with PD. Life will go on for this person after the time for giving care has passed. And he deserves to attend to that life while still attending to your needs. As your relationship adjusts to a new balance of roles, remember that this is the same person who's been right there with you as your *partner*. He's well aware of the emotional and psychological impact these challenging times have on both of you.

Giving care versus partnering in care

Your roles are changing now. More and more it's your care-partner-turned-caregiver who must take charge of decisions and actions that affect your welfare and safety. Decisions that once focused on *your* needs must now increasingly focus on your *caregiver's* needs, abilities, and emotional strength in order to deliver what you need when you need it without sacrificing her normal routine.

Never will it be more tempting to give in to the anger and resentment that this widening chasm can create. Never will your care-partner-turned-caregiver need your love, appreciation, and emotional support more.

And yet an important element of partnering remains. If you and your partner have prepared for this day, discussed the difficult decisions that you knew you might face, and explored options to address your increasing needs, then your partner is simply carrying out the decisions you both made months or even years ago.

Is your care partner a novice or a natural caregiver?

Some people are natural nurturers. Others are not. Some come to the role of caregiver with years of experience already under their belts. Other folks who are new to the role may find themselves entering a strange world that they're not prepared to tackle. But most caregivers have one fact in common: The need to step in sneaks up on them. One day their loved one is managing fairly well, and the next day the caregiver suddenly needs to intervene. The ongoing care becomes not only necessary, but essential.

Keep in mind that not everyone is up to the job. Just because a person is your spouse or adult child and the most obvious candidate, this doesn't mean that he's physically and emotionally prepared to take on increasingly complex caregiving duties. You and your care partner need to keep an open mind and be willing to creatively decide how best to meet your needs as your PD progresses.

It's called the 36-hour day for a reason

Jus how long the need for care will continue is hard to estimate. It can be anywhere from a year to decades. But if the caregiver devotes 20 to 40 hours a week (as statistics indicate) to giving care in addition to the other roles she's juggling, then the idea of a 36-hour day fits.

In addition to selecting the best caregiver for the job, you and your care partner need to get real about how much time it's going to take *and* where that time will come from. Two lives are at stake here — yours and your caregiver's. At this stage (as in the earlier stages), each of you has the right to maintain some semblance of a lifestyle that fills your physical, mental, emotional, and spiritual needs. (For more ideas on how to make your priorities a reality, check out Chapters 7 and 15 for your relationships and Chapters 6, 13, and 17 for physical, emotional, and spiritual suggestions.)

Considering How Your Relationships May Change

If you've prepared for this day, you and your significant other (or adult child or other care partner) have discussed the what-will-happen-when questions.

And you've thought about how to address your increasing need to rely on other people. The most likely candidates for caregiver are pretty obvious, but each situation comes with a history that can affect this shift in roles.

When you rely on your spouse or significant other: A balancing act

"Grow old along with me . . ." the old saying goes.

In a marriage or union between two people, each person settles into a role. She pays the bills and manages the day-to-day budget. He handles their financial and healthcare security. She's the gardener; he's the cook. She's the social butterfly; he prefers staying home with a good book. Through the years, they develop ways of compromising, moving out of their comfort zones, and reinventing themselves individually as they find their way as a couple.

So, what happens if everything shifts? He has advanced PD and can no longer safely prepare the meals. She takes this on. When going out becomes more difficult for him, she adapts by staying home to be with him. He feels guilty that his PD impacts her life so much; she reassures him but can't deny a sense of mourning at how their lives have changed. As the caregiving becomes more intense, perhaps she abandons more and more of those activities that gave her identity.

When one partner becomes the caregiver, both partners need to maintain balance as their duties and responsibilities shift. The best way you and your care partner can accomplish this shift is through your willingness to accept the help of other people. This help can free your partner to pursue (in moderation) her life, and (if she accepts this help as your contribution to the relationship) it can relieve her guilt for wanting a life beyond your PD.

When your adult child steps up: You're still the parent

Sometimes the relationship that comes from an adult child caring for a parent has been called *parenting our parents*. Wrong! Roles may shift as you turn to your child for advice on finances or assistance with daily chores, but the relationship between you and your child has a history. There's no reversal here. (See Chapter 15 for more discussion on this relationship.)

If your adult child becomes your primary caregiver, your history influences the relationship you forge. Although the ways you've communicated (or not) through the years may have mellowed, the base of your relationship doesn't change just because you now need help. And this reality may be good, or it may cause some rough moments.

The key for this caregiving relationship is one of mutual respect. As an adult, your child deserves the same trust and respect that you would extend to any person of maturity and experience. At the same time, that child needs to accept that — regardless of your frailties and even childlike dependencies — you're still a grown-up with a history of managing your own life.

When your sibling comes to your aid: Rivalries remain

Family history plays a part with siblings too. Your position within the family order (eldest, middle, youngest) continues to impact the relationship. "Mom always liked you best" isn't forgotten, although someone may mention it in jest these days. Old jealousies, wounds, and slights that you never addressed as adults can still fester. Labels from when you were small can linger. "Mary was the smart one." "Jim was the family comedian."

If a sibling seems the most likely candidate to become your caregiver and spokesperson, the time to mend fences is way before that day arrives. You also need to set ground rules about the way you live your life and interact with other people. If your sibling can't respect your ways and expects you to adapt to his, the relationship may be under stress from day one. And, trust us, the last thing you need in your life is more stress.

When your friends offer to help: Are they in it for the long haul?

If you're single and have no family member close enough (geographically or emotionally) to consider as your caregiver, you may turn increasingly to a long-time friend for help and support. Although this pattern can and does work for many people, take care. A lifelong friendship can be destroyed if both sides aren't absolutely upfront about giving and receiving care.

Identify the specific ways you anticipate needing help. Start with one task — perhaps transportation to and from doctor appointments or a daily call or visit to be sure you're okay. Friends are usually quite willing (even anxious) to step up, but they need direction. Bottom line: If they need to back off, they need to know you'll understand and can find another source for help.

Exploring Alternative Arrangements

If you've been living alone, you may need to look outside your immediate home for the care partner who's willing to take on caregiving as your PD progresses. In fact, you may want to split the job up and enlist more than one caregiver.

When the most obvious caregiver lives far away

In today's world, family members often scatter across a wide area. The most obvious caregiver may be someone living miles away. Short of you or this person making a major move, what are your choices?

Making a long-distance arrangement

One caregiver in Wisconsin managed care for her parents in Virginia over an eight-year period without anyone having to move. When long-distance caregivers take care of loved ones, the keys are knowledge and preparation.

Take these two steps:

1. **Know ahead of time what programs and services your community has for support and care.**

2. **Prepare for the day that your needs increase:**

    • Establish contacts within those community programs.

    • Identify emergency caregivers who can step in for a short time until the long-distance caregiver can arrive.

Establishing an emergency backup

Emergency caregivers are people who are available to step in when something unforeseen arises. Their role is temporary but important.

Your emergency caregiver may be a neighbor who's home during the day (while your primary caregiver works) or a friend who's agreed to assume this key role. It may be your clergyperson who can marshall the forces of the congregation to step in until more permanent help arrives.

Whoever you identify for this role, you — and especially your long-distance caregiver — need to establish a plan for emergency action sooner rather than later. If you fall and your primary caregiver is miles away, who will come to your aid?

When no one applies

In rare cases, no single person can step in and assume the role of primary caregiver. When that happens, don't despair. You have at least two options for preparing for the day when you need more hands-on care.

The first option

Assess how you can remain in your home and get the help you need. Some aspects of this plan are easier than others. For example,

- Many pharmacies and grocery stores offer a delivery service for medications and food.

- You can address safety issues by installing a phone service and wearing a pager. If you don't contact the service within a specified time each day (or even twice a day), then the service contacts someone to come and check on you. Or if you fall and need help, you can activate the pager.

The second option

Other facets of care are more complex. How are you going to manage routine tasks such as showering, shaving, or shampooing? How are you going to manage financial matters if you begin to experience diminished mental capacity?

Consider a change in residence sooner rather than later. At the very least, community services can be a lifeline for you. Or you may consider an actual move. Options such as assisted living facilities and so-called *step* communities are two possibilities. For a full discussion of care and housing options and how to manage the costs, see Chapters 21 and 22.

Making the Transition

When the transition from partnering to caregiving begins in earnest, you and your caregiver need to be ready for the learning curve. Consider these new challenges:

- Moving from independence to the need for assistance

- Rapidly shifting from partner to caregiver, a seemingly full-time job

- Moving from blind stubbornness to acceptance

- Consciously recognizing the emotional roller coaster you've boarded — right when your physical and emotional defenses are down

Your best tactic is to acknowledge the difficult feelings (see Chapter 24) that come with those challenges and deal with them head on. Get professional help to deal with the transition if you need it.

Just make sure that you understand that accepting help from others — regardless of how independent and self-sufficient you've always tried to be — is simply one more tool you and your primary care partner have. Allowing others (friends, extended family, the community) to provide assistance gives you much needed support in preserving your energy to live life as fully as possible for as long as possible.

Learning to accept help

Humans are by nature fiercely independent and perhaps never more so than when that autonomy is threatened by illness or other circumstances beyond their control.

One of the concepts we try to instill throughout this book is that fighting PD is a team effort. If it takes a village to raise a child properly, it takes a contingent of healthcare professionals, family, and friends to maintain a life with PD. You may be the quarterback, but you need every one of those other players to help you run those plays and live on your own terms.

There's no shame in accepting the help of other people. As a matter of fact, *you're* often helping *them!* You empower them by needing them. And you enrich their lives by giving them a way to tangibly demonstrate their love and respect for you.

You know how much you hate this PD being all about you — the glances, the murmured comments when people think you're out of earshot. You have just one way to change that: Take control, and accept the help you need.

Still not convinced the time has come to seek additional help? Think again. Maybe you're reading this chapter because you already suspect you and your care partner can no longer manage totally on your own. But refusing to acknowledge it (and then make the necessary changes and accept help) can result in serious setbacks for both of you. Some of these can be:

- A toll on your relationship
- Financial costs associated with emergencies brought on by your refusal to accept help
- Isolation that comes from managing your PD to the exclusion of everything and everyone else
- Confusion from managing alone, trying to protect your independence

✔ Ignored warning signs (such as anger, depression, guilt, and other difficult feelings)

✔ Damaged health (physical, mental, emotional) and financial well-being
for you and your care partner

Whether you enlist the help of other people or make a more permanent
change (like moving to a different residence where support and care are readily available), don't be stubborn about this. Don't toy with your life and the
life of your beloved, devoted care partner. Snap out of it!

Take charge by establishing a routine for daily, weekly, and long-term breaks
(be sure you read the section "Dealing with burnout" later in this chapter)
and by accepting the help and support that's within your reach.

Remembering that your PD isn't your caregiver's fault

The song says you always hurt the one you love. And it happens fairly inno-
cently. Your care partner knows you aren't always at your best and doesn't
expect you to be. You can let go of the brave façade, the "I'm doing great"
demeanor, with this person.

But avoid going too far with this. The dark side of being yourself comes out
when you start taking out your anger and frustration on that person. This
emotion may come in the form of a short temper, snappish comments, or
actual physical lashing out. It may also come in more subtle ways, like shutting the person out through silence or isolating the person from his own life
by your neediness.

Your care partner has surrendered a piece of his life to continue this journey
with you. Just how great that sacrifice turns out to be may be up to you.

Dealing with burnout

If you or your care partner were not dealing with the terrible situation, if both
of you were living normal lives, wouldn't you make room for regular breaks
from routine? Consider how most jobs include breaks, holidays, vacation
time, and personal days. You deserve at least that same consideration!

Review your current situation

Burnout is common in the workplace and even more so among caregivers.
However, rarely do you hear about burnout in the person with PD (PWP) or in

people with other chronic, progressive conditions that require constant adjustment and adaptation. Ask yourself and your care partner the following questions:

- ✔ Is it becoming increasingly difficult for each of you to face the daily challenges of your PD?

- ✔ Is your care partner showing signs of health changes — sleeplessness, under-eating or overeating, headaches, or vague complaints of aches and pains?

- ✔ Do you or your care partner react to good news or complaints with irritation, cynicism, or sarcasm? (In other words, has your ability to show interest in or concern for other people been compromised?)

- ✔ Are the two of you often irritable and impatient with each other?

- ✔ Are you seeing signs that you or your care partner is becoming increasingly isolated, sad, lonely, or resentful of others?

Then ask these big questions and be brutally honest in answering:

- ✔ Do you or your care partner reject suggestions and offers of help because you believe other people just don't get it? (They haven't been through this, so they can't possibly understand!)

- ✔ Do you honestly believe that only your care partner and you can make this work?

If you answered "Yes" to two of the first five questions for yourself or your care partner, think *burnout*. If you answered "Yes" to one or both of the last two questions, you need a break, possibly some counseling, and you need it now.

Ask for additional help

Ideally, sit down with your care partner and consider the following ideas together:

- ✔ Identify your personal support network and your care partner's. ***Note:*** They're not necessarily the same people. To do this, list the one or two people that each of you would call if you just needed to vent. Then add the names of three or four people you'd call for specific help or the occasional favor.

- ✔ Of these people, have you or your care partner turned down help from one or more of them?

- ✔ If you've rejected their support, how can you reopen the door and welcome them back as active partners in care?

If the person accepts your overture and asks what you need, be prepared with specifics. For example, "Can you just stop by for a visit while my care partner goes to the store? It's getting harder for her to take me along, and, frankly, the break does us both good."

Consider counseling to get your head and spirit straight

Depending on how far you've distanced yourselves from other people, professional counseling may be necessary. But you have other choices that carry built-in benefits of community and social interaction. Check out these three possibilities:

✔ **Support group:** Okay, you may have resisted this option up until now, but get over it — if not for yourself, then for your care partner. Properly facilitated support groups can be a real source of new ideas, local information and updates, and even inspiration for managing your PD more effectively.

You may need to visit more than one group to find a good match, but smaller communities may not have a group specifically for PD. To find support groups in your area, go to the National Parkinson Foundation Web site (www.parkinson.org), or, for more general information, go to the Web site of the National Family Caregivers Association (www.nfcacares.org).

✔ **Community:** Every community has counseling resources for low or even no cost. For example:

- Religious communities have one or two clergypersons well known for providing comfort and counsel. The clergyperson doesn't need to be yours (or even of your faith).

- Hospitals, your local library, and civic groups may offer community programs with experienced speakers addressing topics of loss, aging, living with chronic illness, and so forth.

- Funeral homes often offer grief counseling by a professional who's trained in helping people work through a loss. Certainly you and your care partner have suffered loss as your PD's progressed.

✔ **Professional:** At some point you or your care partner may benefit from the guidance of a professional. There's no shame in this. Your physician, hospital or home care social worker, and local Office on Aging are good resources for referrals.

Plan for the healing power of R&R

Good news: You can avoid much of the damage caused by burnout if you build regular respite into your routine — early on. This means planning daily and weekly breaks as well as the occasional (but just as regular) longer hiatus, as we describe in the following:

✔ **Daily short-term respite** means at least two timeouts — separately or together. Perhaps your care partner takes a walk while you watch a sports event on television, or you call a friend while she takes a long, hot bath, or the two of you order takeout from a favorite restaurant, or you watch a favorite movie together. Whatever the respite, be sure you plan it, schedule it, and don't cancel it (okay, short postponements are acceptable).

✔ **Weekly breaks** may include trips to the beauty salon or manicurist, card night, choir practice, a movie, or a club meeting. These breaks last a couple of hours, and support group meetings don't count because *respite* means getting away from *everything* to do with PD. Plan the breaks, write them on the calendar in ink, and make them non-negotiable — unless the house is on fire.

✔ **The longer hiatus** can take many forms but usually lasts several hours to several days. Only you and your care partner can best identify the rest and relaxation you need. It may be a trip to the city for shopping, dining out, and seeing a play. It may be a place without a phone that gives you time to unwind with a book, take a walk in the woods, stroll along a beach, and so on. Such breaks take careful planning but they're doable. And the pay-off can be enormous for you as individuals and for your relationship.

If your care partner receives vacation, holiday, and personal time from work, it's not *respite* if he spends it catching up with a household, a family, and your PD. Respite isn't about labeling time; it's about how time is used. It's taking a break and getting away from everything to do with giving or receiving care.

Recruiting Secondary Caregivers

Okay, your chronic PD has progressed. Little tasks that once were doable are now nearly exhausting — and frankly not always worth the effort. Spending the day in your pj's is easier than the hassle of getting dressed. Brushing or styling your hair is a joke, and shaving or trying to apply make-up? Forget it!

Now you carefully time your appointments or activities to your on-off cycles. Your concentration isn't what it once was, and you're beginning to worry that you may be letting important details (like paying the light bill) slip.

On top of all this, you're seriously worried about your partner — the worry lines around her eyes and mouth, the constant exhaustion, and the lack of attention to personal needs, activities, and grooming. Your partner needs some help — and so do you.

Calling another meeting

We hope you and your family met soon after your diagnosis to talk about the ways PD was likely going to impact your lives (see Chapter 7). Now, as the symptoms worsen and new symptoms seem inevitable, you need to gather the troops once again. This time the agenda is different.

In some cases your adult children may bring everyone together. This family meeting may take on the trappings of an intervention if your family believes that you and your care partner are being overly stubborn about asking for and accepting help. Far better for you to acknowledge early on that you need additional help and take charge of the meeting on your terms.

Extending the invitation

Woody Allen once said that 80 percent of success is simply showing up. And that comment is especially true when you have a family meeting to discuss help and support — you need the family to actually show up. Their good intentions just won't cut it. Although we don't suggest subterfuge for getting family members on board, you need to do what you can to gather the family in one place at one time. If that plan's next to impossible, then choose a family holiday when you plan to be together — Thanksgiving or a major birthday for you or your care partner.

Consider these suggestions to help organize this meeting:

✔ Make it clear to family members that the day will include a discussion of the future for you and your care partner.

✔ If the gathering involves young children, make plans to occupy them for two to three hours. Ideally, arrange for them to be at another site so they don't interrupt the meeting.

✔ If a family member refuses to attend the meeting, assure the other family members that you'll speak with this person privately about a commitment to your care. And if that person clearly isn't on board with this arrangement, then drop it for now. Perhaps down the road (maybe when someone else is burning out) this person may step up.

Preparing the agenda

For this meeting, you have three goals:

✔ You and your roster of care partners need to face facts. Your PD has advanced, and your spouse, significant other, adult child, or other rock you've been leaning on can't do it all.

✔ You now need more hands-on and supportive care for you and your primary care partner.

✔ Everyone needs to understand the situation and figure out how to make some definitive contribution.

Initially you and your care partner will approach family for this care and support. But in some situations the family is either unwilling or unavailable. In that case you can follow a similar guide for a meeting with friends and neighbors who have expressed a desire to help. Just keep in mind that your friends and neighbors aren't family — they don't owe you anything.

The meeting will outline the following details:

✔ Help that you need now (chores, bathing, transportation, and so forth)

  • Specifically name the task; quantify how often you need the help and when you need it. (Some tasks are seasonal, like putting up screens and cleaning out gutters; others are regular, like helping you shower or staying with you once a week while your care partner is out.)

  • Indicate community services (and their costs) that can provide the assistance

✔ Help that you'll likely need within the coming year

  • How often and when

  • Availability and cost of community or paid services

You probably won't need help with everything — at least not all at once. But identify all the areas you may need assistance as your PD progresses. The following is a partial list to get you started:

✔ **Hygiene:** Bathing or showering, oral hygiene, dressing, personal grooming (hair, nails, and so on), other personal hygiene such as odor due to urinary incontinence

✔ **Medications:** Organizing and storing, dispensing, refilling prescriptions

✔ **Transportation:** To and from medical appointments, to and from community or social events, to and from shopping

✔ **Exercise and recreation:** Prescribed exercise for flexibility and strengthening, personal exercise preference such as yoga or T'ai Chi, pursuit of hobbies and leisure time activities

✔ **Basic nursing tasks:** Ambulation (walking from room to room), transferring (from bed to chair to car and such), care of medical equipment such as a catheter

✔ **Emergency care** (prepare every caregiver in basic first aid): Wound care, falls, fractures, fainting, choking, adverse reactions to medications

✔ **Household chores:** Exterior home maintenance (regular like grass cutting; seasonal like snow-shoveling), interior home maintenance (regular like weekly cleaning; occasional like changing the furnace filter), errands (like grocery shopping and trips to the post office), meal preparation

✔ **Financial tasks:** Bill paying (like utilities or medical and household bills), taxes (preparing, filing), money management (like investments and pensions)

As you prepare these lists, don't be too quick to surrender a task (such as grocery shopping) if it gives you or your primary care partner a break from confinement to the house. In this case, the opportunity for socialization and being out in the world may have greater value than the assistance. Perhaps someone can stay with you while your partner shops. Then that secondary caregiver can assist in bringing in the groceries and putting them away.

Turning over the meeting

Surprise! We suggest that you open the meeting, lay out the agenda (see the previous section) . . . and then leave. Why should you do this when you and your life are under discussion? Simple. Family members may find it difficult to admit limitations and aversions to giving care; saying this to your face can be even more difficult. When you leave, let your primary care partner take over the facilitation of the meeting, or, better yet, you may want to ask a third party (such as your support group leader or clergyperson) to conduct the meeting. The point is to create an environment where those in attendance feel free to express concerns and limits without hurting your feelings.

Especially in families with a history of discord, asking an objective third party to direct the entire meeting is a good move. A trusted clergyperson, counselors, and the facilitator of your support group are possible candidates. In this case, both you and your primary care partner leave the meeting after the opening.

Getting everyone talking and committing

Open the meeting by stating that you fully intend to manage as much as you can for as long as you can. But you do need their assistance (not control) and patience to accept that tasks may take you longer and require more effort.

Distribute printed copies of the agenda that includes your list of tasks (see the earlier section "Preparing the agenda" for ideas). Then excuse yourself (see the previous section "Turning over the meeting"). Your care partner or third party then facilitates the meeting as follows:

1. **Give everyone time to consider the list and their emotional commitment (10 to 15 minutes should do).**

   Note: Don't try to limit any part of this meeting to a specific schedule. You want to make this meeting an open discussion, not one constrained by time.

2. **Ask everyone to mark tasks that they'll consider taking on.**

   Explain that people won't have to take on every task they mark. You'll use the results of this process to assign specific tasks, establish back-up help for a task, and identify gaps that may need outside help.

3. **Open the floor to questions, discussion, and additional suggestions for the list.**

4. **Go through items one by one and identify coverage (or lack thereof).**

5. **Tally the cost of outside help for the apparent gaps. Ask family members to indicate (in writing for your care partner's eyes only) what amounts they're willing to contribute to that total each month.**

6. **Finally, adjourn the meeting with the assurance that you'll plan a follow-up meeting after you and your care partner have gone over the information and made a tentative schedule.**

After the meeting, you and your care partner can review the information and get actual commitments for hands-on help and financial contributions.

Accepting aid with appreciation and gratitude

Now that you have the commitment of family members, you and your primary care partner have an important task: You need to accept their willingness to help by making specific assignments.

The division of contributions will not be equal or fair. Everyone needs to face that fact from the outset. The physical and emotional toll for a family member living nearby can be very different from a member who lives at some distance. Similarly, one family member may not be able to accept that you need help with such personal tasks as combing your hair, taking a shower, or going to the bathroom.

You and your primary care partner must not pass judgment but must try to find ways each personality can contribute. If hands-on care is beyond a person's capacity, assign them to *outside* tasks, such as home maintenance, shopping, finances, taxes, and so on.

Some individuals are just naturally more nurturing. One of your adult children or siblings may mark practically everything on the list. Resist the urge to take him up on that. The last thing you need is for these secondary caregivers to burn out when you need them most.

Teen-aged children, grandchildren, extended family members, close friends, and other people may welcome the opportunity to help you and your care partner in concrete ways. Don't leave them out of the discussion, although you may want to approach them separately. If so, do that shortly after the meeting with adults in your family — perhaps that same afternoon.

You and your care partner probably have a realistic idea of the time and effort each task takes (especially the ones involving personal, hands-on care). You also understand the emotional toll of dealing with PD better than these relative newbies. Keep all these concerns in mind as you consider who may be the best provider for each task.

Whatever the contribution, as long as the provider gives it with love and the best of intentions, accept it and say "Thank you."

A Word for the PD Care Partner

You didn't ask for this, but here you are. Now you need to find a way to attend to the needs of the PWP in addition to other facets of your life. Many of those facets may be (probably are) vital to the situation. For example, your work may be the prime source of income these days. It also may provide the insurance that both you and the PWP need.

Your health is also a factor. You can hardly manage the escalating tasks of a caregiver if your own health is compromised. So, good eating habits, daily physical exercise, and adequate rest are more than good ideas — they make a huge difference in your overall ability to tackle this new challenge.

Get real about the time this is going to take

The Family Caregiver Alliance estimates that the average caregiver spends 18 to 20 hours each week giving care. One-fifth of family caregivers provide 40 or more hours of care per week. Even if you don't work outside the home or work part-time, you have other facets of your life that need your attention. You have *you* that needs and deserves your attention.

You don't have PD — your partner does. And you won't have PD after your partner moves beyond your ability to provide full-time, hands-on attention. You'll have a life — and we hope it's still filled with the people and activities that have sustained you since before PD became a part of it.

Consider the roles you play now: spouse or significant other, adult child, parent, sibling, employee (or employer), homemaker, civic or community leader (in your town, religious community, or such), volunteer. Add to these official roles a list of the activities you enjoy, such as reading, biking, traveling, gardening, and so on. Finally, add any additional hobbies you enjoy (and don't necessarily share with the PWP), such as needlework, photography, sports, playing cards, and such.

Wow! When you write it all down, chances are good that you have a life that's pretty full. Add one more item: Besides the PWP, do you have other family members, such as an aging parent or in-law, who will likely need your care and support in the next few years?

The big question is: How are you going to fit caregiving into that busy life? Put another way, what will you have to put aside or give up altogether to be an effective caregiver over possibly several years?

Get creative about finding the time

Time management experts advise you to look at time as blocks. Start with your five weekdays — that's five 24-hour blocks. Block out the non-negotiables: work (hours per day) and sleep (at least 7 hours a night). What's left on a normal weekday? Full-time work and sleep account for 15 hours, leaving 9 hours available. Okay, so far.

Now add time to get ready for work, travel to and from work, shopping and errands, laundry and other housework, and meals. Whew! Chances are you just knocked off another two hours a day and you still have to find time for meal preparation, eating those meals, laundry and housework, checking up on other family members, catching up with friends, making time for choir practice or a workout — and oh yes, partnering in care. Where does the time go? Better question: Where will the time come from?

America as a society has gotten very good at multi-tasking, and that practice may save you time in a few places. For example, can you make phone calls while preparing a meal or doing the laundry? Can you work part of your week from home so you can do the actual job in the evening and open up the day for something like a doctor's appointment, grocery shopping, and that workout?

How about taking advantage of available community services such as adult day care (see Chapter 21)? Can they provide the PWP some of the care you currently give (such as a hot meal or hair care) in order to free up time for you?

The options are out there. You and the PWP just have to be willing to accept the help and accept the fact that it may not be done your way or as well as you do it. But if these options can give you back the time you've surrendered to mundane tasks so you can once again enjoy a quiet evening of television or visiting with friends, then they're certainly worth considering.

Be prepared to delegate

The temptation in giving care is to simply do it yourself. Maybe it seems faster and easier than trying to explain what you need. And maybe you get energy from the praise and admiration you receive when you handle everything on your own.

The world has its super-moms. Are you becoming super-caregiver, trapped into believing (and convincing other people) that you and the PWP are managing fine? Are you sending signals that these people can go about their lives with no guilt or concern? *Whoa!*

In the early and mid-stages of PD, you and the PWP managed for some time without relying on others. Then one day you realize that the PD, its physical demands, and its mental and emotional demands are falling squarely on your shoulders.

The point is:

- ✔ If you haven't already opened the door (and your mind) to accept the help of other people (see the previous section "Recruiting Secondary Caregivers"), this is the moment.
- ✔ If you haven't held a family meeting, do it now.
- ✔ If you've had the meeting, call the family together and let them know the need for help and support has reached another level.

  Review what else they can do and what they can add to their present financial contributions.

In the process of taking on more care responsibilities, don't make the mistake of ignoring the PWP. Ask yourself these questions:

- ✔ Are you (or others) assuming that the PWP can't perform tasks or make decisions that are in fact still possible?
- ✔ Are you making sure that the PWP is still part of the discussion and decision-making?
- ✔ Are you keeping in mind that, for your loved one, this is another loss in the battle to maintain autonomy and independence?

Bill of Rights for the PD care partner

As the care partner for someone with PD, you perform an incredibly valuable and loving service. Anyone willing to put his life on hold in order to make the life of another better deserves the respect and appreciation of everyone involved. Just in case you have days when you feel as if that respect is not forthcoming (and you will have such days), make a copy of the following Bill of Rights for care partners, carry it with you, and take it out now and then to read through.

I have the right

🖒 To take proper care of myself because doing so will make me a better care partner for the PWP

🖒 To seek the help and support of others and to have the PWP accept that such support is necessary

🖒 To maintain certain facets of my life beyond the PWP, just as I would have if that person didn't have PD

🖒 To occasionally (and humanely) express anger, sadness, and other difficult feelings

🖒 To reject any attempt by others (including the PWP) to manipulate me (either consciously or unconsciously) through guilt

🖒 To receive respect, appreciation, and acceptance for the support and care I provide, knowing that I am giving it my best possible effort

🖒 To take pride in my efforts and to recognize the courage and sacrifice required to provide that support and care

🖒 To protect my individuality and my right to make a life for myself beyond the support and care the PWP needs

🖒 To expect and demand that, even as new strides are made toward the treatment and cure of PD, similar strides be made toward aiding and caring for those of us who partner in care

This isn't about you. Presumably you have years ahead of you, but your PWP faces a progressive decline. And you still have choices that the PWP no longer has. On the other hand, no one expects you to martyr yourself in the cause of giving care. That's where respite comes in — for you and your loved one. If you haven't read it yet, be sure you check out the earlier section "Dealing with burnout" for specifics on healthy respites.

Chapter 20

Putting Your Financial and Legal House in Order

. . . .

In This Chapter

▶ Organizing: A place for everything

▶ Checking the pulse of your financial health

▶ Maneuvering through the insurance maze

▶ Making your choices known — and legal

. . . .

Managing long-term illnesses like Parkinson's disease (PD) has more than a physical, mental, and spiritual price tag. The financial cost is also significant. And closely related to financial considerations are the legal issues that need your attention throughout the journey.

As with the rest of this book, in this chapter we preach planning and preparation. Chances are good that before receiving the PD diagnosis, you had made financial plans for your future, so you already have a lot in place. If not, you need to attend to these matters sooner rather than later because PD can progressively affect your capacity for decision-making. The information in this chapter gets you through the financial and legal red tape of protecting your assets and the futures of loved ones.

Gathering Important Information

The first step in managing your financial and legal affairs is to gather all the information and documents in one place. Some people are already terrifically organized; they can put their hands on key documents from three years ago in a flash. But a lot of people don't do as well. Some of these folks think nothing of showing up at the tax auditor's office with shoeboxes stuffed with receipts, cancelled checks, and handwritten notes; they dump it all on the poor auditor's desk and then assume that the auditor can make sense of it.

Whichever group you fall into, set aside some time, get a notebook and pen (or work off your computer if that's preferable), and find a place to work on this important piece of preserving your security.

Inventorying legal and financial documents

You need a clear inventory of key identity information, like Social Security number, insurance numbers, bank account numbers, and so on. Also, if you've appointed a power of attorney for legal or health matters, that document (and copies of it) must be readily available. Your health history is also a vital piece of this inventory. In fact, everything that may be needed — when you're unable to provide it or give its location — needs to be a part of this inventory.

Prepare a document in your computer files or make a list in a notebook with the following information. Then carefully store this information where it's secure from theft or fire (such as in a home safe) and be sure your care partner and others you trust can readily access it.

- ✔ **Access to personal information:** For each of the following include pin number and password clue (or actual password); contact name and phone number for technical support; online addresses as appropriate:

  - E-mail account

  - Voicemail

  - Personal and business Web sites

  - Online banking and shopping accounts (such as credit cards, electronic transfer accounts [ETA], or bills paid automatically or online)

- ✔ **Personal documents:** Record the location of each of the following:

  - Medical history and records

  - Family history

  - Birth certificate

  - Adoption documents

  - Naturalization papers

  - Marriage license

  - Divorce decree

  - School records

  - Employment history

- Social Security card (including the number)
- Driver's license (including number and expiration date)
- Income tax filings
- Savings certificates and bonds
- Stock certificates
- Safe deposit box (including information about location of the key)
- Military discharge information (including branch of service and service ID number)
- Passport (including number and expiration date)
- Religious papers (including names of preferred place of worship; clergy person and phone number; important religious records)
- List of memberships (including names of organizations; contact information; membership numbers)
- Organ donor wishes (give a copy to your physicians for your medical records)
- End of life and funeral instructions (including funeral home and cemetery names; contact names and numbers; location of original documents — especially if you pre-pay)
- Name of your favorite charity (for donations in lieu of flowers)

✔ **Information for dependents:** List their names, birth dates, and contact information.

✔ **Inventories:** List all of the following items. In addition to this list, consider taking photos of the items. Store the list and photos in an online file and keep a copy in your safe deposit box. For especially valuable items, get appraisals and keep the appraisals with a photo of the item in your safe deposit box.

- Home inventory including fixtures, furnishings, appliances, equipment, and so on
- Personal valuables including jewelry, artwork, antiques, books, clothes, mementos, and so on
- Business inventory including fixtures, furniture, stock, and so on

✔ **Personal bank and credit union accounts:** For each of the following entries include name of company or institution; contact name and phone number; account or file identity number(s); name(s) on the account and location of documents.

- Personal loans
- Liens against property

- Paid liens against property

- Loans paid on installment

- Business accounts

- Business loans

- Pension and retirement accounts

✔ **Insurance:** For each of the following entries, include name of company or institution; contact name and phone number; policy and any group number; name(s) on the policy and location of documents:

- Health insurance and Medicare

- Vehicle insurance (including registration number and location of the title)

- Other insurance (life, disability, long-term care, homeowner's, renter's, business, liability, valuables, and so on)

✔ **Legal papers:** Record the location of the original for each of the following:

- Will and living will, including name and phone number of attorney and other people with copies

- Durable power of attorney (finance and healthcare), including name and phone number of the person appointed, the attorney, and other people with copies

✔ **A list of contents of your safe deposit box:** Be sure to include the following items in your safe deposit box:

- Copies (possibly photos) of your home, personal, and business inventories (see these categories earlier in this list)

- Appraisals and photos of especially valuable items

- Original documents and files

- Original Social Security card

- A copy of your driver's license

- A copy of your health insurance and Medicare cards

- A copy of other insurance (life, disability, long-term care, homeowner's, renter's, business, liability, valuables, and so on)

✔ **Miscellaneous:** Record the location of each of the following:

- Storage units' contracts (including location of unit; name and phone number of company; unit number; location of key or combination)

- Home and business safe (including key or combination)

Getting the info into the right hands

You aren't finished yet. In addition to completing the inventory, you need to tie up these other loose strings:

- ✔ Make sure your care partner and other trusted family or friends are aware of this inventory and how to access it.

- ✔ Place all of the documents and files in a safe deposit box (keeping a copy at home) or in a fireproof file container at home.

- ✔ Be sure someone other than you and your care partner knows where you store the documents and files. As an alternative, file a copy of key documents with your physician, attorney, or financial advisor as appropriate.

- ✔ Make sure that your care partner and one other trusted family member or friend has copies of your medical information (your Social Security number, insurance cards, list of medications, and so on).

- ✔ Be sure that your checking and savings accounts are accessible (if you're incapacitated) by putting your care partner's name on the accounts.

- ✔ Be sure your safe deposit box is accessible by putting your care partner's name on the account (especially if you're going to store key documents like your will or living will or the originals of your power of attorney documents there).

- ✔ Make sure you give your doctor(s) copies of any advanced directives (like Do Not Resuscitate [DNR] orders); also, have a copy available to hand to the admissions representative any time you check in to the hospital or the emergency room.

- ✔ Give your doctor(s) written permission to discuss your health with your care partner.

Assessing Your Financial Health

Your ability to orchestrate your healthcare and solid financial future for you and your family is tied to your ability to understand the complexities of healthcare in America today. In many cases, the decisions that insurance companies and government programs make are based on generalizations, not your specific situation.

So, getting a handle on your specific economic well-being is a wise move. The information you put together in the following sections can provide a better idea of your financial health at this stage of your life, and this understanding can help you and your care partner make the best decisions to protect your futures.

Tracking income and out-go

In addition to an inventory, you need a clear idea of your resources versus your expenses. In your notebook or on your computer, set up a table with two columns, one titled *Resources* and the other *Expenses*. The information you enter under each column is pretty self-explanatory. Under Resources, list:

- ✔ Cash on hand (in checking and savings accounts as well as literal cash on hand)

- ✔ Annual income (from salary, trusts, royalties, dividends, property rental, and so on)

- ✔ Pay-outs due you (from pensions, investments, and so on)

- ✔ Property value (home, car, antiques, jewelry, land, and so on)

For Expenses, enter annual data for:

- ✔ Standard household expenses (food, utilities, rent or mortgage, insurance payments, payments on loans, and so on)

- ✔ Medical expenses (doctor visits, medications, medical equipment, therapy sessions, and so on)

- ✔ Occasional but regular expenses (clothing, household items, service for the car, and such)

Projecting costs over the long term

You have a condition that is progressive and will change over time. Predicting how that will translate into dollars and cents is difficult, to say the least. But you do know that costs will increase as your income decreases. What to do?

Yep, you need to make another list. So get out your trusty notebook or open a file on your computer and enter your best estimates for the following additional expenses you can anticipate as your PD progresses. Estimate the cost per month for each item.

- ✔ Lost wages
- ✔ Lost benefits
- ✔ House changes or remodeling

- ✔ Transportation expenses
- ✔ Medical expenses
    - Medications
    - In-home assistance (aides)
    - Medical equipment (walker, wheelchair, hospital bed)
    - Therapy not covered by insurance (physical, occupational, speech)
    - Medical bills not covered by insurance
- ✔ Respite costs (for you and your care partner)
    - Day care
    - Vacation care
    - Weekly in-home relief
    - Counseling

Using your assets to cover medical expenses

A home or other real estate can be a financial asset to cover the escalating costs of medical care. If you're still making payments on your home, you may be able to get a second or a refinanced mortgage. If you own your home outright, a reverse mortgage may be an option.

With a reverse mortgage, you receive monthly payments from a lender (usually the bank) while you continue to own and live in the property. The amount of cash you receive is based on your equity in the home, your age, current interest rates, the value of the property, and its location. You can receive payments in one of three ways:

- ✔ **Term plan:** Fixed monthly payments over a specific time period
- ✔ **Tenure plan:** Fixed monthly payments for as long as you continue to live in the house
- ✔ **Line-of-credit plan:** Cash advance withdrawals from a fixed total sum

Eligibility requirements for a reverse mortgage don't include income limits but

- ✔ You must be at least age 62.
- ✔ You must own the home outright.
- ✔ The home must be your principal residence based on voter registration information.

Do reverse mortgages have a downside? Yep. Two of the significant downers are the following:

- ✔ Up-front fees can be steep for insuring and administering the reverse mortgage.

- ✔ If you choose to use part of your cash advances from the reverse mortgage to pay those fees, those sums plus interest are added to the bottom line of those fees.

How do you repay the loan? After the borrower moves out of the home or dies, the home can be sold to repay the loan, or family members can retain the home and repay the loan in other ways.

The good news? The total of the reverse mortgage loan can never be greater than the value of the home at the time the loan is repaid, even if the loan balance is greater than the home's value at that time.

Deciding to take a second or reverse mortgage isn't as simple as it may appear. Before you take such a step, engage the services of a professional counselor (such as your financial planner, your attorney, the bank's reverse loan officer, or all three).

For more information, check out the U.S. Department of Housing and Urban Development (HUD) Web site at www.hud.gov.

Understanding the Intricacies of Insurance

With the seemingly gazillion insurance products on the market, figuring out which product best meets your needs can be a full-time job. For people diagnosed with young onset PD (YOPD) or people with PD (PWP) who are still working and receiving employee benefits, check out the section on insurance in Chapter 8.

Before choosing an insurance policy of any type, go online to www.ambest.com, the Web site of A.M. Best, a company that rates insurance companies. You want to see a rating of at least A+, preferably A++. A high rating assures you that this company is financially stable and likely to be around when you actually need the benefits.

You also want to check whether the company has raised premiums on existing policies. When an insurance company's management has to make this move, one or two reasons are behind the raise:

- ✔ They didn't do their homework before setting the premium.

- ✔ They're planning to raise rates on a regular basis; unfortunately, just when a person needs the benefits, he drops the policy because he can't afford the high premiums any longer.

For most people 60 years and over, the insurance game is a little more straightforward. Although you may have trouble taking out certain types of insurance because of your PD, other options exist. For example, if you're a veteran, you may qualify for veterans' benefits that include insurance. Or your state may offer a special state health insurance plan to cover people with pre-existing conditions that aren't covered by other insurers.

Whatever your options, your goal is pretty clear: You want to work with your insurance advisor to protect you and your family against the ravages of long-term illness on your financial security.

Qualifying for federally funded programs

This is the good news: Federally funded healthcare programs provide health insurance for some Americans; Medicare and its sister program, Medicaid, are the two most prominent. But as the section below explains, all federally funded programs aren't created equal, and although they're certainly a big help, they're simply not going to pay all your healthcare costs.

Be sure your doctors accept Medicare — not every doctor does.

Medicare

Medicare is a federally funded and administered national health insurance program available to any American citizen who is age 65 and older or who is eligible for Social Security disability benefits. Enrollment is automatic regardless of health, income, or political persuasion.

But all is not rosy. The original Medicare program was designed in 1965, when the goal was to provide financial help for seniors due to the rising costs of *acute* (immediate) care. In other words, the program was intended to help pay for care following a catastrophic event such as a heart attack, a fall that results in a hip fracture, and so on. Unfortunately, the program can be confusing in terms of what it covers and what it doesn't cover. (See the sidebar, "Medicare: A primer.")

The Medicare program works on a system of *assignment,* which means the government assigns the number of days you can be hospitalized and the payment levels for each service. So, if your final hospitalization bill reads $75,247.63 and Medicare has assigned only $50,000 to the procedure, a $25,247.63 shortfall exists. Whoa! What happens then? (See "Medigap" in this section for more info on this equation.)

For more information on Medicare coverage, you can call 800-MEDICARE (800-633-4227) or go to www.medicare.gov and request publication #CMS-10050-28, the annual update on Medicare programs and coverage.

Medigap

Medigap is the slang expression for Medicare supplemental insurance policies. You need one of these policies if you're receiving Medicare benefits because — drum roll, please — a gap (sometimes a cavern) exists between the cost of medical care and Medicare's payments. A gap also exists between the services Medicare covers and the services you need.

As a minimum, you need a Medigap policy to cover the 20 percent remainder of charges that Medicare covers at 80 percent. But beyond that, look for a policy that covers what Medicare doesn't cover at all:

- ✔ Hospitalization expenses for a year or more past the Medicare allowance
- ✔ Coverage for most excess charges not covered by Medicare (such as doctor bills beyond allowable fees)
- ✔ Coverage for care received outside the United States or Canada

Fortunately, several policies are available, and these companies must accept anyone who's eligible for Medicare. The concept of pre-existing condition is not part of their vocabulary and you have no wait period. For more information on selecting a policy, call 800-MEDICARE (800-633-4227) and ask for CMS publication #02110, "Choosing a Medigap Policy."

Medicaid

Medicaid is another federal healthcare program with a twist. Although the funding comes from the federal government, each state runs its own programs. And the rules can vary wildly. However, all programs base eligibility on income, and that amount is very close to the federally determined poverty level. Income is the only factor in Medicaid; age doesn't affect eligibility.

When you're at a certain level of income (and remain there), Medicaid covers care costs for the rest of your life. What's the catch? Most states get to decide where, when, and from whom you receive that care.

For more information about your state's requirements for Medicaid eligibility, contact your state Office on Aging.

Looking into long-term care insurance — Not just for old folks

We hope you've already looked into a long-term care (LTC) policy well before being diagnosed with PD (either because you're reaching the age where people consider such issues or because your employer offers a plan). In some cases, pre-existing conditions (such as PD) can disqualify you automatically (or seriously limit your options). If it's too late for you, definitely look into a long-term care policy for your care partner because it may have secondary benefits that help you if your partner becomes unable to provide the care you need.

Although many people can benefit from LTC coverage, two instances where LTC insurance isn't essential are:

✔ When your income is low (or you're willing to spend down your assets as discussed in the earlier section "Medicaid")

✔ When you will likely qualify for Medicaid

At the other end of the spectrum, perhaps you're in the Fortune 400 crowd of multimillionaires, in which case your assets are such that you can afford to cover the costs of your care without seriously impacting your lifestyle. Just remember: Some estimates place annual costs of managing healthcare with a chronic progressive condition between $65,000 and $100,000. Did you catch that? That's the per-year cost. If your assets need to stretch to cover 10, 15, or 20 years, you do the math.

Using private health insurance, disability benefits, HIPAA, and COBRA

For many people, health insurance is a benefit offered by their employer, but too many people fail to examine the actual benefits of their coverage until they need it. Don't make that mistake. Take a look at your current coverage and identify where it may be leaving you exposed. For example, does it include coverage for medications? If not, is there a rider or supplemental policy you can add to help cover those costs? Review the following discussion of health insurance basics; then you (or your partner if she has the policy) may want to sit down with someone in Human Resources and review the gaps in your coverage.

✔ **Private health insurance** comes in two forms:

- *Individual policies* that you purchase on your own give you choices and coverage that last until age 65. These policies can't be cancelled, and premiums can't increase on the basis of your health condition.

  Coverage can be expensive, and at the outset, you can be turned down or denied coverage for treatment for PD or other pre-existing conditions.

- *Group policies* are funded at least in part through your employer. You may have little or no choice on features, but the coverage is usually available with no penalties for pre-existing conditions when you start a job.

✔ **Long- and short-term disability coverage** is available through many employers or as an individual product. The ground rules are essentially the same as for health coverage:

- For individual policies, you need to be in good health when you apply.

- The group policy may require a period of employment (typically 6 to 12 months) and a waiting period of several months during which the employee has not sought treatment for the condition before being eligible for disability benefits.

  Benefits are based on a percentage of base salary, but that salary is still taxable. No adjustments are available for inflation or cost-of-living increases. For more information on disability benefits, see Chapter 8.

✔ **HIPAA** is a government acronym for the **Health Insurance Portability and Accountability Act,** a relatively new program designed to protect working people.

In a nutshell, HIPAA requires states to make all health insurance portable. This means that if you leave one job for another or to start your own business, you can't be denied coverage regardless of health as long as you're under age 65. Each state decides which carrier provides this portable product, but you can't be denied coverage. For a fact sheet on HIPAA check out www.dol.gov/ebsa/newsroom/fshipaa.html.

✔ **COBRA,** another federal government alphabet-soup acronym, stands for **Consolidated Omnibus Budget Reconciliation Act.** This program protects and benefits the employee, giving you the option to continue your employer's group insurance for up to 18 months at your expense after leaving your job.

This option guarantees that your coverage isn't interrupted. You pay the group rate (including what your employer was contributing on your behalf), which is usually far less expensive than the same coverage in an individual policy (if you can even get an individual policy).

Relying on other resources to pay for care

As the government continues to wrestle with the issue of affordable health insurance, Congress and many states continue to enact legislation that partially addresses the problem.

For example, a growing number of states have established health insurance co-ops or pools for people who are denied coverage (usually due to a pre-existing condition). *Note:* Such programs usually have a residency requirement, and the cost of coverage runs higher than similar coverage if you were completely healthy. To find out whether your state offers such a program, contact your State Insurance Department.

Check that medical bill *before* you pay up

How many times have you gotten a statement from your insurance provider that shows the name of a doctor you never saw or heard of? How many times has payment by your insurer been denied because the billed service duplicates coverage already paid? How many times have you called the hospital or lab and been told the strange doctor was the one who read the results? Since when is reading the results not part of the lab work? Your insurance carrier is likely to catch such double-billing practices and decline to pay. Not to worry. The purpose is to try and get a higher insurance payment. If that's declined, the provider usually drops the matter rather than bill you out-of-pocket.

According to Medical Billing Advocates of America (an advocacy organization), every hospital Web site and lobby proudly posts a list of patient rights. Included in that list is the right to request an itemized statement or explanation of items on your bill that you don't understand or believe you didn't receive. Unfortunately most patients never take advantage of this right, so medical billing errors go undetected. Either the insurance company pays them (adding to the spiraling costs of health care across America) or the patient pays.

An itemized bill may be overwhelming at first (some can run on for 20 to 30 pages), but every

time you catch an error, you put the billing office and the insurance company on notice. For example:

- ✔ Administration of oxygen may be a common protocol for the procedure you had, but if you didn't need or didn't received that oxygen, you shouldn't pay for it.

- ✔ Maybe your doctor ordered a pain medicine on an as-needed (or as-requested) basis. You know you never requested that medicine, yet it's on the bill.

- ✔ A scan through an itemized bill may reveal outlandish charges such as $10 for a cotton swab. Go to the discount store and buy a package of a thousand swabs for a couple of bucks. Take them with you when you go to question the bill. It'll make your point.

Managing your medical costs is one way you can maintain control as your PD progresses. Requesting an itemized statement and questioning services you didn't receive or were overcharged for delivers the message loud and clear: You may have PD, but you're still in charge. By the way, the billing office isn't allowed to charge you for making a copy of the bill even if it runs into a couple hundred of pages.

In 2004, Congress created Health Savings Accounts (HSA) for people who purchase a government-approved, high-deductible health plan (HDHP). The buyer pre-funds a substantial percentage of the deductible each year in a tax-deductible savings account similar to an IRA. Funds deposited in the account can be used to

✔ Pay the deductible

✔ Cover the costs of medical and dental services not covered under your policy including alternative medical treatment

Any part of the deposit not used in a given year carries forward. As your PD progresses, you're likely to meet or exceed the deductible in any given year, but this plan may be an option for your care partner.

To find additional information about programs and disability coverage, check out Chapter 8 or go online to www.socialsecurity.gov.

Making Sure Your Wishes Are Sacrosanct

One key to good long-term-planning is to put certain documents in place well before you or your care partner needs to access them. These documents include:

✔ A will, of course

✔ Trusts in your children's names if you have children to protect

✔ A durable power of attorney for finances and healthcare if your state has provisions for them

✔ Your end-of-life wishes

✔ Advance directives (make sure you've shared those wishes in writing with your doctor[s] and your family)

Durable power of attorney

Appointing someone to act on your behalf is the purpose of a *power of attorney* or simple POA. The standard document allows you to assign someone the right to manage financial and personal matters for you. The catch is that this person's appointment only lasts as long as you remain capable of making those decisions yourself.

For the time when you can't make decisions known, you still need a spokesperson you can trust to move forward as you want. At this point, the *durable* POA comes into play. Two types exist:

- ✔ **Durable power of attorney:** You appoint someone to speak on your behalf for financial and other non-healthcare matters when you no longer can.

- ✔ **Durable power of attorney for healthcare**: You appoint someone to make medical and healthcare decisions for you when you're unable to make them yourself.

Not all states recognize the same documents. Check with your attorney to understand your state's laws on these issues. If these documents are available, don't put off officially naming your non-healthcare and healthcare representative.

Whether you're living with PD or you're perfectly health, stuff happens and none of us can guarantee that we won't end up unconscious in an emergency room, unable to make our wishes known.

Advance directives and living wills

The trend in medical care today has moved away from the paternalistic model where the doctor made decisions for the patient. Today the patient has the autonomy to state medical and end-of-life choices and to expect that those choices will be honored. But what happens when you can't speak up for yourself?

Give advance consent to all your doctors as well as your lawyer to talk with your care partner as needed. The rules and forms for doing this will vary from one state to another, so ask your lawyer to make sure this consent is a part of your legal portfolio.

Advance directives and living wills are tools for stating your desires regarding decisions the doctors and your family are facing when you're unable to participate in the decision. This concept has dual benefits:

- ✔ You take the pressure off your doctors and family members from making emotional and tough decisions when they're under enormous stress.

- ✔ You can make your exact choices clear in a legally binding document.

For example, the choice of terminal sedation is legal in most states. Terminal sedation isn't considered assisted suicide or euthanasia because the goal is to ease suffering, not to induce death. You (or your healthcare power of attorney) can ask the doctor to order medication at the end of your life to ease pain or difficult breathing.

Another specific to consider is whether you want an autopsy that can help researchers understand more how PD affects the brain. If terminal sedation, autopsy, or a procedure equally specific is part of your decision, you need to state this in your living will and make sure that a copy is on file with each doctor likely to treat you.

Last will and testament

A *will* states your choices regarding the distribution of your property and mementos after you die. This is a legal document, and although you may believe writing down your wishes (or telling them to your care partner) is enough, you can save everyone headaches (and probably a good measure of trauma) after you're gone if you take the time to create a legally witnessed and signed document that makes your wishes binding for your survivors. To help you in that, the Funeral Consumers Alliance offers a packet of materials entitled *Before I Go, You Should Know* available through their Web site at www.funerals.org.

Tough stuff, but even the healthiest of people need to address these seemingly gloomy issues. Getting on top of them early on is just one more way you can take control and move forward with your life — on *your* terms.

Chapter 21

It's Just Bricks and Mortar: Housing Options You Can Live With

*I*n times of personal crisis, *home* often becomes a synonym for refuge or safe harbor. It's the one place most people can go and be themselves without feeling the need to keep up appearances or a brave front. It's also the place where people surround themselves with items that bring back memories of good times, successes, and even trials endured through the years.

The day will come when you and your care partner need to reassess your current living situation in terms of its safety and practicality. As time and your Parkinson's disease (PD) progress, you may develop balance problems that result in falls and fractures. In many cases, you can make adjustments to your present home that allow you to remain there in comfort. However, you may eventually need to choose between a building that represents your past and a place where you have the assistance you need for a productive and satisfying future.

And in the spirit of our mantra — prepare, don't project — you can get to work on these housing issues well before the need is imminent. This chapter helps you do just that. We first guide you through the safety issues of your present home and cover the community services that enable you to remain there. Then we take you through the tough steps of deciding to move. Finally the chapter breaks down the variety of residences you can choose from when you've decided the time is right.

Making Your Home PD User-Friendly

Your first step in thinking through this whole nest quest is to take a good look at your current residence. You may be surprised to discover how even small changes can give you additional months, if not years, to enjoy your current home.

Safety first: Assessing your home

Accidents in the home are one of the most common causes of injury and death in America. With your PD and the meds that can make you more prone to falling (see Chapter 18 for more on this), a check of your home is imperative. You may want to schedule one as often as you check the batteries in your smoke detectors — which is at least once a year, right?

Your local fire or police department may offer a home safety assessment at no cost. If so, take advantage of this great community service. There are also home safety assessments offered by trained nurses, and this service is usually covered by Medicare and some insurance companies. If neither of those professional surveys is available for you, you can also go through the following checklist to get started on your own home safety assessment:

✔ **Oh say, can you see?**

- Make sure lighting is adequate both inside and outside the home.

- Pay special attention to lighting in stairways and hallways.

- Place nightlights in the bathroom and along the path from bedroom to bathroom.

- Check lamps and electrical appliances. Do the cords and wiring show wear and need for repairs?

- Avoid using extension cords if at all possible; when they're absolutely necessary, anchor them to the wall (not the floor) to prevent tripping.

- Bundle and tie up excess footage on computer and other electronics cords; then anchor them safely under the desk or along the baseboard.

✔ **Underfoot stuff can be dangerous!**

- Get rid of all scatter rugs (even those with rubber backing) and carefully check for worn carpeting or edges that are coming free of their tacking; make necessary repairs.

- Make sure floors (tiled, wood, or uncarpeted flooring) aren't slippery.

Test floors in a pair of socks. If you can do the slide, the floors need to be stripped of the wax or compound that's making them slippery.

- Remove any raised threshold strip that separates one room from another; make the transition smooth.

- Install nonskid runners on uncarpeted stairways. Each stairway needs a sturdy handrail on at least one side and light controls at the top and bottom of the stairway. Use bright neon tape to mark stairs in especially dark places.

- Shop for shoes with nonskid soles and no laces, the kind boaters prefer.

✔ **Two key spaces are accidents waiting to happen.**

- In the kitchen: Standard safety rules apply. Keep curtains or flammable materials away from the stove and make sure all appliances are in good working order. Assess whether items in the kitchen are convenient for you. For example, are glasses better on a lower shelf? Can you move the skillet from the drawer under the oven to a hook or a higher cabinet?

- In the bathroom: Place nonskid strips in the bathtub and shower; install grab bars wherever they make life easier — bathtub, shower, and toilet. Set the hot water heater at 110 degrees or lower to prevent accidental burning.

✔ **Don't forget:**

- Place emergency and other medical contact numbers next to every phone.

- Install smoke detectors (or check present ones) in every stairway and in the kitchen; place fire extinguishers in an accessible place on every floor level including the basement; determine an escape route in the event of fire.

- Check for needed repairs to sidewalks and driveways: broken asphalt or concrete, uneven brickwork in paths and sidewalks, and so on. Consider installing ramps for the time when managing even a few stairs becomes difficult.

- Double-check your house's security. Are all locks on windows and doors working properly? Be sure screens, storm windows, and doors are properly and securely installed. Get to know your neighbors and let one or two trusted neighbors know who to contact if they have concerns about your safety or the security of the property.

Got your to-do list ready? Great. Time to get busy!

If possible, make this a family project. List everything that needs attention and then subdivide that list into large and small jobs. Tackle any fairly extensive changes for improving movement (such as removing threshold strips) first. Such structural barriers — usually in multiple places in your home — may put you in the greatest danger for falling.

De-cluttering and hazard-proofing

Take a good, long look at the contents of your residence. Address the clutter that may be hazardous and clean out unnecessary *stuff*. For example, does your son still play that drum set, or could it be moved into the attic or better yet sent to his house for the grandkids to use?

Rearranging to go with the (traffic) flow

You've de-cluttered your living space, so now you're ready to consider repositioning your furnishings. You want to create the best traffic flow, meet your needs for comfort, and still have some design appeal. (Wedging your television in the far corner may offer more space, but not a whole lot more!)

Some people seem to have an eye for positioning furnishings for maximum convenience and visual appeal. The rest of the world needs help — a decorator, a particular family member, a friend, or a friend of a friend who has a real knack.

But you can do a little preliminary evaluating on your own. What suggestions can you incorporate from your assessment (see the previous section, "Safety first: Assessing your home") and from the safety check by the police or fire department? For example, would a simple change in the placement of the sofa make it easier to access the doorway in the event of a fire or other emergency?

 How can you put the rooms of your home to better use — not just because you have PD but because they may serve everyone better? Forget those room labels and think outside the box. If you're going to be spending more time on the computer — checking out information and staying in touch with — maybe that little-used guest room could become your headquarters. Even if you didn't have PD, chances are the rooms of your home could be far more user-friendly for the real life you lead. Besides, change and playing around with new ideas can be fun!

Taking Advantage of Community Care Programs

If you choose to remain in your own home for as long as possible, you have some options for extending that timetable even after your PD begins to put you at risk for falls or other traumas. But staying at home and bringing in care services has financial considerations. Most services — even if your insurance or Medicare covers part of them — are for a limited period of time and focus on a higher level of care, such as the services of a nurse or physical therapist. The following sections help you weigh your options.

In-home services

In-home help may be your first line of defense against moving because it can provide two significant services:

- ✔ Household help, such as meal preparation, shopping, and home maintenance
- ✔ Personal and medical assistance, such as help with personal hygiene, dressing, or medications

Most large communities have agencies that offer in-home care-assessment services at no cost. They can suggest support options for you and your care partner. Smaller communities or rural areas likely have a well-known network of independent contractors — people experienced in offering the elementary services you may need at some stage of your PD.

To find independent contractors and community services, consider the following strategies:

- ✔ Talk to neighbors, friends, and the nurse or office manager in your physician's office for references.
- ✔ Check with your local librarian or search your telephone directory's business listings for agencies offering services.
- ✔ Call the local hospital's social services department or your regional Office on Aging (in the phone book under *state* or *county government offices*).
- ✔ Use a computer to check out several sites that may be helpful such as www.eldercare.gov. Search the Internet using key words like *home care* and your community's name.

Expand your search to the county level and surrounding communities if you live in a smaller community.

Even if these people can't offer the answers you need, don't stop there. Ask them for other people to contact. Thank them for their help and follow their suggestions for that next contact.

Consider exploring the types of services in Table 21-1 for your area and file the information for when you may need it down the road.

Table 21-1	Services for In-Home Assistance		
Service	*Contact Name and Number*	*Cost*	*Notes*
Errand services			
Home repairs			
Transportation			
Meal programs			
Medical equipment and supplies			
Delivery: Meds			
Delivery: Groceries			
Housekeeping			

Some programs may involve little or no cost. For example, youth groups may offer snow-shoveling or routine home maintenance. Grocery stores and pharmacies may offer free delivery. Government-funded meal programs for seniors can provide not only a hot, nutritious meal but also the opportunity to get out and interact socially with other people.

On the other hand, some services may come with sticker shock that has you reeling and saying, "Are you kidding? I'll do it myself," or "If I can't, my care partner will!" But take care not to burn those bridges too quickly. What happens when you can't manage some tasks on your own? What happens when your care partner is ill, needs to go away, or has to work overtime and can't be there when you need the help? What about your escalating need for care? Are you really prepared to ask your care partner to assume all the household and personal care tasks that the two of you may have shared up to now?

Don't be stubborn about accepting care from other people — even when you have to pay for it. If the service provides help for you *and* extra time for your enjoyable activities (not to mention independence!), it may seem downright priceless.

Home healthcare services

Home healthcare is a higher level of medical assistance that isn't part of the normal services offered through either your doctor's office or the hospital. At the same time it includes services that your doctor or the hospital's social worker and discharge planner might *prescribe* for you (such as a visiting nurse to come to your home and check up on you after you've had a fall).

The good news: If your physician orders or prescribes professional in-home care, your insurance or Medicare pays most, if not all, of the bill. After the professional (a nurse or physical therapist, for example) is approved, you may also become eligible for personal-hygiene care and housekeeping services you've needed.

The not-so-great news: Such home health-services are finite — they continue for as long as medically necessary. After the need for professional service is over, the personal care also ends. Likewise, when you can reasonably travel to the site of the professional services (like physical therapy), the home delivery ends.

The most common situation for home healthcare is following a hospitalization, often because of a fall that causes a hip fracture or other broken bones. Check out Chapter 6 for a full discussion on what to expect (and do) if you've been discharged from the hospital and still need extra care. Such services — whether they follow a hospitalization or another scenario — are finite and short-term, but they are available. *Note:* The downside is that you have to demonstrate your knowledge of them and then ask for them.

Adult day care

Adult day care is relatively new in the United States and therefore not as geographically widespread as the need is. Day care programs for adults can offer an array of services in a variety of settings — from community rooms in religious or senior centers to free-standing facilities.

In most cases, day care programs focus on socialization rather than health-care services. Still, they offer more health support than traditional senior centers because day care programs have staff trained to provide nursing assistance and routine medical support (such as overseeing medication dosages, assistance with transferring from one position to another, and, in some instances, personal care services such as bathing and barber or beautician services).

Day care can bridge an important gap in the continuum of care services. When your PD symptoms keep you from safely getting out and about on your own or when your care partner needs to work, day care offers an opportunity for you to be with other people and remain active.

Keep the following facts in mind:

✔ Not all states license or certify day care centers for adults. This means safety, cleanliness, and regular reviews of staffing and program standards aren't regulated.

✔ Because programs can vary greatly, be sure you understand what services are included in the fee and what services you pay for on an as-needed basis.

✔ Some centers may offer a free trial day; if they don't, then visit the center (if possible, more than once) before making your decision.

Adult day care isn't for everyone and may not be right for you if you're still an active participant in other social and community circles. But it's an option to consider as your PD progresses. Adult day care can lengthen the time you're able to remain in your own home, and it can provide occasional respite for your care partner.

Respite care

The concept of respite isn't just for your care partner. (Review Chapter 19 for this discussion.) When you have a chronic, progressive condition like PD, you too need time off. Trying to keep up that brave and optimistic demeanor can be enormousiy exhausting. Managing symptoms and fighting for every bit of function and independence can sap the energy of even the strongest PWP.

You deserve a break — a regular timeout from thinking about PD at least once a week. (Although we cover this more completely in Chapter 19, the routine's important enough to reinforce here.) You also need (and deserve) the occasional longer R&R to

- ✔ Take a deep breath and be cared for without feeling as if you're imposing on your family or under their watchful eye
- ✔ Come to terms with the progression of your PD

Believe it or not, such places exist. In the early stages of your PD when your symptoms are well managed by your treatment plan, consider traveling to:

- ✔ A retreat center that offers rejuvenation, often at a reasonable cost.
- ✔ A cabin or lodge in a state park where you can spend a few days or a week for a reasonable cost in settings that inspire introspection.
- ✔ A major city if you really can't deal with all that quiet time. Treat yourself to a stay in a hotel, tickets to a play or sporting event, shopping, dining (as opposed to simply *eating*), and letting strangers pamper you.

As your PD progresses, options for respite are available in an environment of safety and care appropriate to your needs. For example,

- ✔ Adult day care programs (see the earlier section "Adult day care") can give you and your care partner a few hours of respite.
- ✔ Hospitals, step-care communities (see the section "Communities of care" later in this chapter), rehabilitation centers, and dedicated Parkinson's centers on medical-center campuses may offer overnight, weekend, or vacation *respite care.*

 Even if you're not ready to make use of such programs right now, gather information about the ones in your area. You may find that such a service is handy when an emergency arises (such as your care partner's mother needs help in another state) and your care partner worries about leaving you.

Deciding When It's Time to Move

One day in the future, your current residence may simply not work for you. (Frankly that day comes for a lot of folks who aren't even dealing with PD!) Certainly you've had other life passages when change wasn't necessarily welcomed, but required. You managed then — and perhaps you even thrived in the new setting. You can certainly do it again — especially if the move simplifies your care and frees you to enjoy other activities.

Bidding your abode adieu

The truth is that you're going to know in your heart of hearts when your home is no longer practical. You can't climb the stairs. Your bathroom — in spite of its maze of grab bars and safety features — is too small or difficult to use. Your wheelchair doesn't fit through the doorways or roll easily across the carpeted floors. You and your care partner are becoming isolated from friends, family, and the community activities you love.

The only problem is if you refuse to admit that the time is right. If you've prepared for this day (as we've been known to preach), the struggle can be far less distressing. The decision won't be easy, but you can skip the panic and anxiety of not knowing where to turn because you already know your options. You're ready to pick one and get on with your life.

Weighing the pros and cons of moving

Certainly you don't want to move before you're ready, but you do need to let go of any fantasies about the future and face reality. Is it practical and safe to continue living in your home? More to the point, can your life, routine, and ease of functioning improve if you move?

One person with Parkinson's (PWP) didn't leave his home without a fight. Before he was willing to admit it was time, he tried everything — an alert necklace so he could call for help if he fell (which he did frequently), a hospital bed for his living room so he didn't have to go to the upstairs bedrooms, a portable commode next to the bed so he didn't have go to the bathroom during the night, and a private-duty aide at night so his wife could get her rest.

One day he looked around the house and realized that it wasn't the refuge he had loved for so many years. The memories it held had been pushed aside to make room for the trappings of his illness — his home had become one giant sick-room. And he didn't want that for himself or his wife.

Moving is 90 percent attitude

However you come to the decision — willingly or kicking and screaming — moving day is tough. It's tough on you and on the people who love you and share the memories that made your house a home.

Further, this is a major step in the progression of your PD — the admission that you need to (rather than *choose to*) move. This is the time to talk about your feelings with a counselor or trusted friend — one who has no stake in the emotional real estate of the home itself. In short, you need to take the time to grieve this passage the same way you mourn any major passage in your life. Talking about your sadness and regrets eventually leads to acceptance and even (perhaps) anticipation of the next step.

Redefining Your Castle

Leaving the old homestead is the end of the world only if you say it is. Remember the discussion of your coping style — the old fight or flight scenario? (Check out Chapter 7 for a refresher if you need one.) Well, in this case, flight is turning your back on the positive possibilities of housing opportunities. Fight, on the other hand, is taking charge of this new challenge by considering the options you've researched and by choosing the best one with your care partner.

Weighing your options

You may be surprised at the possibilities after you begin to consider solutions for moving to a place that will permit you to continue to have as much independence and control over your routine as possible. The following sections describe some of the more common choices.

Moving in with a family member

Okay, stop shuddering. Moving in with a family member can work as long as both parties work through the details of the living arrangements and routines *before* making the decision to share living space. In every household there are routine chores and schedules. What's yours and what's the schedule for the rest of the household? If you're moving in with an adult child, are there also grandchildren in the house? Then their schedules (and rights to privacy and socializing with friends) must also be taken into consideration. Ideally you will have a specific space of your own in the house — your room (hopefully furnished with your things) and possible (hopefully) your own bathroom. And the rules for you? Keep in mind that this is your relative's home — not yours. By all means, state your needs at the outset, but then settle in and do your part to become a welcomed member of the household.

Considering a more practical apartment, condo, or house

Some options aren't as drastic as moving to a care facility. If you're having mobility problems in your current residence, what can make that easier? Perhaps your home is multi-level, or the doorways are too narrow, or the rooms are too small to accommodate a wheelchair or the safe use of your walker. In such cases, consider a house, condominium, or apartment that's on one level and constructed for an aging population. Much new construction today offers wider doorways, smooth thresholds, and safety features in bathrooms as standard fare. Several other options are also available:

- ✔ **Accessory dwelling units (ADUs):** ADUs are living spaces within an existing home or on the same property. (Remember the concept of the mother-in-law apartment?) Can you remodel your present (and beloved) home to include a small apartment where you can live comfortably and safely while your adult child moves into the main house? Can you use the ADU as a residence for a live-in caregiver who, in exchange for room and board, provides care services for you?

  An alternative is to move into an ADU within the home or on the property of your son or daughter whose been encouraging you to move in. An ADU gives you (and your child) privacy and autonomy while relieving the stress of living some distance apart.

  Check local zoning ordinances and assess the practicality of constructing an ADU. If you're determined to stay in your home for as long as possible, the ADU can help lengthen that stay.

- ✔ **Subsidized senior housing:** In many communities, apartment or housing complexes use state and federal funding to accommodate middle- or low-income senior citizens. In such facilities, rents reflect a percentage of income.

- ✔ **Board-and-care homes:** If you have no live-in care partner, a board-and-care home may be an option. Also referred to as *group homes,* these facilities are usually large homes that have been converted to serve people who can no longer manage on their own but who don't need a higher level of care. These homes are in residential neighborhoods, and residents have their own bedrooms and share common areas of the house. Sometimes the makeup of the residents revolves around a common factor such as age, gender, or disability. A paid staff prepares meals, assists with some care, and may engage residents in group activities. *Note:* Such facilities aren't eligible for public funding such as Medicare or Medicaid.

Communities of care

In response to the aging of America (and the rest of the world), the options for long-term care have grown in the last several decades. Today the most common types of services are grouped according to client-ability: independent, needs some assistance, needs major assistance, and end-of-life. The facilities may have different names in different states, and the services and costs vary widely.

To locate services in your area (or in another community closer to adult children or a preferred climate), consider the following:

- ✔ Call the local Area Agency on Aging (look under state- or federal-government listings in your phone directory).

- ✔ Call the Eldercare Locator at 800-677-1116.

- ✔ Go online to `www.eldercare.gov`.

Medicare covers costs on the same basis as medically necessary services in a resident's private home (for example, if the doctor orders physical therapy for you, Medicare might cover such *skilled* home-care with some possibility of personal care as long as such services aren't already provided by the facility).

This section breaks out five basic types of long-term care facilities along with their specific features, pros, and cons.

Continuing care retirement centers (CCRCs or step-care communities)

These facilities offer levels of care from independent through nursing care. The primary advantage is that you don't have to research new facilities, make a major move, or leave behind friends and staff as your needs change. You and your significant other can live together; if one partner needs a higher level of care, the other can remain nearby.

Services, levels of care, and admission procedures and requirements can vary widely in such facilities. Get all the rules up front before you choose. Also, remember that should the time come when you need a higher level of care, you want to be sure that the nursing part of any step community is certified as a *skilled-care* facility (meaning they're qualified to accept Medicare payment for skilled rehabilitative services). The facility should also be certified for Medicaid (see Chapter 20 for more on this federal program). To be thorough, you may want to check their state inspection record. For more information, check out `www.carf.org/aging`.

Some communities may not include a nursing care facility. If this is the case, ask whether they have an association with a nursing facility in the community and whether residents of the CCRC get preferential consideration if the nursing facility has a waiting list. The same words of caution apply: Be sure this facility is certified to ensure you receive the best possible care.

Independent apartment with services

Many step-community residents begin by residing in an apartment or cottage with their personal belongings. Such units may tie into the overall community through safety features (such as call bells in bathrooms), activities (such as field trips or book discussion groups), and meals in a common dining room.

Note: This level is similar to traditional freestanding apartment or condominium complexes. Residents come and go as they please, manage their own healthcare, and maintain roles of choice in the larger community.

Assisted living

These facilities can vary greatly in terms of standard services and those services offered at an extra cost. Be sure you ask for the specifics regarding both of them. In general, such facilities include assistance with activities of daily living (ADLs), such as bathing, dressing, and transferring from chair to bed and back.

Standard services may also include the management and administration of medicines, transportation to and from doctor appointments, and most meals. Residents usually live in their own efficiency or one-bedroom apartment within a building or complex of buildings that also houses common areas such as a dining room, chapel, activity room, and library. Most assisted living facilities have a standard monthly fee and then additional services that you can purchase on an as-needed or as-wanted basis.

On the downside, if the facility isn't part of a step community with its on-campus skilled nursing facility and you fall and need extended rehabilitation, that will mean another move (plus having to pay for two places if you intend to return to the assisted living facility).

Skilled nursing facility (SNF) or rehabilitation center

Skilled nursing facilities or rehab centers are facilities that provide *skilled* care and must be specifically licensed to provide these professional rehabilitative services. Nursing facilities that aren't licensed for skilled care (as well as those that are) also offer what is called *non-skilled, custodial,* or *maintenance care.* These non-skilled wings of the facility serve people in the advanced stages of illness or life with a wide range of support, personal care, routine health services, and social opportunities.

SNFs can serve a variety of populations — people of all ages who may reside there for varying lengths of time, including:

✔ People recovering from surgery may spend several weeks in a nursing home or rehabilitation center before returning to more independent living.

✔ People who suffer from dementia, such as Alzheimer's, often live in nursing home care centers when the community or their family can no longer manage the person's care. Often the care centers have special units that maintain the safety and dignity of people suffering from dementia.

✔ People whose care needs exceed the family's or community's ability to meet those needs may live in this type of facility. Many facilities have special units where people who are frail but alert and relatively active can be safe and secure while taking part in the facility's activities and social opportunities.

✔ People in need of care occasionally stay here on a short-term basis to give the caregiver a much-needed break.

The best nursing homes have full occupancy, so visit early on and get your name on the wait list if this is the place you want to be for any future rehab or residency services. *Note:* When your name comes to the top of the list, the administrator calls you. If you're not ready to move to the nursing home, you can request that your name stay on the list.

Hospice

Hospice care is becoming an increasingly preferred option for patients who are clearly coming to the end of life. Hospice programs provide personal care for the patient and also offer counseling for the families and friends. The program may be in a special facility, a hospital, or a nursing home, but in many cases hospice services are also available in your own home. After the program accepts you, a team of doctors, nurses, home health aides, social workers, counselors, and even trained volunteers help you and your family cope with the final days of your illness.

To find a program in your area, ask your hospital social worker, and remember that while Medicare may cover some costs, it won't cover round-the-clock care at home.

Assessing for a perfect fit

Only you and your care partner can describe in detail the needs you have as individuals and as a care team. But as you make that list together and use it to evaluate various housing options, keep these key factors in mind:

✔ Be realistic about your possible future needs and the ability of you and your care partners to meet those needs every day over what could be several years.

✔ List residential care options in your area and in the area of an adult child, friend, or close relative where you may consider moving. Then assess and compare similar facilities for quality and consistency of care.

✔ Visit those facilities (at all levels) that meet your criteria and assess them using the checklist at the end of this chapter.

✔ Talk to people — staff and clients at the facility, people in the community, neighbors, and friends. Ask what they've heard, what they know, and what their Aunt Millie's experience was.

✔ Always choose on the basis of which facility best meets *your* needs.

Making a list, checking it twice: Evaluating the facilities

When you visit a facility, focus on the people in the program and note their interactions with staff. Two words of caution:

✔ Don't let the *window dressing* (beautiful furnishings, plantings, free lattes, treats for prospective clients, and other such details) sway you.

✔ Don't be taken in by an unusually warm welcome or excesses of flattery and interest by your tour guide.

These folks are in business to sell a product and a service. And you, dear reader, are their target audience.

Following is a checklist for your tours of various facilities. In a notebook, record the number of each item and then any notes you have about that service (use a separate page for each facility). Consider placing a numeric value next to each service to reflect your overall observation (for example a 5 is *excellent* and a 1 is *very poor*). Not all items apply to every location, and services offered by one facility and not others may influence your final decision depending on your current idea of what you will need and the reality of what might be needed down the road.

✔ Entrance is user-friendly and attractive.

✔ Staff welcomed and was prepared for appointment or tour.

✔ Light, doorways, and hallways adequate to accommodate people with wheel chair or walker.

✔ Facility is free of any noxious or unpleasant odor; clean and attractively furnished.

✔ Grab bars are in bathrooms and handrails in hallways.

✔ Temperature is comfortable for clients.

✔ Smoking is either not permitted or allowed only in clearly marked, designated areas.

✔ Exits are clearly marked; smoke detectors and sprinklers are throughout the facility.

✔ Furnishings are sturdy and appropriate for people with movement disorders.

✔ If meals are served, clients have choices and special diets are available.

✔ Staff interacts with clients and treats every client as an adult and with respect.

✔ Staff members are certified (where appropriate) or receive ongoing training; hiring includes background checks.

✔ Tour guide calls residents by name and is clearly known to them.

✔ If appropriate, a registered nurse is on staff in addition to the facility administrator.

✔ The ratio of staff to client is reasonable.

✔ Staff takes a team approach with the client and family in developing a plan of care.

✔ The administrative team has been in place at least one year.

✔ Ownership of the facility has not changed more than once in five years.

✔ In a residential facility, residents may bring personal furnishings.

✔ Resident living spaces have adequate and personal closet and dresser space even if room is shared.

✔ If rooms are shared, residents have a voice in choosing a roommate.

✔ Tour guide offers copies of resident-rights documents and any reports of state or facility inspections for review.

✔ Activities are age-appropriate and conducted with respect to the experience and history of the clients.

✔ The facility has an outdoor area for client use; staff is available to assist the residents in accessing that area.

✔ Facility has an emergency evacuation plan that includes plans for unusual events such as tornadoes, hurricanes, and so on if appropriate.

✔ Services alluded to in promotional materials are indeed included in the base cost; extra services and their cost are clearly spelled out.

Certification and licensing isn't a requirement in all states or for all types of care facilities, but facilities that must meet such regulations (either state or federal or both) undergo regular (and unannounced) inspections to ensure compliance.

Certainly any facility that accepts Medicare or Medicaid or both must be licensed and inspected. The results of such inspections are a matter of public record. If you're considering a setting that provides full residential care and is licensed for payment through Medicare or Medicaid, you can view the results of the most recent inspection results online at www.medicare.gov/NHCompare.

A Few Words for You and Your Care Partner

The day may come (or it may never come) when your PD progresses to the point where you need constant round-the-clock care that is beyond the limits of what can be provided to you at home or in a semi-independent setting (such as an assisted living facility). Should that day come and you decide to move to a full-care facility, you and your care partner need to be prepared for some changes.

For example, the PWP must be prepared to accept help from strangers for even his most basic needs including dressing, bathing, getting to and from the bathroom, and such, and he may need to rely on someone else to speak for him and make his wishes known. And the care partner will need to down-shift her role from caregiver back to care partner (Chapter 19 explains the difference), which will involve monitoring the way care is provided by others instead of providing that care herself. The care partner also will need to advocate for the PWP, making sure that the PWP's final wishes are followed.

If the facility isn't used to caring for PWP, the care partner may also need to be firm about the importance of timing in the delivery of medications — even if that means the care partner must lobby for the staff to deliver meds outside of their normal routine rounds. Care partners, be prepared to have these tough conversations and stand your ground.

For both of you, this doesn't have to be a time of sadness. Instead it can be a time to let go of the stresses of the last many years and look back instead to the triumphs of having maintained a full life in spite of having PD.

Part VI
The Part of Tens

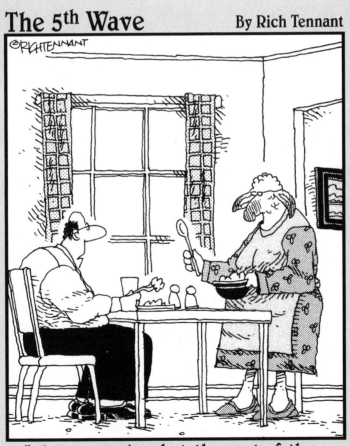

"Tell me again what the goal of the clinical trial is?"

In this part . . .

*E*very *For Dummies* book ends with a few top-ten lists. This one is no exception. We use this part to offer tips for handling the difficult feelings of living with a progressive and incurable condition. We also have a list that gently reminds you that your care partner is living with PD every day too. And finally we reissue our plea for you to get involved in the extraordinary community of people living with Parkinson's around the world. You'll be richer for the experience — we promise!

Chapter 22

Ten Ways to Deal with Difficult Feelings

C oping with feelings has no hard and fast rules. Just like the wild elation of falling in love may seem impossible to control, the bouts of intensely negative feelings that can accompany Parkinson's disease (PD) may also appear beyond your control. Because of the depression, anxiety, and other symptoms of your PD, you may find these feelings more of a challenge over time. To top it off, other people don't easily recognize when you're upset, which only requires more of your limited patience at these troublesome times. Here are ten ideas that may help you begin coping with these feelings.

Banishing the Concept of "Bad"

Placing some sort of value system on feelings is a no-win situation, yet people do it all the time. "I feel bad" doesn't mean that someone's physically ill but rather that he's wrestling with one or more emotions that make him feel out of sorts. By taking the time to examine and name this feeling, a person's more likely to find relief — and minimize the guilt. So, whenever you recognize you're in a funk, consider these two tips:

- ✔ Name the feeling (do *not* judge it as good or bad) by completing this statement: "I am (angry/jealous/sad) because _____."

- ✔ Do not resort to artificial comforts and cover-ups for the pain (like binge-eating, popping a pill, or drowning the feeling in a stiff drink).

Halting the Isolation

Any chronic, progressive illness carries a measure of isolation — for you and your care partner. You get so tired of having to admit that you can't go here or do that. As your illness progresses and you truly have more trouble getting out and about, that sense of isolation can become overwhelming. Heal the feeling by:

- Meeting regularly with other persons with Parkinson's (PWP).
- Encouraging (and accepting) the offers of people to come to you to share an hour, a meal, or an entire evening.
- Connecting through e-mail and phone calls.
- Exercising — take a walk or take part in a sport like golf.
- Tapping into whatever spiritual therapies work for you.

Corralling the Anger

Anger at your PD is one issue, but anger at those who love you and are attempting to meet your needs is quite another. On its own, anger is a completely normal response to living with a condition like PD that hampers your control and freedom. And getting really ticked off once in awhile can even be healthy. But generalized and unidentified anger that festers can do some real damage. So get a handle on your anger from the outset by:

- Recognizing that your mask-like facial expression may compromise your efforts to convey your frustrations and anger.
- Naming the cause and then seizing the moment — rant and rage for a couple of minutes, punch a pillow, or count to ten.
- Putting your anger in perspective — talk it over with someone to look for the actual underlying causes for the outburst.

Taming the Guilt

Guilt is sneaky. It creeps up on you after a jealous, frustrated, or angry reaction. It chafes as you perceive people putting their lives on hold for you. Like anger, guilt can build on other difficult feelings. But, just as you do with anger, you need to name the guilt and nip it in the bud by:

✔ Asking yourself whether you're being fair to people around you by accepting and appreciating their efforts.

✔ Taking stock and reassuring yourself that you're doing all you can to maintain your function in the face of your PD.

Subduing Your Fears

Face it. We live in a pretty scary world, mostly because of the uncertainties that surround us — planes flying into buildings, pandemic threats of famine and contagious disease, and then some. As a PWP, your fears may be far more specific than these world events. You're concerned that you may have passed this disease on to your children; you worry that your PD will incapacitate you before you can achieve certain milestones, such as seeing your daughter married or holding your first grandchild. Face your fears by:

✔ Reviewing the information on anxiety and depression in Chapter 13.

✔ Accepting that life is uncertain. The best anyone can do is to live each day to its fullest and *not* wait to celebrate and appreciate.

Venting Your Frustration

Frustration can arise from many situations. You may get frustrated with your inability to hold a comb or toothbrush. Or you may grit your teeth when you perceive your care partner's taking over tasks you can do for yourself. Or maybe you gag with the lack of straight answers to your questions about PD and its progression. And on and on. Here's an excellent solution: Call or e-mail one of the people in your support group (or go to an online group such as brain.hastypastry.net/forums) and vent! Then get back to life.

Cooling the Jealousy

Jealousy is such a normal human reaction. You've dealt with it your entire life — when a friend got a bigger house or a better car; when a co-worker got the promotion you wanted; when your sister lost 30 pounds without trying (or so she said!). As a PWP, odds are good that your green monster rears its jealous head when your family and friends are free to go and do as they please without even thinking about it. You, on the other hand, have to plan and time activities. Life is *not* fair. You know this one. Face it by:

> ✔ Reminding yourself of *your* successes. Could that co-worker handle the challenge of PD with the kind of grace and humor you do (most of the time)?
>
> ✔ Expressing (in a kind and gentle way) your feelings of jealousy to the person. Chances are good that you'll discover the person is equally jealous of you.

Stopping the Spirals of Sadness

There's a *little* sad and then there's a *lot* sad. A little sad is when you feel sorry for yourself but the feeling passes quickly — usually within a few hours. A lot sad is when sadness spirals into full-blown mourning or grieving, the way you'd feel if you suffered some life-changing event such as the death of a loved one or the break-up of a relationship.

For PWP, intense sadness may be connected to the life they had planned before they heard they had PD. Left to its own devices, sadness of this magnitude can spiral into full-blown depression. You need to nip it in the bud by first acknowledging your right to mourn the life that will no longer be and then by embracing the possibilities that are before you now.

If working your way through the sadness becomes overwhelming, seek professional support by talking to your clergyperson or the counselor you put on your care team to help you through tough times (see Chapter 6).

Caring About Apathy

"I just don't care anymore." "Nothing's going to change." Answers? You care or you wouldn't have made it this far. So start by discussing these feelings with your doctor. If you're not already engaged in some form of talk therapy with a counselor, this is a good time to consider that option.

Dumping Depression

Short spurts of sadness can be healthy reactions as you adapt to life with a chronic and progressive condition. But when such feelings last weeks with no let-up, you may be facing depression. You need to treat it the way you'd treat any physical symptoms that don't go away after a short time. If feelings of helplessness, hopelessness, escalating apathy, or spiraling sadness persist beyond a few days, get help. Start by reading Chapter 13; then talk to your neurologist about treatments for handling depression in PD.

Chapter 23

Ten Ways to Care for Your Care Partner

*L*ife turned an unexpected corner the day you were diagnosed with Parkinson's disease (PD) for at least two people — you and your primary care partner.

Your care partner is your champion — speaking up when you can't, making sure that the medical community focuses on you as an individual and not just as another *case,* and performing the thousand and one tasks that keep life running for both of you. Your care partner deserves not only your empathy and understanding but also your support and attention.

This chapter gives you ten ways to acknowledge the sacrifice and encourage a healthy form of selfishness for your care partner.

Honor the Partnership

A partnership is a two-way street. It's not all about you and your needs. You and your partner honor your partnership by recognizing it as a mutual exchange of ideas as you find your way together through this change in lifestyle. Initially the focus is on you, and that's only right. But eventually you need to get a grip on your own reaction to PD and take a long, hard look at its effect on people around you, especially the person next to you, your partner in care. These are some ideas for doing just that:

✔ In any discussion about adapting to your needs, be sure you address (via words and actions) how those needs will impact your partner's routine.

✔ Be open to the idea of getting support and assistance from someone other than your care partner. For that matter, suggest calling in reinforcements yourself. Perhaps your sister (who's offered to help in the past) can drive you to the hairdresser so your care partner has an afternoon to himself.

✔ Listen to what your partner is really saying. For example, in a discussion about your care partner doing tasks that you can still manage (although it may take you longer), maybe she admits that doing the tasks herself is just easier instead of waiting because of all she has to do. That answer may be a good clue that she's feeling overwhelmed, and you need to discuss ways to get her some help.

Acknowledge Life beyond PD

When every waking moment seems to focus on doctor's appointments, medications, maintaining function, and fighting depression, you need to stop and take a moment to really consider how much of your (healthy) care partner's life has been given over to your PD. How many of your conversations begin and end with PD? How much of your day and your care partner's focus on managing symptoms and maintaining your independence? What facets of your relationship before PD are beginning to slip through the cracks? Address that imbalance right now before it's too late. Talk through just how you can work together to make sure PD doesn't become your and your care partner's life.

One way to remind each other that there's more to life than your PD is to declare certain times of day *no-PD zones*. For example, agree to talk about topics other than your PD during and after dinner. You'll both sleep better if you spend the evening discussing lighter topics and catching up in general.

Accentuate the Positive

Care partners may actually resist talking about pleasurable experiences in their lives. For example, because you can't ride any longer, she may avoid discussing the amazing bike ride she just completed. Or she may feel uncomfortable talking about some political infighting at work because she fears that the details seem so petty and silly to you. Or she may worry that if she talks about a friend's impending vacation, it may just remind you that you'll probably never make that trip to Paris you dreamed of. You have a responsibility to encourage such sharing by making it clear that your partner is in some ways your extended eyes and ears, bringing you news and funny stories that have always entertained you.

Strike a Balance in Caregiving

Surely one of the most exhausting tasks for any care partner is trying to guess how much care is enough and how much is too much. How is your care partner supposed to know whether you're too exhausted to do something for yourself or you're determined to complete a task, even if you take all day? Care partners have many talents and they develop new ones over time, but mind-reading will never be on that list. If your care partner seems to be *doing* rather than *helping*, let that imbalance go for the moment, but find a time later to talk through the problems it may be causing.

Ask, Don't Demand

Listen to yourself. When you need help, do you begin the request with a verb? "Get me the remote." "Come here." "Button this."

Your care partner is not a private in your war against PD. Your care partner is right there in the trenches with you. Show some respect. This advice is not a request — it's a demand!

Use the Magic Words Often

Surely you learned them as kids: *please* and *thank you*. Never have they had more power. In the grown-up version, you need to move beyond simple statements — you need to show as well as tell. The smile, the touch of the hand, the small surprise that focuses just on your care partner are all magic in their own way. And the true magic is that you feel a little more like your old self if you can take care of your partner now and then.

Get Over Yourself

Yes, you've been dealt a really bad hand, but you're still here. For now you have a life that includes this person who has put his life on hold to take this journey with you. You also have a choice: live each day thinking about all the problems you may face as your PD progresses, or *live each day!*

Accept Services as a Gift for Your Care Partner

Asking other people to take care of needs that you once managed is depressing, especially if that person's a stranger who's paid to deliver a service. (And especially if that service is so personal and private that you find it difficult to accept, such as bathing you or helping you to the bathroom.) Try to accept this help as one way of caring for your partner. Does this service free your partner to attend to some other task or simply enjoy a break? Does the help save time that both of you can put to better use?

Find Joy in Life

Caring for someone whose outlook is positive and hopeful — in spite of setbacks — is far less stressful than trying to bolster the spirit of someone constantly seeing the dark side. Your care partner has gone through all of the emotions you have: anger, fear, depression, the gamut. True, PD isn't attacking your care partner's ability to function, but PD is attacking both your lives. Remember, you set the tone for how people respond to your PD. If you've shivered in the shadows for a while, try crossing over to that sunnier side of the street, and take your care partner with you.

Encourage Laughter and Dreams

Your care partner deserves a life beyond your PD, a life as full of pleasure and promise as possible under the circumstances, a life that keeps dreams alive. You can encourage and nurture that life for your partner. Start by flipping to the "Bill of Rights for the PD Care Partner" in Chapter 19. Post the list where you and your care partner see it every day. And when your care partner resists nurturing and caring for herself, ask her to read the list aloud. Then talk about issues that can and must change so you can help care for your partner — physically, mentally, and spiritually.

Chapter 24

Michael J. Fox, Muhammad Ali, and YOU: Ten Ways to Make a Real Difference

. . . .

In This Chapter

▶ Using your *power of one*

▶ Getting out and speaking up

. . . .

*T*he Parkinson's community is unique in that most PD organizations at the national level are super-organized, well-connected, and have earned the respect of the powerbrokers who can affect change. Think of the benefits people with PD (PWP) have gained from the efforts of Michael J. Fox and Muhammad Ali, for example, and then multiply that by 1.5 million — the number of PWP in the United States alone. Wow! There's power in those numbers! But you don't have to be a celebrity to make a huge difference. Here are ten ideas to get you started.

Read More About It

Start by making yourself a local expert on PD. Check out the resources in Appendix B — especially those that offer information to share with other people. Get them on board for a specific issue that needs attention. (See "Get to Know Your Local Officials" a little later in this chapter.)

Vote Early and Often

The shocking fact is that Americans are becoming increasingly apathetic about voting. How often have you heard someone say, "It doesn't matter — politicians are all the same"? Well, if you as a PWP don't care, who *is* going to care? Your elected officials' support for dollars for research and adequate care options is vital for the future of treating and curing PD.

Absentee voting is always an option if getting to the polls is too difficult.

Get to Know Your Local Officials

Local elected officials work for you and often live in your community. Don't hesitate to talk directly to them about key issues that could impact you or others with a chronic progressive condition like PD. For example, if a zoning law is preventing a rehabilitation clinic from locating in your community, let your elected officials know why this clinic is important for you and other people with chronic conditions.

If the issue is a state or national matter, consider making contact (by phone, e-mail, or letter) with an official's senior staff person. Locally or nationally, build relationships with your elected officials — not one of checking up but one of informing that can lead to a difference for many people in the community (and votes for re-election).

Never underestimate the power of a single note or phone call. And don't forget to follow up! If you've written or called an elected official and been told someone will get back to you, but no one has, call again.

Don't Just Be Informed — Pass It On

Okay, you don't want to overdo this but *carpe diem* — seize the day! Say you're at dinner with friends and the conversation has settled on politics. You know a key bill's coming up for a vote that can really impact PD research. Talk about it! Relate its importance to facts that will stick in people's minds and perhaps lead them to contact their congressperson to cast a key vote.

A less in-your-face way to inform people as you go about your daily routine is to stay involved and talk about projects and interests you're involved in even if they're not PD related. Why? Because this is your opportunity to show that PWP can be contributing members to society in spite of PD.

Support Your Local Support Group

Attend meetings and consider getting more involved in the group's effort to influence community leaders (or even national politicians). Even if the support group isn't specifically for PWP, you can find power in numbers. Signing a petition, participating in a charity event, or raising money for research are all ways you can help build a better future for PWP.

Rally Local Support

Consider ways you can build awareness through your local library, employer, and community organizations. For example, encourage your librarian to invest in informative books, videos, and CDs for people with chronic, progressive conditions and their care partners. Ask your employer and community organization leaders to offer literature and seminars that help people with these conditions and their families to manage their time and caregiving. Employers benefit from less absenteeism and a more focused and productive work force, and community groups become more engaged in the needs of the community. (Get things started by ordering a set of the excellent booklets from the National Parkinson Foundation listed in Appendix B.)

Pitch Your Story to Local Media Outlets

People who put together the local news (print, radio, and television) are eager to hear from you. Can you imagine how they would delight in a story about a 60-something doctor with PD performing his first piano recital with a group of kids? What about the young onset Parkinson's disease (YOPD) person's care partner who also works fulltime, cares for their school-aged children, and volunteers?

Before you call your local news desk, check with the person whose story you plan to offer (even if that's your care partner). In telling the story, include:

- A local angle — the story is about a person in your community
- The key that makes it unique and not just another health story — as in the piano-playing doctor mentioned earlier
- The visuals (for print and television; for example, is there a photo op at the recital so a photographer can attend along with the journalist?)

Never forget that your story could help others struggling with chronic illness.

Join the Parkinson's Action Network

Advocacy requires conviction and passion for a cause. The national PD community has banded together (for the most part) and named the Parkinson's Action Network (PAN) to speak in Washington DC for the entire PD community. You can be a part of that national call to action by logging on to the PAN Web site at www.parkinsonsaction.org or calling 800-850-4726 to find a local or area chapter or to get on their mailing list for updates.

Raise Money for Research

Of course, if politics isn't your gig, you can raise awareness as well as dollars for research several other ways. For example, some events (such as a marathon or walkathon) require quite a bit of organization and teamwork. Sign up to volunteer and get your friends and family on board as well.

You also can be effective on your own. How many times have you read of someone biking or walking across America and collecting donations along the way to raise awareness of some cause? Personally taking action doesn't mean you need to plan a trek across America, but what else can you do on your own to raise awareness and financial support? Try holding a yard sale with all the money going to PD research or ask family and friends to make a monetary contribution in your name to a PD organization in lieu of gifts on holidays, birthdays, and other gift occasions. (After all, do you really need another book, t-shirt, or CD?)

Celebrate National PD Month in April

PD gets its own month for national awareness — April (think springtime, renewal, and hope). How appropriate! How can you and your care partner mark this special month? The following are some easy ideas:

- ✔ Donate a copy of this book (or another on PD) to your local library.
- ✔ Plan to schedule one of the events suggested earlier in this chapter during the month of April.
- ✔ Go to New York City and take part in the annual Parkinson's Unity Walk. (Check out www.unitywalk.org for full information.)
- ✔ Buy a couple dozen red tulips (a floral symbol of the fight against PD) and pass them out to your friends, family, and everyone on your health-care team to thank them for making the journey with you.

Part VII

Appendixes

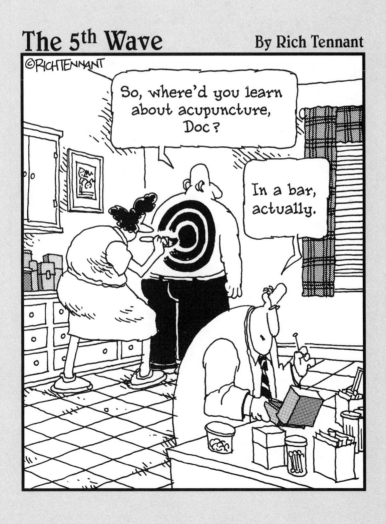

In this part . . .

In Appendix A you find a glossary that defines terms frequently tossed around in the world of Parkinson's disease. These are terms you should get to know because your doctors, other people with PD, and even the journalists who report the latest PD news use them.

Appendix B is a collection of resources that we introduce throughout this guide. The list includes national PD organizations with Web sites that can help in everything, from locating a neurologist or support group to updating you on the latest advances in medicines and treatments. We also include a list of programs and assistive devices that can make your life easier. Even if you don't have access to a computer (or don't know how to use one), get your child, grandchild, or the local librarian to help you discover these resources for enhancing your life.

Appendix A

Glossary

action tremor: An *involuntary*, rhythmic movement of the hand, arm, foot, or leg when a person performs a *voluntary* action such as lifting a fork, writing, or stepping onto a ladder. See *resting tremor.*

activities of daily living (ADLs): Routine activities that are part of a person's normal day (such as dressing, bathing, eating, toileting, transferring from bed to chair, walking from one room to another, participating in social and leisure activities).

advocacy: The process of influencing people via education, group actions, and publicity for a cause.

agonist: A muscle that contracts so the body can perform a specific movement; also a chemical or drug that stimulates a specific receptor to signal a desired action. See *dopamine agonist.*

akinesia: Also called *freezing;* temporary inability to initiate a desired movement.

antioxidants: Body chemicals that neutralize *free radicals.*

antiparkinsonian drugs: Drugs or medicines for the management and control of Parkinson's disease and its symptoms.

apraxia: The inability to execute a voluntary movement despite normal function and mental understanding of the desired action.

ataxia: Loss of balance and coordination.

athetosis: *Involuntary,* repetitive movements, especially with the hands, fingers, and (sometimes) feet.

basal ganglia: Groups of cells deep in the base of the brain that help the cortex in controlling *voluntary* movement and coordination.

bilateral: Occurring on or affecting both sides of the body or organ.

bradykinesia: The gradual slowing or loss of spontaneous movement that results in impaired abilities to perform a task or change positions.

bradyphrenia: The gradual slowing or loss of ability to process information.

carbidopa: A drug that, when combined with *levodopa,* reduces the side effects of levodopa yet improves overall effectiveness of levodopa by allowing more of it to enter the brain.

care partner/caregiver: Usually a family member (spouse, parent, sibling) who provides the emotional (and eventually physical) support and care for a person diagnosed with a chronic, progressive condition.

central nervous system (CNS): The network responsible for cueing the human body's mental and physical actions; consists of the brain and the spinal cord.

clinical trial: The research and testing required by the Food and Drug Administration (FDA) to determine whether new medicines, medical devices, and treatments are safe and effective before approving them for patients.

cognition: Those mental skills necessary to process information (such as perception, memory, reasoning, judgment, intellect, and creativity).

cogwheeling: The slow, jerky, or ratcheting sensation the doctor perceives when moving a patient's rigid limb at the joint.

computerized axial tomography (CAT or CT scan): A diagnostic computer procedure that uses a series of X-rays to produce a two-dimensional image of the body or specific body part.

Catechol O-methyltransferase (COMT) inhibitors: Drugs that block an enzyme that breaks down *levodopa* before the levodopa can convert into *dopamine*, thereby increasing the therapeutic supply of levodopa to the brain.

deep brain stimulation (DBS): A surgical procedure that helps control symptoms of advanced PD; electrodes are implanted in the brain and controlled through a battery-operated device known as an implanted pulse generator (IPG) or pacemaker.

delusion: A fixed belief that is false, not proven by objective evidence.

dementia: The neurological condition or sign of progressive decline in intellectual ability (such as impaired judgment, memory loss, confusion, personality changes, and disorientation) caused by one or a combination of underlying conditions, such as Alzheimer's disease and strokes.

depression: Sustained, prolonged feelings of hopelessness, helplessness, and sadness.

diagnosis: A doctor's conclusions based on a patient's medical history and symptoms as well as the doctor's observations and tests.

dopamine: The natural chemical substance present in areas of the brain that regulate movement, motivation, and feelings of pleasure. See *neurotransmitter.*

dopamine agonist (DA): *Antiparkinsonian drugs* that imitate and supplement the brain's naturally produced *dopamine.*

dysarthria: Difficulties with speech caused by impaired movement of muscles; results in slurred or muffled words or the inability to project one's voice or speak at a normal volume.

dyskinesia: Abnormal *involuntary movements* (examples are sudden muscle contractions; rapid, jerky or lurching movements; fidgeting or restless movements of upper body, arms, legs, or head); may be a response to long-term use of *antiparkinsonian meds* and may worsen with stress.

dysphagia: The impaired ability to swallow.

dystonia: A movement disorder that causes significant and unexpected muscle contractions or spasms that result in abnormal and *involuntary* movement and posture. Can be a symptom of Parkinson's disease.

essential tremor (ET): More common than *primary PD*, this movement disorder causes an uncontrolled *tremor* of the hands, neck, head or voice; most apparent when performing a *voluntary* action, such as lifting a cup. See *action tremor.*

executive function: The intellectual ability to set goals, make decisions, and perform multi-stepped processes such as balancing a checkbook.

festination: A series of progressively quicker, shuffling, almost-running small steps after walking is initiated; sensation of the upper body wanting to move forward but the legs are unable to follow appropriately.

Food and Drug Administration (FDA): The federal body charged with monitoring clinical trials and assuring the safety and effectiveness of a medicine or therapy before it's available to the public.

free radicals: Potentially toxic substances produced by the normal metabolism in all human cells; left uncontrolled, they can damage or destroy vital brain cells.

freezing: The sudden and temporary inability of a *PWP* to initiate a movement such as going through a doorway or exiting a car. See *akinesia.*

gait: Medical term for walking; includes the individual style of walking.

gene: The building block of inheritance contained in every human cell; a change in the gene can predispose the individual to a disease.

genetic: Anything related to genes or inherited characteristics, including diseases.

globus pallidus: One of the areas of the *basal ganglia* most affected by the lack of *dopamine* in Parkinson's disease.

hallucination: Unreal perceptions that a person may experience while awake; hearing or seeing objects or people that are not present. Visual hallucinations may be a side effect of *antiparkinsonian meds.*

hypokinesia: Decreased or reduced movement.

hypomimia: The lack of facial expression and absence of eye-blinking caused by Parkinson's disease. Also called *mask* or "facial mask."

hypophonic: Reduced vocal volume and clarity.

idiopathic: A diagnostic term meaning "of unknown origin or without apparent cause."

involuntary movement: Movement that happens without the person's intention or control.

levodopa (L-dopa): The most commonly used drug for treatment of PD; restores levels of *dopamine* in the brain.

Lewy bodies: Abnormal, round clumps of protein in damaged and dying *dopamine*-producing brain cells.

magnetic resonance imaging (MRI): A noninvasive, diagnostic imaging tool that uses an electromagnetic field to create cross-sectional illustrations of particular organs and systems in the human body.

mask: See *hypomimia.*

micrographia: The small, cramped handwriting due to impaired fine motor skills in some *PWP.*

motor fluctuations: Daily variations of the benefits from *antiparkinsonian drugs*. Usually occur as PD progresses. Also called *on-off phenomenon, wearing off,* and *dyskinesia.*

movement disorders: A category of neurological conditions that impair normal control of movements; includes *Parkinson's disease* and similar disorders (*parkinsonism* disorders), *essential tremor, dystonia,* tics, chorea, and other less common diseases.

multiple system atrophy: A neurological disorder characterized by *parkinsonism* that is poorly responsive to *levodopa;* typically associated early in its progression with other signs of neurological dysfunction including low blood pressure when standing (orthostatic hypotension), impotence, urinary incontinence, severe *gait* imbalance, slurred speech, incoordination, loss of cognitive function, and *dementia.*

National Institutes of Health (NIH): The primary federal agency charged with conducting and supporting medical research.

National Institute of Neurological Disorders and Stroke (NINDS): The branch of *NIH* that focuses on diseases and conditions that affect the brain and *central nervous system.*

neurodegenerative: A neurological disease (such as Alzheimer's and Parkinson's) marked by the progressive loss of *neurons.*

neurologist: A specialist in the diagnosis and treatment of neurological disorders of the brain, spinal cord, nerves, and muscles (such as PD, stroke, Alzheimer, and multiple sclerosis).

neuron: A type of cell (mainly in the nervous system) that processes and transmits information for specific functions.

neuroprotective therapy: Any treatment with the ability to prevent or slow the loss of vital *neurons* affected by a *neurodegenerative* disease.

neurosurgeon: A surgeon specializing in the treatment of neurological disorders.

neurotransmitter: The body's natural chemicals (such as *dopamine*) that send messages from one nerve cell to another or from nerve cells to muscles.

occupational therapy: Skilled rehabilitation techniques that help people with neurological conditions perform routine daily tasks at home; maximizes physical potential through lifestyle adaptations and possible use of assistive devices.

on-off phenomenon: Severe *motor fluctuations* that are particularly frequent, sudden, and unpredictable; also called "yo-yo" syndrome.

pallidotomy: A surgical procedure that lesions (burns) parts of the *globus pallidus* to lessen PD symptoms; now largely replaced by *deep brain stimulation* (DBS).

palsy: Also called "paralysis;" loss of the ability to move a body part. Parkinson's disease was originally called "shaking palsy."

parkinsonism: A group of movement disorders characterized by a variable combination of *tremor, rigidity, bradykenesia,* and *postural instability.*

Parkinson's disease (PD): A slowly progressing neurological disease resulting in the loss of *dopamine*-producing brain cells in the *substantia nigra.* The disease normally responds to the medication *levodopa.*

person (or persons) with Parkinson's disease: See *PWP.*

physical therapy: The use of stretching and strengthening exercises and machines to help *PWP* maintain (or regain) strength, balance, coordination, flexibility, endurance, and function for as long as possible.

pill-rolling: A characteristic finger *tremor* in which the thumb and index finger slowly rub against each other as if rolling something into a small ball. Typically (almost exclusively) seen in patients with *Parkinson's disease.*

placebo effect: A change or improvement (physical or emotional) in a patient who has been given a medication with no therapeutic benefits (as in clinical trials); there is no medical explanation for the change.

positron emission tomography (PET scan): A diagnostic imaging tool that uses an injected radioactive form of various compounds (such as glucose *levodopa*) to produce color maps of the sections of the brain and assist in the diagnosis of Parkinson's disease.

postural instability: A person's lack of balance or coordination when walking; usually results in awkward forward- or backward-leaning that may result in a fall as the person attempts to compensate for lack of balance.

postural tremor: *Tremor* or shaking that occurs when a person's arms are stretched outright to the front.

prognosis: A doctor's prediction of a condition's progression based on the patient's medical history and response to treatment as well as the doctor's knowledge of the disease.

propulsive gait: Also called *parkinsonian gait;* walking that is characterized by a stooped, rigid posture with head and neck bent forward; shorter and faster steps propel the person forward, placing him at risk for falling. See *festination* and *retropulsive gait.*

PWP: Abbreviation for "person (people) with Parkinson's disease;" sometimes appears as "PLWP" for "person (people) living with Parkinson's."

range of motion (ROM): The measurement of a person's ability to fully straighten or bend a joint (knee, elbow, hip, ankle, shoulder, or spine).

receptor: The part of a nerve cell that receives a message from a *neurotransmitter* (*dopamine*, for example).

resting tremor: A *tremor* or shaking that occurs when a body part is relaxed and supported (hand resting on the arm of a chair) but not engaged in activity; typically tremor ceases or lessens if the limb is engaged in activity.

retropulsive gait: A movement characterized by a person propelling herself backward in an attempt to maintain balance, thereby placing herself at risk for falling. See *propulsive gait.*

rigidity: The abnormal stiffness of a joint or limb.

seborrhea: Increased volume of oily perspiration.

sialorrhea: Drooling.

side effects: Undesirable problems a patient experiences when taking a certain medication; prescription meds list major side effects in their printed information and over-the-counter products list them on the packaging.

Sinemet: The brand name for *levodopa/carbidopa*, the most common medication for treating PD symptoms.

speech therapy: Rehabilitative techniques that help restore or strengthen speech and swallowing muscles affected by PD.

stem cell: Undeveloped or undifferentiated cells that can duplicate themselves or become cells of various body tissues; may originate from an adult tissue or an undeveloped embryo. Current studies consider these cells as potential cures for *neurodegenerative* diseases.

striatum: Part of the *basal ganglia* affected by the lack of *dopamine*. See *globus pallidus* and *subthalamic nucleus.*

substantia nigra: The small area of the brain that houses cells that produce the *neurotransmitter dopamine;* specifically affected by Parkinson's disease.

subthalamic nucleus: One of the small groups of cells in the *basal ganglia* primarily affected by PD; the most frequent surgical target for *DBS.* See *deep brain stimulation.*

support group: A gathering of people with a common connection (such as *PWP* or PD *care partners*) who meet regularly to share information, receive education, and sustain one another.

thalamotomy: A surgical procedure intended to relieve *tremor;* now largely replaced by *DBS.* See *deep brain stimulation.*

transcranial magnetic stimulation (TMS): A procedure in which an electromagnetic coil briefly stimulates specific areas of the brain in order to modulate their activity; used experimentally to treat depression and PD.

tremor: A repetitive and involuntary movement such as trembling or shaking; usually in the hands but possible in feet, legs, arms, head, or voice.

trigger event: An event (a fall or head trauma), exposure (to toxins or other environmental materials), or unusual stress (loss of job or death of a loved one) that exposes a condition's previously unrecognized symptoms.

unilateral: Occurring on one side of the body.

voluntary movement: Movement performed with full intention and control.

wearing off: Reappearance of PD symptoms before the next dose of *levodopa* is due. See *motor fluctuations.*

young onset PD: PD diagnosed in people under the age of 50.

Appendix B

Additional Resources

● ●

*E*ven though this handy guide covers Parkinson's disease (PD) from A to Z and offers a world of suggestions in dealing with it, we realize you may not be satisfied with reading just one book. You may want to know everything you can, or you may want more information about a specific topic within this huge subject. So, to round out this all-purpose guide, our appendix highlights other valuable sources for credible information and practical tools. This is by no means an exhaustive list — but it does include some truly valuable *stuff* to broaden your understanding of PD.

Requesting Free Print Materials

The National Parkinson Foundation (www.parkinson.org or 800-327-4545) has a terrific series of booklets about living with PD. Each booklet touches on a specific topic, and the foundation is always coming up with new topics (or revising the current ones). The best news is that these booklets are free. A sampling of the current titles includes:

✔ *Parkinson's Disease: What You and Your Family Should Know*

✔ *Parkinson's Disease: Nutrition Matters*

✔ *Activities of Daily Living: Practical Pointers for Parkinson's Disease*

✔ *Parkinson's Disease: Caring and Coping*

Gathering Free Info Online

As soon as possible, bookmark the following Web sites on your computer. Visit them regularly for updates on the latest treatments, tips on managing symptoms, and suggestions for your care partner. You can even use the Web to locate a neurologist, a local support group, or a medical center that specializes in the treatment of PD.

Don't have a computer? Talk to your local librarian. Better yet, put a child or grandchild on the case. They're the experts at searching the Internet, and when you research a question or topic together, it can be great quality time.

Making national PD organizations your first stop

The PD community is well organized. Each of the following Web sites provides a full range of information from medical updates to tips for coping.

- ✔ **American Parkinson Disease Association Inc.:**
  www.apdaparkinson.org

  Click on *Young Parkinson's* for The Arlette Johnson Young Parkinson Information and Referral Center; also click on *Local Information and Referral Center* on the home page to locate a support group or chapter.

  Also: 135 Parkinson Avenue Staten Island, NY 10305; Phone 800-223-2732 or 718-981-8001

- ✔ **The Bachmann-Strauss Dystonia & Parkinson Foundation:** www.dystonia-parkinsons.org

  This foundation focuses on research updates for dystonia and PD.

  Also: One Gustave L. Levy Place, Box 1490, New York, NY 10029; Phone 212-241-5614

- ✔ **The Michael J. Fox Foundation:** www.michaeljfox.org

  Click on *Sign up for e-mail* on the home page to receive the newsletter plus regular e-mail updates on research and other advances toward a cure.

  Also: 20 Grand Central Station, P.O. Box 4777, New York, NY 10163; Phone 800-708-7644

- ✔ **The Muhammad Ali Parkinson Center:** www.maprc.com

  Click on *Register* to help the center gather data on PD prevalence in the United States.

  Also: 500 W. Thomas Road, Suite 720, Phoenix, Arizona 85013; Phone 602-406-4931

✔ **National Parkinson Foundation:** www.parkinson.org

Click on *Library/Publications* for a complete list and order form for the free publications mentioned at the beginning of this appendix; also click on *Support Groups* to locate a group in your area.

Also: 1501 N.W. 9th Avenue/Bob Hope Road, Miami FL 33136; Phone 800-327-4545

✔ **Parkinson's Action Network:** www.parkinsonsaction.org

Click on *Become an Advocate* and get involved in the fight for a cure.

Also: 1025 Vermont Ave. NW, Suite 1120, Washington, DC 20005; Phone 800-850-4726

✔ **Parkinson's Disease Foundation:** www.pdf.org

Click on *Ask an Expert* to submit a question or to link to expert information.

Also: 1359 Broadway, Suite 1509, New York, NY 10018; Phone 212-923-4700

✔ **Young Onset Parkinson's Association:** www.yopa.org

Click on *YOPA Support* to locate a support group for YOPD in your area.

Also: 22136 Westheimer Parkway #343, Katy, TX 77450; Phone 1-888-WE-R-YOPA (1-888-937-9672)

Locating a neurologist near you

These sites help you find a neurologist or interpret the medical jargon:

✔ **American Academy of Neurology:** www.aan.com

Click on *Contact Us* to ask about a neurologist in your area.

✔ **Cleveland Clinic Foundation:** www.clevelandclinic.org

In the *Search* box, type *Parkinson's* for links to the Center on PD.

✔ **Medline Plus:** www.nia.nih.gov/HealthInformation/Publications

This site provides federal government info on PD, caregiving, and aging.

✔ **Medscape:** www.medscape.com

Click on *Neurology and Neurosurgery* link; then on the *Resource Center* list, click on *Parkinson's disease*.

✔ **NeurologyChannel:** www.neurologychannel.com

Click on *MD Locator* to locate a neurologist in your area.

Connecting with a rehab therapist

Physical, occupational, and speech therapy may be part of your care plan for managing PD symptoms. These national associations can help you locate the appropriate therapist in your area if you doctor hasn't already done so.

- ✔ **American Physical Therapy Association:** www.apta.org or by phone at 800-999-2782
- ✔ **American Occupational Therapy Association, Inc.:** www.aota.org or by phone at 800-377-8555
- ✔ **American Speech-Language-Hearing Association:** www.asha.org or by phone at 800-638-8255

Seeking assistance with your meds

Check out the Pharmaceutical Research and Manufacturers of America (PhRMA) at www.phrma.org. Click on *Patient Assistance Programs* to find out more about financial assistance for meds. Click on *About PhRma* and then *Member List* to locate the manufacturer of any medicine you're taking.

Finding tools that make your life easier

A number of devices are available to make life easier and to prolong independence for people with PD. The following resources offer places to check out as the need arises.

Exercise and speech tools

These resources offer exercise and speech programs you can use at home. They come in a variety of formats from printed booklet with illustrations to videos and audio tapes.

Be sure you show the program to your neurologist or rehab therapist before using any program on your own.

- ✔ *Aquatic Exercises for Parkinson's Disease:* From The American Parkinson Disease Association, Inc.: www.apdaparkinson.org/user/PublicationOrder.asp
- ✔ *Exercise: A Guide from the National Institute on Aging:* www.nia.nih.gov/HealthInformation/Publications/ExerciseGuide
- ✔ *The LSVT (Lee Silverman Voice Treatment):* www.lsvt.org
- ✔ *Motivating Moves for People with Parkinson's:* www.motivatingmoves.com

✔ *The PDF Exercise Program:* www.pdf.org/publications/
brochures

✔ *SIT AND BE FIT:* www.sitandbefit.com

✔ Additional related Web sites at http://parkinsonexercise.com

Clothing, medical alert systems, and other helpful aids

The following sites provide a range of aids from clothing with easy closures
to canes that may help avoid *freezing* (legs locked, unable to step forward) to
medic alert gear. New products come on the market every year.

✔ **Clothing Solutions:** www.clothingsolutions.com

✔ **Exerstrider:** www.exerstrider.com

✔ **Fashion Ease:** www.fashionease.com

✔ **Liberty Cane:** www.libertycane.com

✔ **Philips Lifeline:** www.lifelinesys.com

✔ **Luminaud, Inc.:** www.luminaud.com

✔ **Med-Alert:** www.1800medalert.com

✔ **MedicAlert:** www.medicalert.org

✔ **Sears Health and Wellness:** www.searshealthandwellness.com

✔ **U-Step Walking Stabilizer:** www.ustep.com

Complementary and alternative therapies

If you and your neurologist decide that some form of alternative therapy may
prove helpful, these three resources can help.

✔ **American Massage Therapy Association:** www.amtamassage.org

✔ **National Center for Complementary and Alternative Medicine:**
www.nccam.nih.gov

✔ **Yoga Journal:** www.yogajournal.com

Looking into financial and legal matters

Finances and legal matters are nothing to play around with. You need the
help of (or at least a consultation with) an expert. These resources can help:

✔ **American Institute of Certified Public Accountants:** www.aicpa.org

✔ **American Association of Daily Money Managers:** www.aadmm.com

- **American Association of Retired Persons:** www.aarp.org
- **Financial Planning Association:** www.fpanet.org
- **Medicare:** www.medicare.gov
- **Medicare Rights Center:** www.medicarerights.org

Sharing sites with your care partner

Bookmark these sites for your care partner:

- **CARE:** www.pdcaregiver.org
- **Eldercare Locator:** www.eldercare.gov
- **National Alliance for Caregiving:** www.caregiving.org
- **National Family Caregivers Association:** www.nfcacares.org
- **Parkinson Foundation of the Heartland:** www.parkinson heartland.org
- **Parkinson's Training for Caregivers:** www.parkinsonseducator.com
- **The Parkinson's Web:** http://pdweb.mgh.harvard.edu
- **National Parkinson's Foundation (*Caregiver Resources*):** www.parkinson.org/site

Other Books Worth the $$

New books on living with PD are published every year and your local library may have these recent works. If it doesn't, suggest the librarian add it to the library's wish list, or consider donating a copy yourself.

- ***100 Questions and Answers about Parkinson Disease*** by Abraham Lieberman, MD with Marcia McCall (Jones and Barlett Publishing)
- ***A Life Shaken: My Encounter with Parkinson's Disease*** by Joel Havermann (Johns Hopkins University Press)
- ***Lucky Man: A Memoir*** by Michael J. Fox (Hyperion)
- ***Parkinson's Disease: A Guide for Patient and Family*** (Fifth Edition) by Roger C. Duvosin and Jacob Sage (Lippincott Williams & Wilkins)
- ***Parkinson's Disease and the Family: A New Guide*** by Nutan Sharma and Elaine Richman (Harvard University Press)

Index

BUSINESS, CAREERS & PERSONAL FINANCE

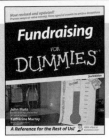

0-7645-9847-3

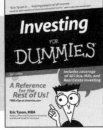

0-7645-2431-3

Also available:

- Business Plans Kit For Dummies
  0-7645-9794-9
- Economics For Dummies
  0-7645-5726-2
- Grant Writing For Dummies
  0-7645-8416-2
- Home Buying For Dummies
  0-7645-5331-3
- Managing For Dummies
  0-7645-1771-6
- Marketing For Dummies
  0-7645-5600-2

- Personal Finance For Dummies
  0-7645-2590-5*
- Resumes For Dummies
  0-7645-5471-9
- Selling For Dummies
  0-7645-5363-1
- Six Sigma For Dummies
  0-7645-6798-5
- Small Business Kit For Dummies
  0-7645-5984-2
- Starting an eBay Business For Dummies
  0-7645-6924-4
- Your Dream Career For Dummies
  0-7645-9795-7

HOME & BUSINESS COMPUTER BASICS

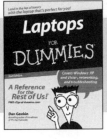

0-470-05432-8

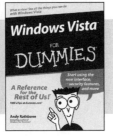

0-471-75421-8

Also available:

- Cleaning Windows Vista For Dummies
  0-471-78293-9
- Excel 2007 For Dummies
  0-470-03737-7
- Mac OS X Tiger For Dummies
  0-7645-7675-5
- MacBook For Dummies
  0-470-04859-X
- Macs For Dummies
  0-470-04849-2
- Office 2007 For Dummies
  0-470-00923-3

- Outlook 2007 For Dummies
  0-470-03830-6
- PCs For Dummies
  0-7645-8958-X
- Salesforce.com For Dummies
  0-470-04893-X
- Upgrading & Fixing Laptops For
  Dummies
  0-7645-8959-8
- Word 2007 For Dummies
  0-470-03658-3
- Quicken 2007 For Dummies
  0-470-04600-7

FOOD, HOME, GARDEN, HOBBIES, MUSIC & PETS

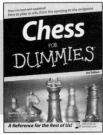

0-7645-8404-9

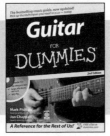

0-7645-9904-6

Also available:

- Candy Making For Dummies
  0-7645-9734-5
- Card Games For Dummies
  0-7645-9910-0
- Crocheting For Dummies
  0-7645-4151-X
- Dog Training For Dummies
  0-7645-8418-9
- Healthy Carb Cookbook For Dummies
  0-7645-8476-6
- Home Maintenance For Dummies
  0-7645-5215-5

- Horses For Dummies
  0-7645-9797-3
- Jewelry Making & Beading
  For Dummies
  0-7645-2571-9
- Orchids For Dummies
  0-7645-6759-4
- Puppies For Dummies
  0-7645-5255-4
- Rock Guitar For Dummies
  0-7645-5356-9
- Sewing For Dummies
  0-7645-6847-7
- Singing For Dummies
  0-7645-2475-5

INTERNET & DIGITAL MEDIA

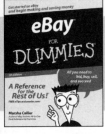

0-470-04529-9

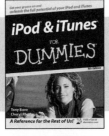

0-470-04894-8

Also available:

- Blogging For Dummies
  0-471-77084-1
- Digital Photography For Dummies
  0-7645-9802-3
- Digital Photography All-in-One Desk
  Reference For Dummies
  0-470-03743-1
- Digital SLR Cameras and Photography
  For Dummies
  0-7645-9803-1
- eBay Business All-in-One Desk
  Reference For Dummies
  0-7645-8438-3
- HDTV For Dummies
  0-470-09673-X

- Home Entertainment PCs For Dummies
  0-470-05523-5
- MySpace For Dummies
  0-470-09529-6
- Search Engine Optimization For
  Dummies
  0-471-97998-8
- Skype For Dummies
  0-470-04891-3
- The Internet For Dummies
  0-7645-8996-2
- Wiring Your Digital Home For Dummies
  0-471-91830-X

* Separate Canadian edition also available
* Separate U.K. edition also available

Available wherever books are sold. For more information or to order direct: U.S. customers visit www.dummies.com or call 1-877-762-2974.
U.K. customers visit www.wileyeurope.com or call 0800 243407. Canadian customers visit www.wiley.ca or call 1-800-567-4797.

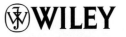 **WILEY**

SPORTS, FITNESS, PARENTING, RELIGION & SPIRITUALITY

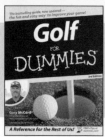

0-471-76871-5

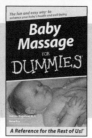

0-7645-7841-3

Also available:
- Catholicism For Dummies
  0-7645-5391-7
- Exercise Balls For Dummies
  0-7645-5623-1
- Fitness For Dummies
  0-7645-7851-0
- Football For Dummies
  0-7645-3936-1
- Judaism For Dummies
  0-7645-5299-6
- Potty Training For Dummies
  0-7645-5417-4
- Buddhism For Dummies
  0-7645-5359-3

- Pregnancy For Dummies
  0-7645-4483-7 †
- Ten Minute Tone-Ups For Dummies
  0-7645-7207-5
- NASCAR For Dummies
  0-7645-7681-X
- Religion For Dummies
  0-7645-5264-3
- Soccer For Dummies
  0-7645-5229-5
- Women in the Bible For Dummies
  0-7645-8475-8

TRAVEL

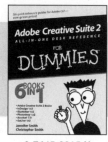

0-7645-7749-2

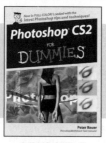

0-7645-6945-7

Also available:
- Alaska For Dummies
  0-7645-7746-8
- Cruise Vacations For Dummies
  0-7645-6941-4
- England For Dummies
  0-7645-4276-1
- Europe For Dummies
  0-7645-7529-5
- Germany For Dummies
  0-7645-7823-5
- Hawaii For Dummies
  0-7645-7402-7

- Italy For Dummies
  0-7645-7386-1
- Las Vegas For Dummies
  0-7645-7382-9
- London For Dummies
  0-7645-4277-X
- Paris For Dummies
  0-7645-7630-5
- RV Vacations For Dummies
  0-7645-4442-X
- Walt Disney World & Orlando
  For Dummies
  0-7645-9660-8

GRAPHICS, DESIGN & WEB DEVELOPMENT

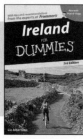

0-7645-8815-X

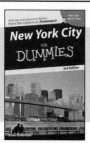

0-7645-9571-7

Also available:
- 3D Game Animation For Dummies
  0-7645-8789-7
- AutoCAD 2006 For Dummies
  0-7645-8925-3
- Building a Web Site For Dummies
  0-7645-7144-3
- Creating Web Pages For Dummies
  0-470-08030-2
- Creating Web Pages All-in-One Desk
  Reference For Dummies
  0-7645-4345-8
- Dreamweaver 8 For Dummies
  0-7645-9649-7

- InDesign CS2 For Dummies
  0-7645-9572-5
- Macromedia Flash 8 For Dummies
  0-7645-9691-8
- Photoshop CS2 and Digital
  Photography For Dummies
  0-7645-9580-6
- Photoshop Elements 4 For Dummies
  0-471-77483-9
- Syndicating Web Sites with RSS Feeds
  For Dummies
  0-7645-8848-6
- Yahoo! SiteBuilder For Dummies
  0-7645-9800-7

NETWORKING, SECURITY, PROGRAMMING & DATABASES

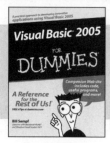

0-7645-7728-X

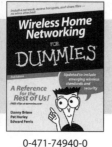

0-471-74940-0

Also available:
- Access 2007 For Dummies
  0-470-04612-0
- ASP.NET 2 For Dummies
  0-7645-7907-X
- C# 2005 For Dummies
  0-7645-9704-3
- Hacking For Dummies
  0-470-05235-X
- Hacking Wireless Networks
  For Dummies
  0-7645-9730-2
- Java For Dummies
  0-470-08716-1

- Microsoft SQL Server 2005 For Dummie
  0-7645-7755-7
- Networking All-in-One Desk Referenc
  For Dummies
  0-7645-9939-9
- Preventing Identity Theft For Dummies
  0-7645-7336-5
- Telecom For Dummies
  0-471-77085-X
- Visual Studio 2005 All-in-One Desk
  Reference For Dummies
  0-7645-9775-2
- XML For Dummies
  0-7645-8845-1

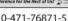